2-Deoxy-D-Glucose: Chemistry and Biology

Editors

Raman Singh

Department of Applied Chemistry
Amity University, Madhya Pradesh, Gwalior
India

Antresh Kumar

Department of Biochemistry
Central University of Haryana
Mahendergarh-123031, India

&

Kuldeep Singh

Department of Applied Chemistry
Amity University, Madhya Pradesh, Gwalior
India

2-Deoxy-D-Glucose: Chemistry and Biology

Editors: Raman Singh, Antresh Kumar and Kuldeep Singh

ISBN (Online): 978-981-5305-15-9

ISBN (Print): 978-981-5305-16-6

ISBN (Paperback): 978-981-5305-17-3

First published in 2024.

need for a court order if at any point you breach any terms of this License Agreement. In no event will any delay or failure by Bentham Science Publishers in enforcing your compliance with this License Agreement constitute a waiver of any of its rights.

3. You acknowledge that you have read this License Agreement, and agree to be bound by its terms and conditions. To the extent that any other terms and conditions presented on any website of Bentham Science Publishers conflict with, or are inconsistent with, the terms and conditions set out in this License Agreement, you acknowledge that the terms and conditions set out in this License Agreement shall prevail.

Bentham Science Publishers Pte. Ltd.
80 Robinson Road #02-00
Singapore 068898
Singapore
Email: subscriptions@benthamscience.net

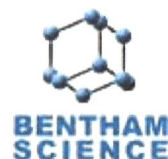

BENTHAM SCIENCE

CONTENTS

FOREWORD

It is with great pleasure that I compose the Foreword for this timely and insightful publication on the 'Chemistry and Biology of 2-Deoxy-D-Glucose (2-DG)'. As comprehensively outlined throughout the chapters, 2-DG is emerging as a versatile molecule with vast therapeutic potential in the fields of antiviral, anti-cancer, and neurological research.

This publication provides an exceptional overview of the medicinal chemistry that underlies 2-DG, encompassing its structure, synthesis, analytical characterization, and pharmacological actions along with its role in diagnostics and therapeutics. The chapters delve into the various synthetic pathways for producing 2-DG, elucidating the advantages and limitations of each method. Additionally, the text thoroughly discusses spectroscopic, chromatographic, and optical techniques for the analysis of 2-DG. These sections offer invaluable insights into optimizing the production and analysis of this crucial pharmaceutical intermediate.

Of particular interest are the mechanistic investigations into the biological effects of 2-DG. As explained, 2-DG acts as a glycolytic inhibitor and glycosylation modulator, selectively disrupting pathological metabolism in viruses, cancers, and seizures. The publication compiles compelling evidence from preclinical and clinical studies that highlight the therapeutic potential of 2-DG in these disease contexts. Furthermore, ongoing research on enhancing the delivery and efficacy of 2-DG through medicinal chemistry approaches is also prominently featured.

In conclusion, this publication provides a comprehensive and well-rounded overview of an exciting molecule that bridges the realms of chemistry and biomedicine. The chapters draw upon essential perspectives from synthetic organic chemistry, analytical methods, pharmacology, and molecular medicine to shed light on the diverse aspects of 2-DG research and applications, including prospects for cancer diagnosis, treatment, and surveillance. This interdisciplinary knowledge equips readers with a solid foundation to advance the potential of 2-DG and related compounds as diagnostic and therapeutic agents.

I commend the editors and authors for creating an outstanding reference that will educate, inspire, and guide future interdisciplinary endeavors in this medically relevant field.

Ravi Bhushan
Central Libr Adv Comm
Founder Coordinator IPR-Cell
Indian Institute of Technology Roorkee
Roorkee - 247667, India

PREFACE

2-Deoxy-D-glucose (2-DG) is a modified molecule of glucose that has garnered significant interest in research in recent years due to its potential for therapy in various diseases. As outlined in this book, 2-DG and its derivatives have shown promise as agents against viruses, cancer, seizures, and COVID-19.

The book provides a comprehensive overview of the chemistry and biology of 2-DG. It delves into the structure, properties, and methods of synthesis of 2-DG, providing important insight into this pharmaceutical intermediate. Analytical techniques for characterizing and establishing the purity of 2-DG are also discussed.

A key highlight of the book is the exploration of the mechanisms and applications of 2-DG in biomedicine. As an inhibitor of glycolysis, 2-DG displays broad antiviral activity by disrupting the supply of energy and replication of viruses. Chapters outline evidence for the effectiveness of 2-DG against herpes simplex virus, influenza, Ebola, and SARS-CoV-2. The book also extensively covers the use of 2-DG and its analogs in cancer therapy, given their ability to selectively target tumor metabolism.

Beyond its roles in antiviral and anticancer applications, the book examines the emerging potential of 2-DG in the management of seizures and neurological conditions. Contradictory effects as anticonvulsant and proconvulsant are elucidated across different models. Therapeutic possibilities in Alzheimer's, aging, and stroke are discussed.

The book emphasizes how the unique properties of 2-DG and its derivatives enable their dual application in medical diagnostics and therapy. Radio-labeled 2-DG offers enhanced imaging, while functionalized analogs may improve drug delivery. This integrated approach can pave the way for more precise and personalized medicine.

Overall, this book provides a comprehensive reference on the chemistry and biology of 2-DG. It compiles essential insights from interdisciplinary research to offer a well-rounded perspective on this versatile molecule. The collective knowledge presented here will equip readers to further explore the therapeutic applications of 2-DG and related compounds. I hope this book serves as a valuable addition to the scientific literature, inspiring further advancement in this medically relevant field.

Raman Singh
Department of Applied Chemistry
Amity University, Madhya Pradesh, Gwalior
India

Antresh Kumar
Department of Biochemistry
Central University of Haryana
Mahendergarh-123031, India

&

Kuldeep Singh
Department of Applied Chemistry
Amity University, Madhya Pradesh, Gwalior
India

List of Contributors

Antresh Kumar	Department of Biochemistry, Central University of Haryana, Mahendergarh-123031, India
Arunagiri Sivanesan Aruna Poorani	Supramolecular and Catalysis Lab, Dept. of Natural Products Chemistry, School of Chemistry, Madurai Kamaraj University, Madurai-625021, Tamilnadu, India
Ashutosh Singh	Department of Life Science, Central University of South Bihar, Gaya–824236, India
Amrita Srivastava	Department of Life Science, Central University of South Bihar, Gaya–824236, India
Hemlata Kumari	Department of Biochemistry, Central University of Haryana, Mahendergarh-123031, India
Juhi Rais	Department of Nuclear Medicine, Sanjay Gandhi Postgraduate Institute of Medical Sciences, Lucknow-226014, Uttar Pradesh, India
Kumar	Analytical Research & Development, Mankind Research Centre, IMT Manesar, Gurugram, Haryana-122052, India
Kuldeep Singh	Department of Applied Chemistry, Amity University, Madhya Pradesh, Gwalior-474005, India
Krishnendu Barik	Department of Bioinformatics, Central University of South Bihar, Gaya-824236, India
Minakshi	Department of Biochemistry, Central University of Haryana, Mahendergarh-123031, India
Mohamed Ibrahim Mohamed Ismail	Supramolecular and Catalysis Lab, Dept. of Natural Products Chemistry, School of Chemistry, Madurai Kamaraj University, Madurai-625021, Tamilnadu, India
Manish Ora	Department of Nuclear Medicine, Sanjay Gandhi Postgraduate Institute of Medical Sciences, Lucknow-226014, Uttar Pradesh, India
Manish Dixit	Department of Nuclear Medicine, Sanjay Gandhi Postgraduate Institute of Medical Sciences, Lucknow-226014, Uttar Pradesh, India
Mohd Faheem	Department of Nuclear Medicine, Sanjay Gandhi Postgraduate Institute of Medical Sciences, Lucknow, Uttar Pradesh, India
Neeru Singh	Analytical Research & Development, Mankind Research Centre, IMT Manesar, Gurugram, Haryana-122052, India
Pandeeswaran Santhoshkumar	Supramolecular and Catalysis Lab, Dept. of Natural Products Chemistry, School of Chemistry, Madurai Kamaraj University, Madurai-625021, Tamilnadu, India
Palaniswamy Suresh	Supramolecular and Catalysis Lab, Dept. of Natural Products Chemistry, School of Chemistry, Madurai Kamaraj University, Madurai-625021, Tamilnadu, India

Ravinsh Kumar	Department of Life Science, Central University of South Bihar, Gaya–824236, India
Rahul Dev	Analytical Research & Development, Mankind Research Centre, IMT Manesar, Gurugram, Haryana-122052, India
Raman Singh	Department of Applied Chemistry, Amity University, Madhya Pradesh, Gwalior-474005, India
Ramji Lal Yadav	Analytical Research & Development, Mankind Research Centre, IMT Manesar, Gurugram, Haryana-122052, India
S. N. Karaiya	Analytical Research & Development, Mankind Research Centre, IMT Manesar, Gurugram, Haryana-122052, India
Shaurya Prakash	Department of Biochemistry, Central University of Haryana, Mahendergarh-123031, India
Vidushi Gupta	Department of Chemistry, Indian Institute of Science Education and Research, Mohali, Punjab, India
Vaibhav Pandey	Department of Nuclear Medicine, Sanjay Gandhi Postgraduate Institute of Medical Sciences, Lucknow, Uttar Pradesh, India

CHAPTER 1

2-Deoxy-D-Glucose: Chemical Structure and Properties

Raman Singh[1] and **Kuldeep Singh**[1,*]

[1] *Department of Applied Chemistry, Amity University, Madhya Pradesh, Gwalior-474005, India*

Abstract: 2-Deoxy-D-glucose (2DG) is a variant of glucose lacking the 2-hydroxyl group. This minor alteration has significant biological and pharmacological implications, enhancing its therapeutic value and necessitating evaluations of its safety and efficacy in clinical environments. This chapter delves into the chemical composition of different deoxy-D-glucose molecules, focusing on the structure and characteristics of 2DG.

Keywords: Analysis, Deoxy-D-glucose, Property, Structure, Toxicity.

1. INTRODUCTION

Deoxy sugars are sugars in which a hydroxyl group (-OH) on the carbon ring is substituted with a hydrogen atom. Deoxyribose, a prominent deoxy sugar, constitutes the sugar-phosphate backbone of DNA, bearing the molecular formula $C_5H_{10}O_4$. Other notable deoxy sugars are detailed in Table **1**. Sugars undergoing the replacement of two hydroxyl groups with hydrogen are classified as dideoxy sugars, with colitose and abequose being instances [1].

1.2. Nomenclature

Traditionally, many deoxy sugars were given trivial or common names. However, a systematic nomenclature system has been developed to name these compounds more precisely. This system uses the prefix 'deoxy' followed by the position number indicating which carbon atom has the hydroxyl group replaced by a hydrogen. The stem name of the parent sugar is then included, along with any necessary configurational prefixes to specify the stereochemistry at the remaining chiral centers of the deoxy sugar molecule.

---

[*] **Corresponding author Kuldeep Singh:** Department of Applied Chemistry, Amity University, Madhya Pradesh, Gwalior-474005, India; E-mail: singh@orgsyn.in

Table 1. Examples of deoxy sugars.

Entry	Trivial Name	Systematic Name	Use/Presence
1.	L-fucose	6-deoxy-L-galactose	Primary constituent of fucoidan found in brown algae and occurs within N-linked glycans.
2.	D-Quinovose	6-deoxy-D-glucose	Component of the sulfolipid known as sulfoquinovosyl diacylglycerol.
3.	L-Rhamnose	6-deoxy-L-mannose	Present in plant glycosides [2].
4.	Deoxyribose	2-deoxy-D-ribose,	Forms the sugar-phosphate backbone of DNA.
5.	Fuculose	6-deoxy-L-tagatose	A significant component of avian influenza virus particles.
6.	L-Pneumose	6-deoxy-l-talose	-
7.	Colitose	3,6-dideoxy-L-xylo-hexose	Present in the O-antigen of certain Gram-negative bacteria.
8.	Abequose	3,6-Dideoxy-D-xylo-hexos	Found within the O-specific chains of lipopolysaccharides present in specific serotypes of Salmonella and Citrobacter bacteria [3].

2. DEOXY-GLUCOSE

When a hydroxyl group in D-glucose is substituted with a hydrogen atom, the result is deoxy-D-glucose, a molecule that possesses one less oxygen atom than D-glucose. Various deoxy-D-glucose types can be produced based on which carbon's attached oxygen is eliminated. Illustrations of these molecular structures arc provided in Fig. (**1**) and Table **2**.

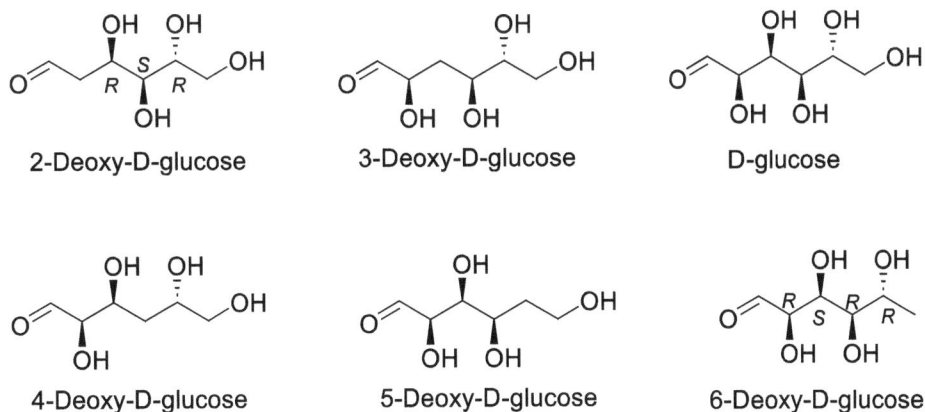

Fig. (1). Various deoxy sugars originating from D-Glucose.

Table 2. Different deoxy sugars derived from D-Glucose.

Entry	CAS	Deoxy-D-glucose	MP (°C)	$[\alpha]^{T}_{D}$
1.	154-17-6	2-Deoxy-D-glucose	146.5 [4]	$[\alpha]^{23}_{D}$ + 48.8° (c 0.13, water) [4].
2.	4005-35-0	3-Deoxy-D-glucose	120 [5]	$[\alpha]^{23}_{D}$ + 6.3° (c 1.2, water) [5].
3.	7286-46-6	4-Deoxy-D-glucose	131-132 [6]	$[\alpha]^{23}_{D}$ + 60.3° (c 2.4, water) [6].
4.	7640-19-9	5-Deoxy-D-glucose	Pail-yellow oil	$[\alpha]^{18}_{D}$ + 24.1° (c 7.8, water) [7].
5.	7658-08-4	6-Deoxy-D-glucose D-quionovose	139.5 [8]	-

Based on data available at AS Common Chemistry. CAS, a division of the American Chemical Society. https://commonchemistry.cas.org/

2-Deoxy-D-glucose (2DG) is the most common but other deoxy positions and substitutions can alter potency, metabolism, and effects. 2DG has become an important research tool and leads to potential therapeutic applications.

3. 2-DEOXY-D-GLUCOSE (2DG)

2DG is a synthetic compound [9], however, α and β D-glucopyranose forms (2-deoxy-α-D-*arabino*-hexopyranose, and 2-deoxy-β-D-*arabino*-hexopyranose) were extracted from the carbohydrate fraction of the solid-state fermentation product of *Actinosynnema pretiosum* ssp. *auranticum* ATCC 31565 [10, 11]. 2DG, has been assigned with the CAS registry number 154-17-6, and its structure has been depicted in Fig. (**2**). This compound is also known by the synonyms 2-deoxy-D-arabino-hexose and D-arabino-2-deoxyhexose. The α-pyranose form of the reducing aldose 2-deoxy-D-arabino-hexose (2-deoxy-D-*arabino*-hexopyranose) adopts a $^{4}C_{1}$ conformation, where the anomeric hydroxyl group is positioned axially, and the remaining substituents align equatorially. In the crystalline state, the four hydroxyl groups participate in an intricate three-dimensional hydrogen-bonding network, each acting as an intermolecular hydrogen-bond donor [12].

4. PHYSICAL PROPERTIES

2-Deoxy-D-glucose (2DG) exists as a crystalline solid with a white to off-white appearance [13]. Its melting point has been reported as 146°C [13]. However, when recrystallized from methanol, it forms colorless needle-like crystals with a melting range of 151-154°C and a specific optical rotation value of +43.0° (c=1.0, H_2O, 15°C) [11]. Under different conditions, such as in a 0.13 concentration aqueous solution, the specific rotation value for 2DG has been documented as +48.8° at 23°c [4]. These physical properties, including the melting behavior and optical activity, can aid in characterizing and identifying the 2DG compound.

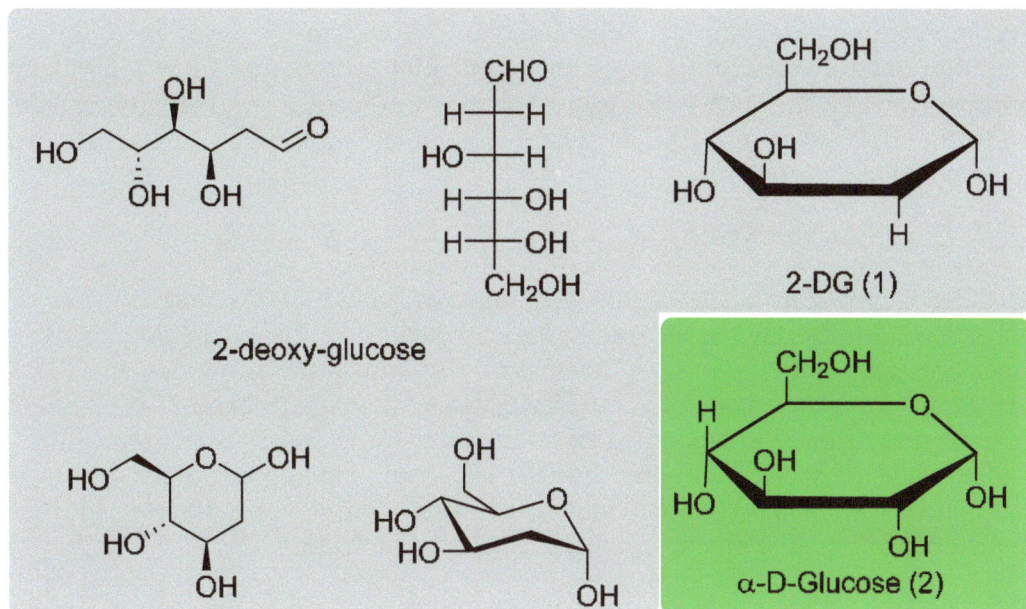

Fig. (2). Structure of 2-deoxy-D-Glucose.

5. ANALYTICAL CHARACTERIZATION

Analytical characterization and confirmation of the precise compound identity and purity of 2DG is crucial for both basic research studies and therapeutic development efforts. Spectroscopic techniques like nuclear magnetic resonance (NMR) spectroscopy [8, 14 - 16], infra-red (IR) spectroscopy [17], and mass spectrometry are used to confirm the core compound structure and distinguish it from similar glucose derivatives [18]. Techniques including capillary electrophoresis (CE), high-performance liquid chromatography (HPLC), and gas chromatography (GC), when linked with appropriate detection systems, are utilized for measuring the relative amounts of 2DG and assessing its purity [19].

5.1. Spectral Characterization

5.1.1. UV-VIS Spectrum

The 2DG molecule shows an absorption maxima at 279 nm in water and 277 nm in DMSO [20].

5.1.2. Mass Spectrum

Mass spectrometric analysis of 2-deoxy-D-glucose (2DG) reveals a prominent fragmentation pathway involving the initial loss of a water molecule, resulting in the formation of an ion with m/z of 119. Concurrently, an alternative decomposition route emerges, characterized by the formal loss of hydrogen peroxide, which proceeds through the sequential elimination of two hydroxyl groups. Notably, this latter pathway precludes the formation of the ion species typically observed at m/z 107, suggesting a compete inhibition of that particular fragmentation channel [21].

5.1.3. IR and Raman Spectrum

The 2-deoxy-D-glucose molecule is composed of 23 atoms and exhibits 63 normal vibrational modes. Venkatesh and colleagues conducted a comprehensive study on the vibrational assignments of the fundamental modes in 2-DG, including calculated (scaled) infrared (IR) and Raman bands, as well as descriptions of the corresponding normal modes [20]. The IR spectrum of 2DG displays a characteristic carbonyl band at 1722 cm^{-1} and an enediol band at 1658 cm^{-1} [22]. These distinct vibrational features provide valuable insights into the structural and bonding characteristics of the 2-DG molecule.

5.1.4. NMR

Table **3** lists ^{1}H-NMR peaks. ^{13}C NMR shows signals at δ 93.61, 95.73 (C-1), 74.31, 73.50, 78.31, 73.17, 72.77, 70.26, 63.27, 63.02, (C-3,4,5,6), 41.77, 39.53 (C-2) [24]. ^{1}H and ^{13}C spectra of 2-deoxy-β-D-glucose were recently captured using a 600 MHz instrument in C_5D_5N (Table **3**) [23]. Fig. (**3**) depicts anomeric sugar signals (600 MHz ^{1}H-NMR; 2 M D_2SO_4/D_2O; 30 °C) [8] for D-glucose, D-mannose and 2DG.

Table 3. NMR Data of 2DG.

^{13}C NMR		^{1}H NMR		
β-pyranose	-	β-pyranose	β-pyranose	α-pyranose
C_5D_5N, 2D HSQC, 150 MHz [23]	-	C_5D_5N (600 MHz) [23]	D_2O [24]	D_2O [24]
95.4	H-1	5.41, dd (*J* 9.7, 1.9 Hz)	4.94 (dd, *J* 9.7 Hz, 1.1Hz)	5.39 (broad d, *J* 3.6 Hz)
43	H-2a	2.79, ddd (*J* 12.4, 4.9, 1.9 Hz)	1.29-1.87 m	-
-	H-2e	2.30, td (*J* 12.0, 9.7 Hz)	2.03-2.40 m	-
72.9	H-3	4.25, ddd (*J* 11.8, 8.6, 4.9 Hz)	3.26-4.12 m	-
73.8	H-4	4.09, t (*J* 8.9 Hz)	-	-
78.7	H-5	3.92, ddd (*J* 9.4, 5.6, 2.7 Hz)	-	-
63.4	H-6a	4.59, dd (11.6, 2.7)	-	-
-	H-6e	4.42, dd (11.6, 5.6)	-	-

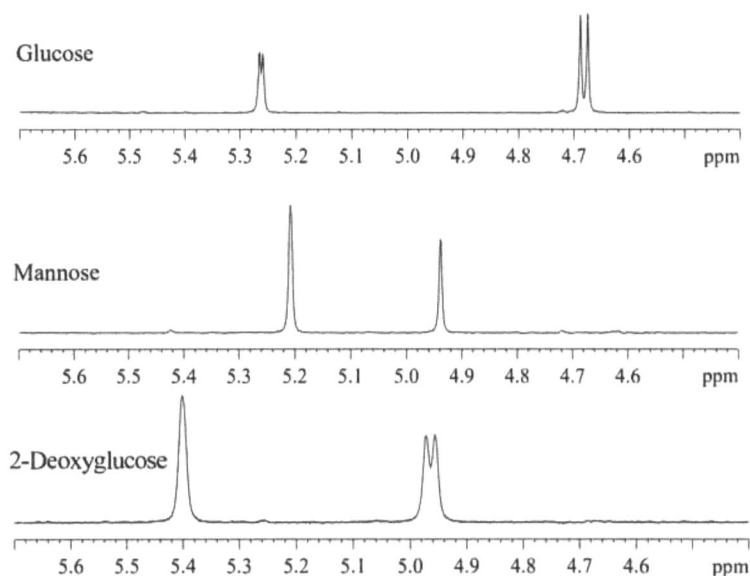

Fig. (3). Anomeric Sugar Signals (600 MHz 1H-NMR; 2 M D2SO4/D2O; 30 °C) [8].

6. ANALYSIS OF 2-DEOXY-D-GLUCOSE

2DG exhibits reducing properties, as evidenced by its ability to reduce Fehling's solution [11] and yields a positive result in the Keller-Kiliani reaction [11], which is a test for identifying reducing sugars. The concentration and purity of 2DG in crystalline or liquid samples can be accurately and precisely determined using high-performance liquid chromatography (HPLC) analysis, a technique suitable for the analysis of active pharmaceutical ingredients and drug products [25]. This method is applicable for the standardization and quality control of 2DG-based active pharmaceutical ingredients and drug formulations. Ultraviolet (UV) detection at 195 nm, coupled with HPLC using μBondapak 10 μm NH^2 or Varian Micropak 10 μm NH_2 columns, has been employed for the detection and quantification of 2DG, with a typical retention time of around four minutes when using an 85% acetonitrile/water mobile phase. Additionally, polymer-based amino columns (*e.g.*, HILICpak VG-50 4E) and Shodex SUGAR SC1011 columns have been utilized for the separation of 2DG and glucose [26]. In pharmacokinetic studies involving 2DG, the estimation of 2-deoxyglucose in plasma is crucial. To facilitate this, a precolumn fluorescent derivatization technique has been developed, which involves reductive amination of 2DG using sodium cyanoborohydride and 2-aminobenzoic acid [27].

7. DRUGABILITY OF 2DG

2DG exerts its effects by inhibiting various enzymes involved in the glycolytic pathway, ultimately leading to cell death. 2DG is also a mannose-mimetic that interferes with protein glycosylation. This molecule has a molecular weight of 164.158 Daltons, a calculated logP value of -1.525, five hydrogen bond acceptors (HBA), and four hydrogen bond donors (HBD). Consequently, it satisfies four out of the five Lipinski rules for drug-likeness. Additionally, 2DG has a polar surface area (PSA) of 90.15 $\mathring{A}^2$ and a single rotatable bond (RotB), thereby meeting two of the Veber criteria. The approval of 2DG for emergency use in Indian hospitals to treat COVID-19 patients requiring supplemental oxygen has highlighted the potential of this compound and ignited hope for the development of a safe drug to combat the current pandemic [28]. Viral mutations, which can render existing drugs and monoclonal vaccines ineffective, are a significant concern. Targeting the glycolytic pathway, a process essential for energy production in infected cells, represents a promising strategy as it is less susceptible to viral mutations [29 - 32]. Various studies have explored the use of varying doses of 2DG, with the maximum tolerable dose reported to be 250 mg/kg body weight [33].

8. TOXICOLOGY AND HANDLING OF 2DG

2-Deoxyglucose (2DG) is a toxic glucose analog that operates through a pleiotropic mechanism [34 - 36]. Its molecular structure bears resemblance to both glucose and mannose. Due to its similarity with mannose, 2DG significantly disrupts the N-linked glycosylation process [34], leading to the inhibition of protein synthesis and inducing endoplasmic reticulum (ER) stress within cells [34, 37]. Reports indicate that 2DG can stimulate autophagy, increase oxidative stress levels, and impair the N-linked glycosylation pathway [38]. Following a ketogenic diet has been shown to enhance tolerance to glycolysis inhibitors [39]. When handling 2DG, proper safety precautions should be taken, including wearing hand protection and a mask, as well as avoiding exposure to moisture [40].

CONCLUSION

2-Deoxy-D-glucose, a molecule that resembles D-glucose and D-mannose, complies with Lipinski's rule of five, indicative of promising drug-like characteristics. It demonstrates a range of activities, such as an inhibitor of glycolysis, impacting metabolic pathways, signaling pathways like AMPK and mTORC1, biosynthesis processes such as lipid and protein-N-glycosylation and its use as a tracer compound. Its potential application in treating COVID-19 has sparked heightened interest, potentially paving the way for novel antiviral medications and therapeutic approaches for individuals experiencing hyper-glycemia.

LIST OF ABBREVIATIONS

2DG   2-Deoxy-D-Glucose

BW   Body Weight

ER   Endoplasmic Reticulum

HBA   Hydrogen Bond Acceptors

HBD   Hydrogen Bond Donors

PSA   Polar Surface Area

RotB   Rotatable Bond

ACKNOWLEDGEMENTS

The authors extend their heartfelt gratitude to the management of Amity University Madhya Pradesh, Gwalior, Madhya Pradesh, India, for offering the necessary facilities that enabled the writing and submission of the book chapter for publication.

REFERENCES

[1]   Singh, R.; Gupta, V.; Singh, K. A review on synthetic methods for 2-deoxy-D-glucose. *ARKIVOC,* **2023**, *2022*(6), 199-219.
[http://dx.doi.org/10.24820/ark.5550190.p011.946]

[2]   Brown, M.R. The amino-acid and sugar composition of 16 species of microalgae used in mariculture. *J. Exp. Mar. Biol. Ecol.,* **1991**, *145*(1), 79-99.
[http://dx.doi.org/10.1016/0022-0981(91)90007-J]

[3]   Katzenellenbogen, E.; Kocharova, N.A.; Toukach, P.V.; Górska, S.; Korzeniowska-Kowal, A.; Bogulska, M.; Gamian, A.; Knirel, Y.A. Structure of an abequose-containing O-polysaccharide from Citrobacter freundii O22 strain PCM 1555. *Carbohydr. Res.,* **2009**, *344*(13), 1724-1728.
[http://dx.doi.org/10.1016/j.carres.2009.06.005] [PMID: 19576576]

[4]   Yaylayan, V.A.; Ismail, A.A. Investigation of the enolization and carbonyl group migration in reducing sugars by FTIR spectroscopy. *Carbohydr. Res.,* **1995**, *276*(2), 253-265.
[http://dx.doi.org/10.1016/0008-6215(95)00188-Y]

[5]   Prokop, J.; Murray, D.H. Synthesis of 3'-Deoxynucleosides I. *J. Pharm. Sci.,* **1965**, *54*(3), 359-365.
[http://dx.doi.org/10.1002/jps.2600540304] [PMID: 14301563]

[6]   Hedgley, E.J.; Overend, W.G.; Rennie, R.A.C. 900. Structure and reactivity of anhydro-sugars. Part V. 3-Deoxy-D-ribo-hexopyranose and 4-deoxy-D-xylo-hexopyranose. *J. Chem. Soc.,* **1963**, *4701*, 4701.
[http://dx.doi.org/10.1039/jr9630004701]

[7]   Durrwachter, J.R.; Drueckhammer, D.G.; Nozaki, K.; Sweers, H.M.; Wong, C.H. Enzymic aldol condensation/isomerization as a route to unusual sugar derivatives. *J. Am. Chem. Soc.,* **1986**, *108*(24), 7812-7818.
[http://dx.doi.org/10.1021/ja00284a053] [PMID: 22283291]

[8]   Giner, J.L.; Feng, J.; Kiemle, D.J. NMR tube degradation method for sugar analysis of glycosides. *J. Nat. Prod.,* **2016**, *79*(9), 2413-2417.
[http://dx.doi.org/10.1021/acs.jnatprod.6b00180] [PMID: 27603739]

[9]   Pajak, B.; Siwiak, E.; Sołtyka, M.; Priebe, A.; Zieliński, R.; Fokt, I.; Ziemniak, M.; Jaśkiewicz, A.; Borowski, R.; Domoradzki, T.; Priebe, W. 2-Deoxy-d-Glucose and its analogs: From diagnostic to

therapeutic agents. *Int. J. Mol. Sci.,* **2019**, *21*(1), 234.
[http://dx.doi.org/10.3390/ijms21010234] [PMID: 31905745]

[10]   Lu, C.; Bai, L.; Shen, Y. Five unusual natural carbohydrates from Actinosynnema pretiosum. *Chem. Nat. Compd.,* **2008**, *44*(5), 594-597.
[http://dx.doi.org/10.1007/s10600-008-9140-x]

[11]   Murakami, T.; Tanaka, N.; Tezuka, T.; Chen, C. Chemische unterschungen der inhaltsstoffe von pteris inaequalis baker var. aequata (Miq.) Tagawa. *Chem. Pharm. Bull. (Tokyo),* **1975**, *23*(7), 1634-1637.
[http://dx.doi.org/10.1248/cpb.23.1634]

[12]   Hess, D.; Klüfers, P. 2-Deoxy-α- D-*arabino* -hexopyranose. *Acta Crystallogr. Sect. E Struct. Rep. Online,* **2011**, *67*(10), o2615-o2615.
[http://dx.doi.org/10.1107/S1600536811035264] [PMID: 22058760]

[13]   Overend, W.G.; Stacey, M.; Staněk, J. 598. Deoxy-sugars. Part VII. A study of the reactions of some derivatives of 2-deoxy- D -glucose. *J. Chem. Soc.,* **1949**, *0*(0), 2841-2845.
[http://dx.doi.org/10.1039/JR9490002841]

[14]   Fontana, C.; Widmalm, G. Primary Structure of Glycans by NMR Spectroscopy. *Chem. Rev.,* **2023**, *123*(3), 1040-1102.
[http://dx.doi.org/10.1021/acs.chemrev.2c00580] [PMID: 36622423]

[15]   Inagaki, M.; Iwakuma, R.; Kawakami, S.; Otsuka, H.; Rakotondraibe, H.L. Detecting and differentiating monosaccharide enantiomers by [1] H NMR spectroscopy. *J. Nat. Prod.,* **2021**, *84*(7), 1863-1869.
[http://dx.doi.org/10.1021/acs.jnatprod.0c01120] [PMID: 34191514]

[16]   Duus, J.Ø.; Gotfredsen, C.H.; Bock, K. Carbohydrate structural determination by NMR spectroscopy: modern methods and limitations. *Chem. Rev.,* **2000**, *100*(12), 4589-4614.
[http://dx.doi.org/10.1021/cr990302n] [PMID: 11749359]

[17]   Mucha, E.; Stuckmann, A.; Marianski, M.; Struwe, W.B.; Meijer, G.; Pagel, K. In-depth structural analysis of glycans in the gas phase. *Chem. Sci. (Camb.),* **2019**, *10*(5), 1272-1284.
[http://dx.doi.org/10.1039/C8SC05426F] [PMID: 30809341]

[18]   Alley, W.R., Jr; Mann, B.F.; Novotny, M.V. High-sensitivity analytical approaches for the structural characterization of glycoproteins. *Chem. Rev.,* **2013**, *113*(4), 2668-2732.
[http://dx.doi.org/10.1021/cr3003714] [PMID: 23531120]

[19]   Lu, G.; Crihfield, C.L.; Gattu, S.; Veltri, L.M.; Holland, L.A. Capillary electrophoresis separations of glycans. *Chem. Rev.,* **2018**, *118*(17), 7867-7885.
[http://dx.doi.org/10.1021/acs.chemrev.7b00669] [PMID: 29528644]

[20]   Venkatesh, G.; Sixto-López, Y.; Vennila, P.; Mary, Y.S.; Correa-Basurto, J.; Mary, Y.S.; Manikandan, A. An investigation on the molecular structure, interaction with metal clusters, anti-Covid-19 ability of 2-deoxy-D-glucose: DFT calculations, MD and docking simulations. *J. Mol. Struct.,* **2022**, *1258.* , 132678.
[http://dx.doi.org/10.1016/j.molstruc.2022.132678]

[21]   Coppola, M.; Favretto, D.; Traldi, P.; Resnati, G. Negative-ion fast atom bombardment mass spectrometry in the characterization of deoxyfluorinated sugars. *Org. Mass Spectrom.,* **1994**, *29*(10), 553-555.
[http://dx.doi.org/10.1002/oms.1210291007]

[22]   Parker, F.S.; Ans, R. Infrared spectra of carbohydrates (700–250 cm $^{-1}$) determined by both attenuated total reflectance and transmission techniques. *Appl. Spectrosc.,* **1966**, *20*(6), 384-388.
[http://dx.doi.org/10.1366/000370266774386542]

[23]   Pieri, V.; Schwaiger, S.; Ellmerer, E.P.; Stuppner, H. Iridoid glycosides from the leaves of Sambucus ebulus. *J. Nat. Prod.,* **2009**, *72*(10), 1798-1803.
[http://dx.doi.org/10.1021/np900373u] [PMID: 19795902]

[24]   Wong, M.Y.H.; Gray, G.R. 2-deoxy-d-arabino-hexose, 2-deoxy-d-lyxo-hexose, and their (2R)-2-deuterio analogs. *Carbohydr. Res.,* **1980,** *80*(1), 87-98.
[http://dx.doi.org/10.1016/S0008-6215(00)85317-3]

[25]   Li, M. Analytical Methods for Polynuclear. WO2006002323A1, **2005**.

[26]   Hughes, D.E. Determination of α-2-deoxy-d-glucose in topical formulations by high-performance liquid chromatography with ultraviolet detection. *J. Chromatogr. A,* **1985,** *331*(1), 183-186.
[http://dx.doi.org/10.1016/0021-9673(85)80020-0] [PMID: 4044738]

[27]   Gounder, M.K.; Lin, H.; Stein, M.; Goodin, S.; Bertino, J.R.; Kong, A.N.T.; DiPaola, R.S. A validated bioanalytical HPLC method for pharmacokinetic evaluation of 2-deoxyglucose in human plasma. *Biomed. Chromatogr.,* **2012,** *26*(5), 650-654.
[http://dx.doi.org/10.1002/bmc.1710] [PMID: 21932382]

[28]   Aiestaran-Zelaia, I.; Sánchez-Guisado, M.J.; Villar-Fernandez, M.; Azkargorta, M.; Fadon-Padilla, L.; Fernandez-Pelayo, U.; Perez-Rodriguez, D.; Ramos-Cabrer, P.; Spinazzola, A.; Elortza, F.; Ruíz-Cabello, J.; Holt, I.J. 2 deoxy-D-glucose augments the mitochondrial respiratory chain in heart. *Sci. Rep.,* **2022,** *12*(1), 6890.
[http://dx.doi.org/10.1038/s41598-022-10168-1] [PMID: 35478201]

[29]   Bhatt, A.N.; Shenoy, S.; Munjal, S.; Chinnadurai, V.; Agarwal, A.; Vinoth Kumar, A.; Shanavas, A.; Kanwar, R.; Chandna, S. 2-deoxy-d-glucose as an adjunct to standard of care in the medical management of COVID-19: a proof-of-concept and dose-ranging randomised phase II clinical trial. *BMC Infect. Dis.,* **2022,** *22*(1), 669.
[http://dx.doi.org/10.1186/s12879-022-07642-6] [PMID: 35927676]

[30]   Codo, A.C.; Davanzo, G.G.; Monteiro, L.B.; de Souza, G.F.; Muraro, S.P.; Virgilio-da-Silva, J.V.; Prodonoff, J.S.; Carregari, V.C.; de Biagi Junior, C.A.O.; Crunfli, F.; Jimenez Restrepo, J.L.; Vendramini, P.H.; Reis-de-Oliveira, G.; Bispo dos Santos, K.; Toledo-Teixeira, D.A.; Parise, P.L.; Martini, M.C.; Marques, R.E.; Carmo, H.R.; Borin, A.; Coimbra, L.D.; Boldrini, V.O.; Brunetti, N.S.; Vieira, A.S.; Mansour, E.; Ulaf, R.G.; Bernardes, A.F.; Nunes, T.A.; Ribeiro, L.C.; Palma, A.C.; Agrela, M.V.; Moretti, M.L.; Sposito, A.C.; Pereira, F.B.; Velloso, L.A.; Vinolo, M.A.R.; Damasio, A.; Proença-Módena, J.L.; Carvalho, R.F.; Mori, M.A.; Martins-de-Souza, D.; Nakaya, H.I.; Farias, A.S.; Moraes-Vieira, P.M. Elevated Glucose Levels Favor SARS-CoV-2 Infection and Monocyte Response through a HIF-1α/Glycolysis-Dependent Axis. *Cell Metab.,* **2020,** *32*(3), 498-499.
[http://dx.doi.org/10.1016/j.cmet.2020.07.015] [PMID: 32877692]

[31]   Zhu, J.; Wang, G.; Huang, X.; Lee, H.; Lee, J.G.; Yang, P.; van de Leemput, J.; Huang, W.; Kane, M.A.; Yang, P.; Han, Z. SARS-CoV-2 Nsp6 damages Drosophila heart and mouse cardiomyocytes through MGA/MAX complex-mediated increased glycolysis. *Commun. Biol.,* **2022,** *5*(1), 1039.
[http://dx.doi.org/10.1038/s42003-022-03986-6] [PMID: 36180527]

[32]   Chavda, V.P.; Pandya, R.; Apostolopoulos, V. DNA vaccines for SARS-CoV-2: toward third-generation vaccination era. *Expert Rev. Vaccines,* **2021,** *20*(12), 1549-1560.
[http://dx.doi.org/10.1080/14760584.2021.1987223] [PMID: 34582298]

[33]   Singh, D.; Banerji, A.K.; Dwarakanath, B.S.; Tripathi, R.P.; Gupta, J.P.; Mathew, T.L.; Ravindranath, T.; Jain, V. Optimizing cancer radiotherapy with 2-deoxy-d-glucose dose escalation studies in patients with glioblastoma multiforme. *Strahlenther. Onkol.,* **2005,** *181*(8), 507-514.
[http://dx.doi.org/10.1007/s00066-005-1320-z] [PMID: 16044218]

[34]   Fokt, I.; Skora, S.; Conrad, C.; Madden, T.; Emmett, M.; Priebe, W. d-Glucose and d-mannose-based metabolic probes. Part 3: Synthesis of specifically deuterated d-glucose, d-mannose, and 2-deoxy-d-glucose. *Carbohydr. Res.,* **2013,** *368*, 111-119.
[http://dx.doi.org/10.1016/j.carres.2012.11.021] [PMID: 23376241]

[35]   Budikhina, A.S.; Pashenkov, M.V. The role of glycolysis in immune response. *Immunologiya,* **2021,** *42*(1), 5-20.
[http://dx.doi.org/10.33029/0206-4952-2021-42-1-5-20]

[36]   Reiter, R.J.; Sharma, R.; Rosales-Corral, S. Anti-warburg effect of melatonin: a proposed mechanism to explain its inhibition of multiple diseases. *Int. J. Mol. Sci.,* **2021**, *22*(2), 764.
[http://dx.doi.org/10.3390/ijms22020764] [PMID: 33466614]

[37]   Zhang, J.; Yang, J.; Lin, C.; Liu, W.; Huo, Y.; Yang, M.; Jiang, S.H.; Sun, Y.; Hua, R. Endoplasmic reticulum stress-dependent expression of ero11 promotes aerobic glycolysis in pancreatic cancer. *Theranostics,* **2020**, *10*(18), 8400-8414.
[http://dx.doi.org/10.7150/thno.45124] [PMID: 32724477]

[38]   Zhang, D.; Li, J.; Wang, F.; Hu, J.; Wang, S.; Sun, Y. 2-Deoxy-D-glucose targeting of glucose metabolism in cancer cells as a potential therapy. *Cancer Lett.,* **2014**, *355*(2), 176-183.
[http://dx.doi.org/10.1016/j.canlet.2014.09.003] [PMID: 25218591]

[39]   Voss, M.; Lorenz, N.I.; Luger, A.L.; Steinbach, J.P.; Rieger, J.; Ronellenfitsch, M.W. Rescue of 2-deoxyglucose side effects by ketogenic diet. *Int. J. Mol. Sci.,* **2018**, *19*(8), 2462.
[http://dx.doi.org/10.3390/ijms19082462] [PMID: 30127309]

[40]   Singh, R.; Gupta, V.; Kumar, A.; Singh, K. 2-Deoxy-D-Glucose: A novel pharmacological agent for killing hypoxic tumor cells, oxygen dependence-lowering in Covid-19, and other pharmacological activities. *Adv. Pharmacol. Pharm. Sci.,* **2023**, *2023*, 1-15.
[http://dx.doi.org/10.1155/2023/9993386] [PMID: 36911357]

CHAPTER 2

Methods and Procedures for the Synthesis of 2-Deoxy-D-Glucose

Raman Singh[1], **Vidushi Gupta**[2] and **Kuldeep Singh**[1,*]

[1] *Department of Applied Chemistry, Amity University, Madhya Pradesh, Gwalior-474005, India*

[2] *Department of Chemistry, Indian Institute of Science Education and Research, Mohali, Punjab, India*

Abstract: Many synthetic procedures for preparing 2-deoxy-D-glucose (2DG) are available in the literature. The synthesis of 2DG involves the modification of glucose at 2-position. Several methods to synthesize 2DG include glucose nitrosation and reductive amination of 2-deoxy-D-arabinose. These methods are highly efficient and produce high yields of 2DG. This chapter discusses various methods for synthesizing 2DG and their advantages and disadvantages. This chapter describes the different approaches for synthesizing 2DG and how the choice of method affects its purity, yield, and properties.

Keywords: Deoxy-D-glucose, Synthetic procedures.

1. INTRODUCTION

Although several methods have been published for the synthesis of 2DG, many have significant limitations that constrain their utility [1, 2]. Classical procedures often suffer from issues such as low yields, cumbersome workup or purification steps, and the formation of impure diastereomeric or racemic mixtures. This limits the accessibility, scalability, and stereochemical control of the current 2DG synthetic routes. There is a need for optimized and practical synthetic methods that improve the yield, simplicity, and stereoselectivity to support the research, development, and eventual production of 2DG. Overcoming these challenges in 2DG synthesis will facilitate its study and therapeutic applications. One or more methods could solve some of these problems, and reviewing these methods could provide insight into the issues to be addressed while developing new methods.

* **Corresponding author Kuldeep Singh:** Department of Applied Chemistry, Amity University, Madhya Pradesh, Gwalior-474005, India; E-mail: singh@orgsyn.in

2. SYNTHETIC METHODS

This section summarizes the various synthetic methodologies reported in the literature for the preparation of the important compound, 2-deoxy-D-glucose (2DG). As illustrated in Fig. (**1**), 2DG is a C-2 epimer of both D-glucose and D-mannose [3]. Therefore, the deoxygenation reaction at the C-2 position of D-glucose or D-mannose produced the same final product, 2DG. Consequently, synthetic routes starting from D-glucose, D-mannose, or derivatives of these two hexose sugars have been widely explored as potential approaches to accessing 2DG.

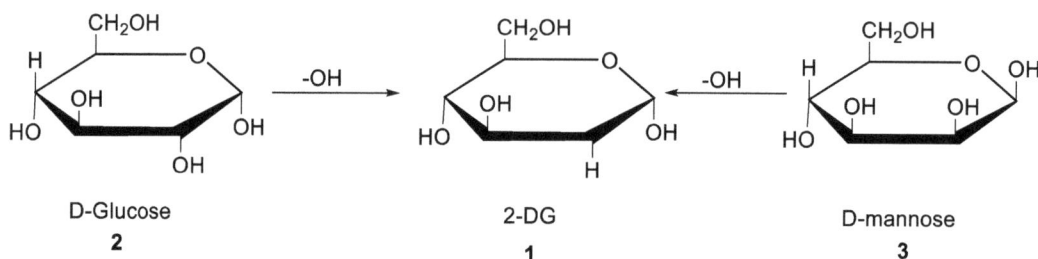

Fig. (1). DG from D-glucose and D-mannose.

2.1. From Glucal and its Derivatives

Glucal, a glycal derived from glucose, served as the standard starting material for the synthesis of 2DG. A commonly employed method for preparing glucal involves the classical Fischer–Zach reductive elimination reaction, which utilizes zinc dust in acetic acid to reduce 2,3,4,6-tetra-O-acetyl-D-glucopyranosyl bromide [4]. The general conversion process for synthesizing 2DG involves the initial bromination (or halogenation) of glucal at the C-2 position, followed by the subsequent replacement of bromine atom with a hydrogen atom. Bromination is typically carried out in a nucleophilic solvent using molecular bromine. Various reagents have been explored for the second step, which involves substituting the bromine attached to the C-2 carbon with hydrogen, as summarized in Table **1**.

Table 1. Reagents used to replace bromine attached to C-2 with a hydrogen.

S. No.	Catalyst/Reagent or Condition	References
1.	Photolysis	Binkley & Bankaitis, 1982 [5]
2.	Raney nickel/ H_2	Monneret, 1983 [6]
3.	Pd/C	Mereyala & Mamidyala, 2004 [7]
4.	Zn/NaH_2PO_4	Xu *et al.*, 2017 [8]
5.	Benzene, Bu_3SnH, MeCN, Et_2O, KF	Hakamata and co-workers [9]

In addition to chemical methods, enzymatic halohydration of glycals has been reported in the literature as an alternative approach for synthesizing 2-deoxy-D-glucose (2DG) [10]. Binkley and colleagues described a photolytic method involving the treatment of α and β anomers of compound **7** to yield the corresponding α and β anomers of compound 8. Subsequently, compound **8** was subjected to an ion-exchange resin, Baker's ANGA-542, in methanol, resulting in the formation of 2DG with a 78% yield. Precursor compound **7** was synthesized through a multi-Step process involving the nucleophilic bromination of compound **4**, followed by hydrolysis and acetylation reactions (Scheme **1**). This photochemical approach, coupled with the ion-exchange resin treatment, represents an alternative synthetic strategy for obtaining 2DG from glycal-derived intermediates [5].

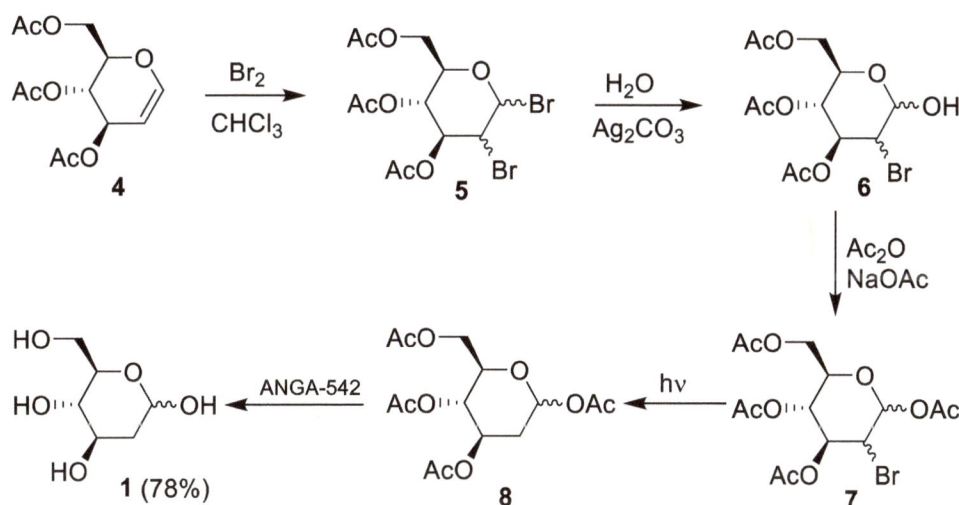

Scheme (1). Preparation of 2DG by photolysis coupled with ion-exchange resin treatment.

Monneret *et al.* reported a high-yielding synthetic method for producing 2DG from the precursor compound 3,4,6-tri-O-acetyl-1,5-anhydro-2-deoxy-D-*arabino*-hex-1-enitol. Their approach involved two key steps: 1) bromination of the precursor using N-bromosuccinimide as the brominating agent and 2) subsequent debromination achieved by catalytic hydrogenation over Raney nickel under 1 bar of hydrogen pressure. This two-step sequence afforded 2DG with an impressive 95% overall yield, making it an efficient synthetic route for obtaining this important glucose analog [6].

Mereyala and colleagues reported an economical and high-yielding synthetic process for the production of high-purity 2DG starting from (R)-D-Glycal

(Scheme **2**) [7]. Starting from D-Galactose, Hakamata and co-workers synthesized derivatives of *p*-nitrophenyl (PNP) α-D-galactopyranoside by treating **8** with p-nitrophenol in the presence of BF$_3$Et$_2$O, followed by ZnCl$_2$/AcOH [9].

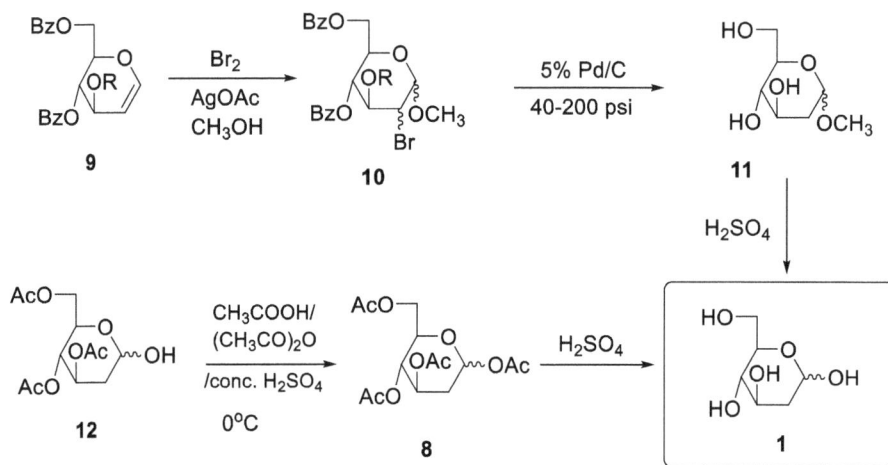

Scheme (2). Synthesis of 2DG from D-glucal.

The synthesis of 2-deoxy-D-glucose involves the hydrolysis of an alkyl 2-deoxy-α/β-D-glucopyranoside intermediate. This intermediate is prepared through a multi-step sequence beginning with the haloalkoxylation of R-D-glucal (R = H, 3,4,6-tri-O-benzyl) to yield alkyl 2-deoxy-2-halo-R-α/β-D-gluco/mannopyranoside, which is then reduced to form the desired alkyl 2-deoxy-2-halo-R-α/ β-D-gluco/mannopyranoside [7]. In a similar strategy, Fokt *et al.* reported the synthesis of 2-deutero-2DG **15** in 42% yield by debenzylation of **14** (Scheme **3**) [11]. The incorporation of deuterium at the 2-position of the glucose analog was a key aspect of their synthetic approach.

Interestingly, Yadav and co-workers reported the highly stereoselective addition of an alcohol to compound **4** in the presence of a CeCl$_3$·7H$_2$O–NaI reagent system in refluxing acetonitrile under neutral conditions. This reaction afforded the corresponding 2-deoxy-α-glycopyranosides in high yields [12]. However, in the absence of NaI, the glycals underwent a Ferrier rearrangement, leading to the formation of 2,3-unsaturated glycosides (Scheme **4**). Although this methodology has not been extended to the production of 2-deoxy-D-glucose (2DG) thus far, it presents a potentially straightforward approach. The deprotection of the C-1 alcohol in the 2-deoxy-α-glycopyranosides can be achieved through various procedures reported in the literature [13 - 16]. Subsequently, these deprotected compounds can be reduced to obtain 2DG [7].

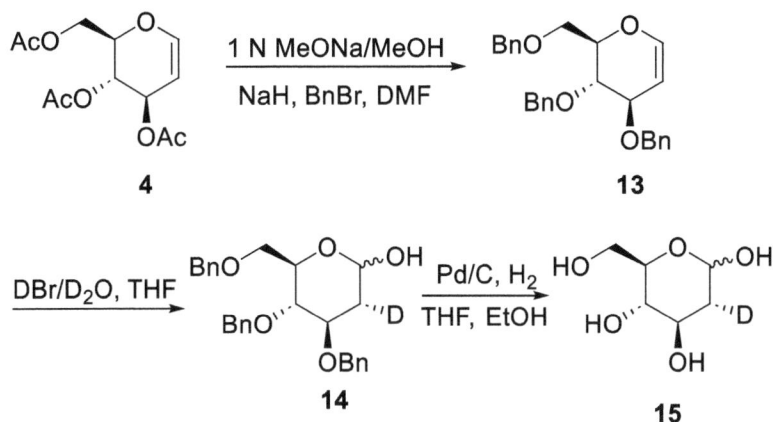

Scheme (3). Synthesis of 2-deoxy-2-deutero-D-glucose.

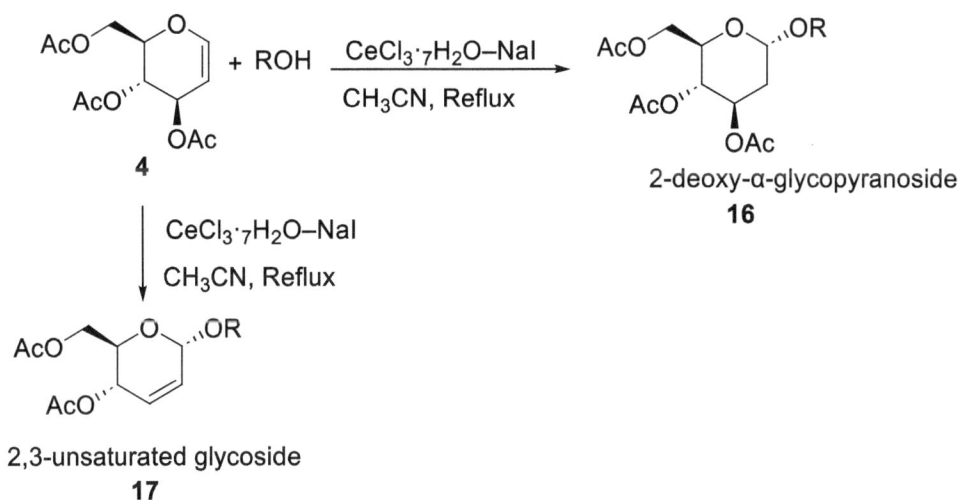

Scheme (4). Methodology for the preparation of 2-deoxy-α-glycopyranoside.

The use of N-iodosuccinimide (NIS) as an iodinating agent, coupled with the subsequent reduction and deprotection steps, provides a viable synthetic pathway for accessing 2-deoxyglucopyranose derivatives from suitably protected glucal precursors. A stereoisomeric mixture of 2-deoxy-2-iodoglucopyranose was obtained when 3,4,6-tri-O-benzyl-D-glucal or 3,4-di-O-benzyl-6-O-TIPS-D-glucal was treated with NIS. Subsequent reduction of these iodinated intermediates with sodium dithionite, followed by a debenzylation step, generates 2-deoxyglucopyranose as the desired product [17].

Watanabe and colleagues reported the synthesis of caged-2-deoxyglucose compounds **21** and **22** starting from precursor **4**. Their synthetic approach yielded caged products in moderate to good overall yields. Notably, the reaction afforded a mixture of anomeric isomers, with an α/β ratio of 7:3 for compound **21** and 4:1 for compound **22**. (Scheme **5**) [18].

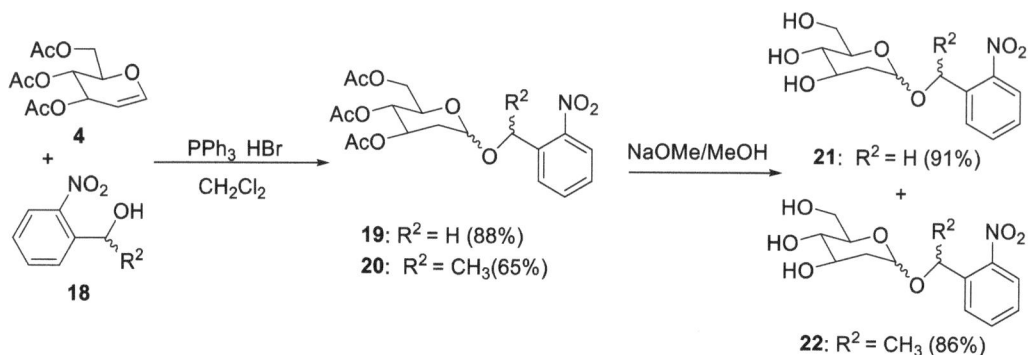

Scheme (5). Synthesis of caged-2-deoxyglucoses **21** & **22** from **4**.

2.2. Preparation of 2DG from D-glucose

Xu and colleagues reported a synthetic approach for the preparation of 2DG directly from D-glucose as the starting material. Their methodology involved a multistep sequence (Scheme **6**). Notably, this synthetic route afforded 2DG an overall yield of 62%, which is a decent yield for such a transformation starting from the natural glucose precursor [8].

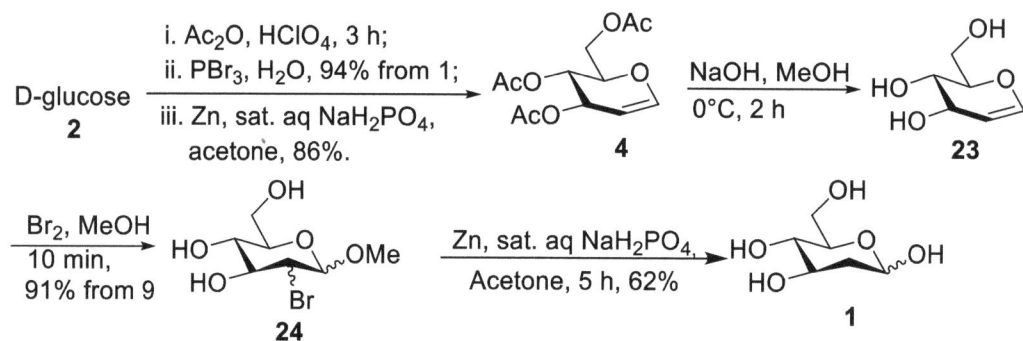

Scheme (6). D-glucose as a starting material for the synthesis of 2DG.

Masuda and colleagues reported a three-Step synthetic route for converting naturally occurring D-glucose directly into 2DG. Their approach circumvented the need for protection/deprotection steps typically involved in carbohydrate synthesis. This streamlined procedure afforded 2DG an overall yield of 48% from the D-glucose starting material (Scheme **7**) [19].

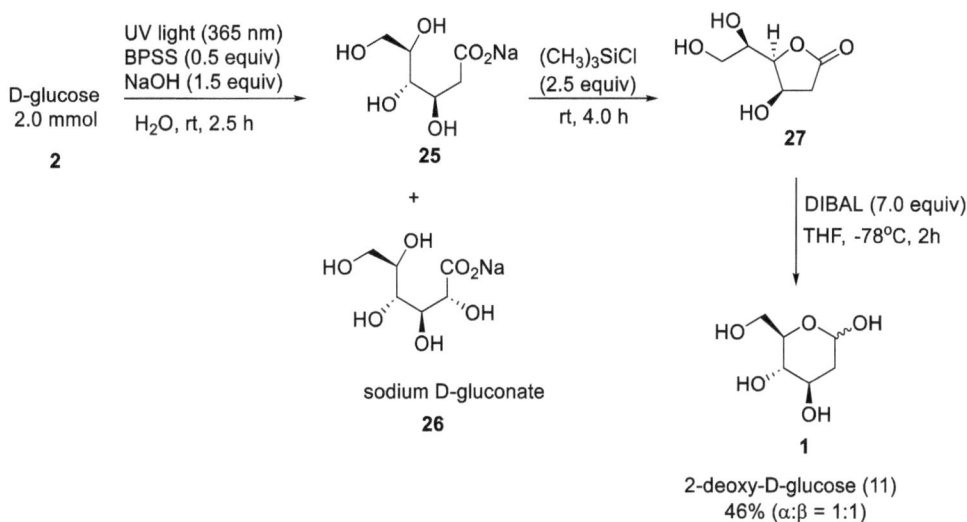

Scheme (7). Synthesis of 2-deoxy-D-glucose (1).

Cramer and colleagues reported a synthetic route for preparing 2-deoxy-D-glucose (2DG) starting from D-glucose **2**. However, their approach suffered from two major drawbacks: low product yields and the presence of impurities in the final product. (Scheme **8**) [20, 21].

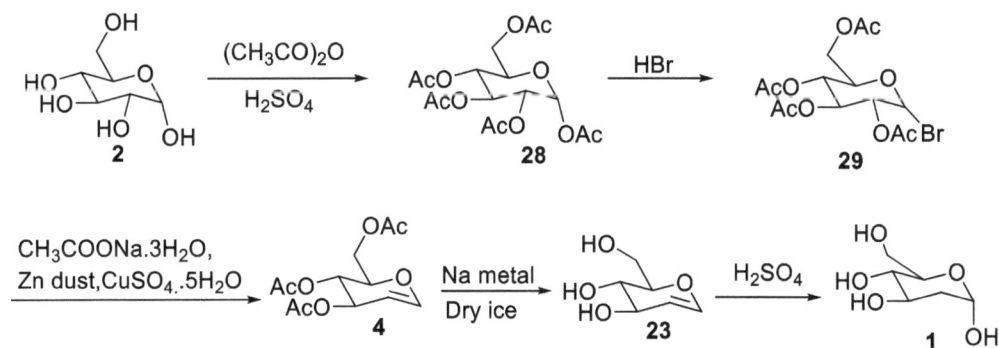

Scheme (8). Synthesis of 2DG from D-glucose.

2.3. Preparation of 2DG from Phenylhydrazone of D-Mannose

Jogersen and co-workers synthesized 2DG **1** and its epimer **29** from the phenylhydrazone of D-mannose. Their synthetic approach afforded a mixture of the two epimeric products in a 13:7 ratio, favoring the formation of 2DG. The use of D-mannose as the starting material is noteworthy, as it is an epimer of D-glucose and a readily available natural sugar. (Scheme **9**) [22].

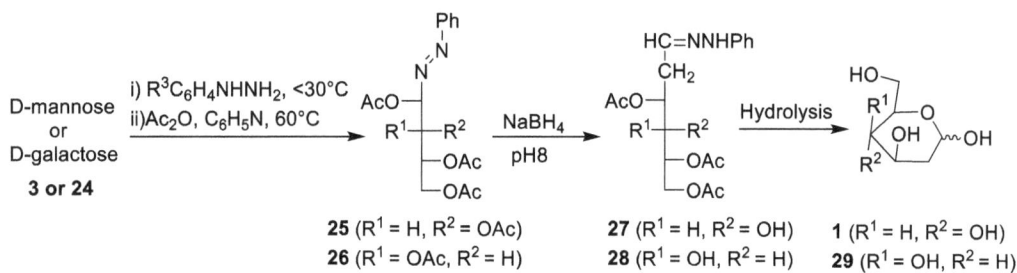

Scheme (9). Synthesis of 2DG from D-mannose.

2.4. Preparation of 2DG from D-*arabino*se

Sowden *et al.* described the synthesis of D-arabo-2-desoxyhexose from ribose (Scheme **10**, **30** → (**31**+**32**) → **33** →**34** → **1**) [23]. In a separate study, Koos *et al.* reported a synthetic route to obtain 2DG from tetraacetoxy-D-*arabino*-1-nitro-1-hexene **33** (Scheme **10**) in 73% yield as a diastereomeric mixture. Their approach involved reducing the nitro group using tin(II) chloride, followed by an acidic workup, with the reaction proceeding at room temperature [24].

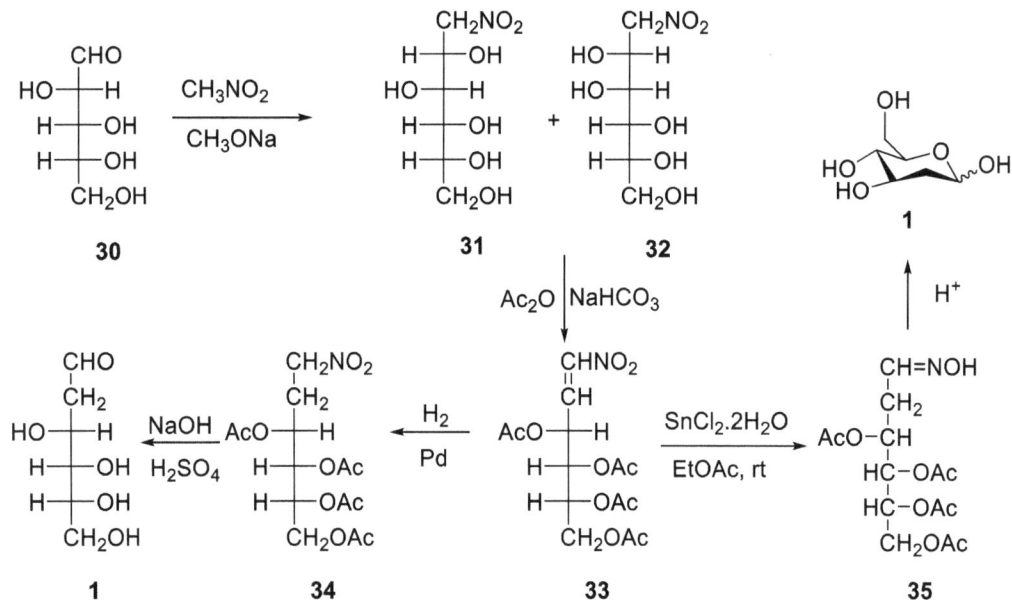

Scheme (10). Synthesis of 2-desoxy-D-*arabino*-hexose from D-*arabino*se.

2.5. Synthesis of 2DG by Ozonolysis of Tetrols

In their research, Roush and collaborators developed a synthetic pathway to 2DG that involved ozonolysis of tetrol intermediates **36**. These tetrol compounds **36** were themselves produced by methanolysis of the corresponding tetraacetate precursors, (Scheme **11**) [25]. However, the diastereoselectivity of this route was restricted by the enantiomeric purity of the epoxy aldehyde starting materials employed.

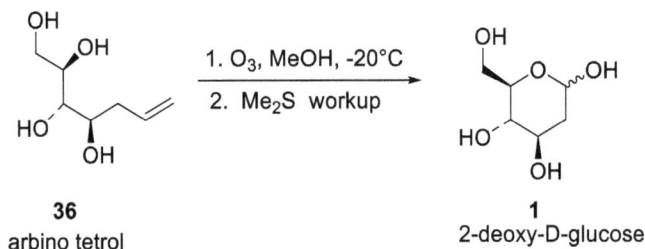

36
arbino tetrol

1
2-deoxy-D-glucose

Scheme (11). Synthesis of 2DG by ozonolysis of Tetrols **36**.

Regeling and colleagues reported a synthetic approach to produce 2-deoxy-D-glucose using D-glucono-1,5-lactone 37 as the starting material (Scheme **12**) [26]. Their synthetic sequence provided an efficient and high-yielding route to this important 2-deoxy sugar derivative, taking advantage of the readily available and inexpensive D-glucono-1,5-lactone precursor.

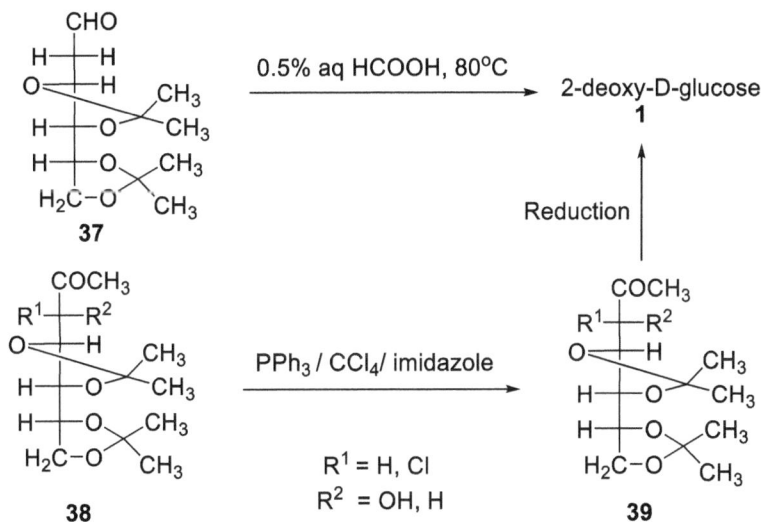

Scheme (12). Synthesis of 2-deoxy-D-glucose.

2.6. Synthesis of Labelled 2DG

Researchers have explored various synthetic routes to produce labeled versions of 2-deoxy-D-glucose (2DG), a glucose analog with applications in medical imaging and therapy.

Van Haver and co-workers reported the synthesis of 2-deoxy-D-[1-^{11}C]-glucose. The intermediate **11** was purified by HPLC before reduction to yield the final radiolabeled product (Scheme **13**) [27].

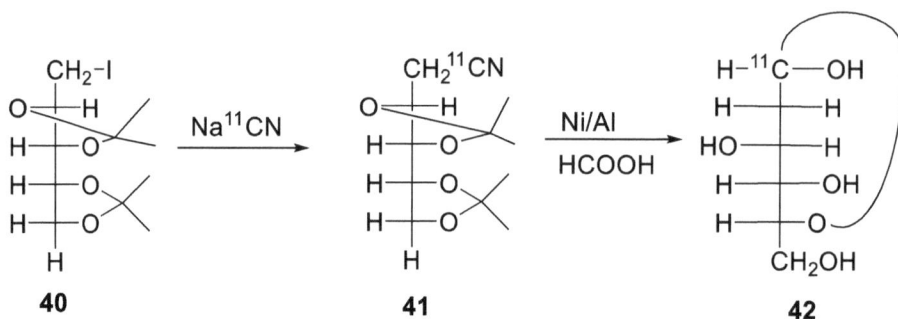

Scheme (13). Synthetic route to 2-deoxy-D- [1-^{11}C] glucose.

Yorimitsu *et al.* devised a rapid, automated synthesis of 6-[^{15}O]-2DG starting from **43** leveraging computer control for an efficient synthetic sequence and purification process. (Scheme **14**) [28].

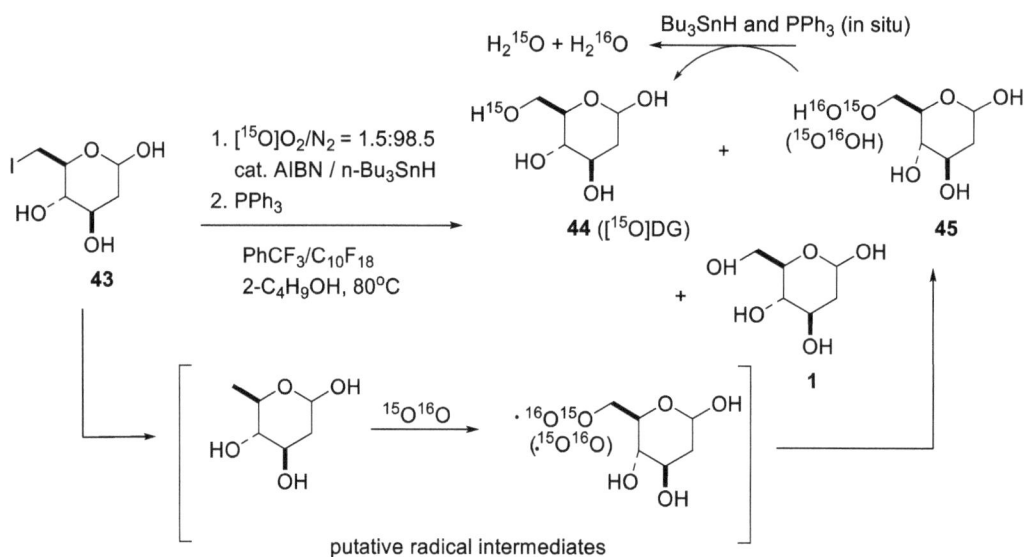

Scheme (14). Rapid synthesis of 6-[^{15}O]-2-deoxy-D-glucose.

Beyond radiolabeling, platinum(II) complexes derived from 2DG have also been prepared. These involved initial acetylation of 2DG followed by a platination reaction with a platinum diamine salt (Pt(DACH)SO$_4$) in the presence of barium hydroxide [29]. Synthesis of the deuterated analog 2-deutero-2DG **15** was reported by Fokt *et al.*, who employed a debenzylation strategy on a precursor molecule to install the deuterium label (Scheme **3**) [11]. While tritium-labeled [1,2-³H]-2DG has shown utility as a radiotracer for bacterial imaging, details on its radiosynthesis were not provided in the literature discussed [30].

The variety of labeled 2DG molecules accessible through these synthetic efforts highlights the significance of this glucose mimic and the desire to functionalize it for different biomedical applications.

2.7. Preparation of 2-deoxyglucoses from γ-lactones

Sala and coworkers described a synthetic approach to access 2-deoxyglucose (2DG) by employing a γ-lactone precursor **46** as the starting material (Scheme **15**) [31].

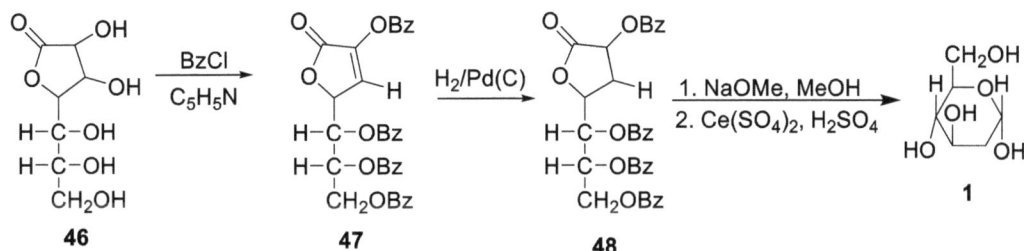

Scheme (15). Synthesis of 2DG from γ-lactone **46**.

2.8. Preparation of 2DG from 6,8-Dioxabicyclo[3.2.1]oct-2-ene

Murray *et al.* described a synthetic sequence where compound 49 was first converted into 1,6-anhydro-2-deoxy-β-DL-arabino-hexopyranose through an oxidation using meta-chloroperoxybenzoic acid (m-CPBA), followed by alkaline hydrolysis. The bicyclic intermediate 52, formed during this process, subsequently underwent acid-catalyzed hydrolysis to furnish compound **1** (Scheme **16**) [32]. However, a major drawback of this synthetic approach was the multi-Step preparation required to access the key starting material 49 [33].

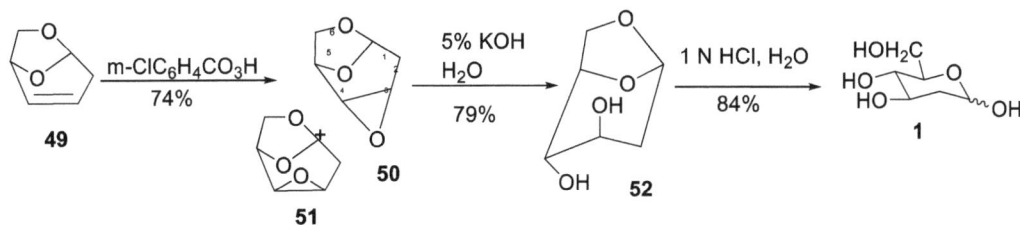

Scheme (16). Synthesis of 2DG by hydrolysis of bicyclic compound **49**.

3. MODERN METHODS TO IMPROVE YIELDS AND REDUCE PROCEDURAL COMPLEXITIES

3.1. Enzymatic Syntheses of 2DG

Researchers have explored alternative synthetic routes to 2DG that can provide improvements over traditional approaches in terms of higher product yields, improved purity profiles, and greater overall efficiency, while also addressing some of the practical limitations associated with conventional methods. A promising direction has been the development of enzymatic strategies for 2DG synthesis, which leverage the benefits of using biocatalysts such as high product yields, high levels of purity, and mild reaction conditions. These enzymatic pathways typically involve a few chemical synthesis steps in combination with enzymatic transformations, an approach sometimes referred to as a chemoenzymatic method. The key advantages of such chemoenzymatic routes include high product yields, high purity of the final product, and the ability to conduct the synthesis under mild conditions compatible with enzymatic catalysis.

Lee and coworkers described a synthetic approach to produce 2-deoxy-D-glucose-containing maltooligosaccharides (2DG-MOs). Their method involved using a pre-warmed mixture of Tris-HCl buffer (pH 7.0), 2DG, and sucrose as the substrate. This substrate mixture was incubated at 35°C and aliquots were taken at different time points. The reaction was carried out using purified recombinant amylosucrase (AS) and terminated by heating in a boiling water bath [34]. Liu and co-workers reported enzymatic halo hydration reactions of D-galactal, D-glucal, and L-Fucal glycals. They were able to synthesize 2-halo-2-deoxy sugars in good yields by employing chloroperoxidase to catalyze the bromohydration and iodohydration of these three glycal substrates. (Scheme **17**) [10].

Percival and co-workers compound **61** was converted into intermediate **64** through an enzymatic process. This key transformation enabled the formation of compound **63** as part of their synthetic efforts. (Scheme **18**) [35].

Kim and colleagues developed a synthetic methodology for 2-deoxy-D-glucose (2DG) and alkyl α-D-2-deoxyglucosides (A2DGs) that relied on the use of α-glucosidase from Aspergillus niger (ANGase) as the key biocatalyst (Scheme **19**) [36].

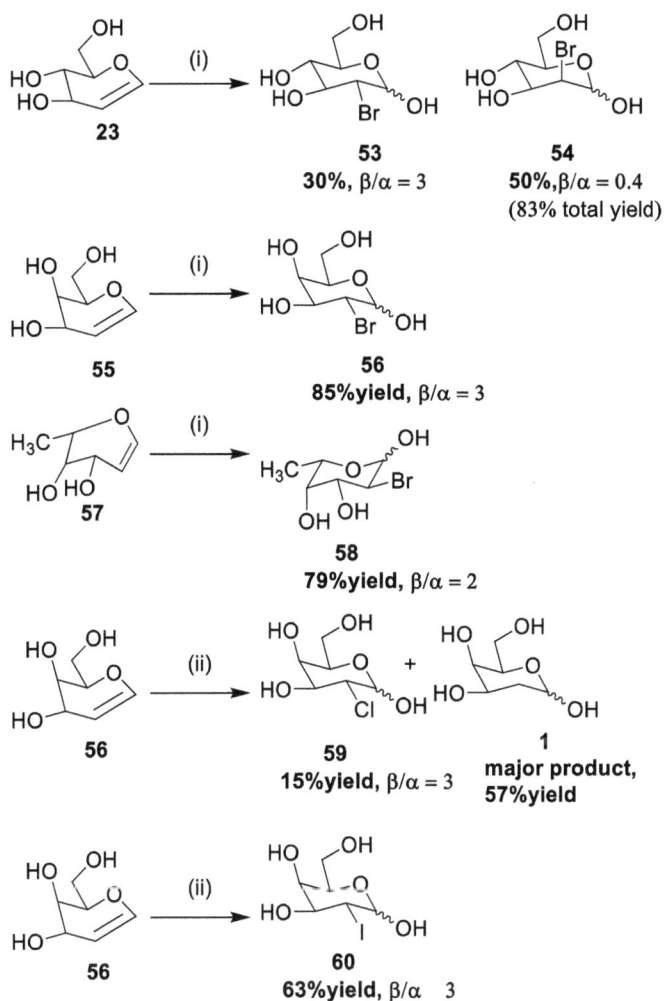

Scheme (17). Reagent and reaction conditions: (**i**) Chloroperoxidase, KBr, H₂O₂, pH 3 buffer solution, 2 h; (**ii**) Chloroperoxidase, H₂O₂, KCl, pH 3, 3 days; (**iii**) H₂O₂, KCl, pH 3, 30 min, with or without chloroperoxidase.

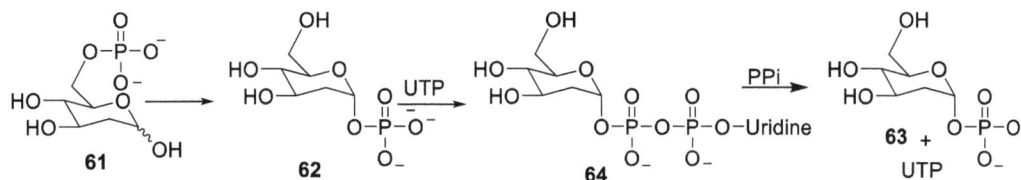

Scheme (18). Synthesis of 2-deoxy-alpha-D-glucopyranosyl phosphate.

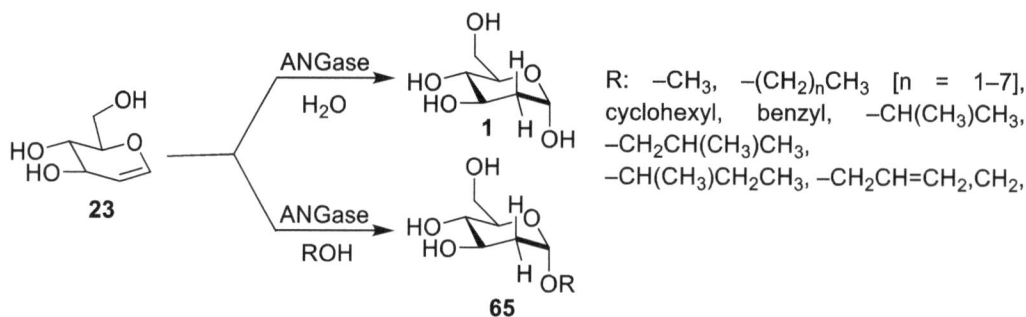

R: $-CH_3$, $-(CH_2)_nCH_3$ [n = 1–7], cyclohexyl, benzyl, $-CH(CH_3)CH_3$, $-CH_2CH(CH_3)CH_3$, $-CH(CH_3)CH_2CH_3$, $-CH_2CH=CH_2,CH_2,$

Scheme (19). Synthesis of alkyl α-D-2-deoxyglucosides by using *Aspergillus niger* α-glucosidase.

A high 95% yield of 2DG was obtained through a multi-Step procedure that employed rabbit muscle aldolase (RAMA; D-Fructose-1,6-diphosphate aldolase) as a biocatalyst. The key step involved the RAMA-catalyzed aldol addition of 1,3-dioxane-2-acetaldehyde to dihydroxyacetone phosphate (DHAP), followed by dephosphorylation using alkaline phosphatase (AP) to afford a ketone intermediate. Subsequent reduction of this ketone with sodium triacetoxyborohydride gave a 2:1 mixture of diastereomers in 75% yield. The desired 5S diastereomer was then resolved and converted into the corresponding acetal in 55% yield. Finally, deprotection of the acetal using aqueous hydrochloric acid in tetrahydrofuran provided 2-deoxy-D-arabino-hexose (95% yield from the acetal) [37].

CONCLUSION

2-deoxy-D-glucose (2DG) is a promising drug candidate that adheres to Lipinski's guidelines for drug-likeness. It exhibits diverse biological activities like glucose metabolism antagonism, sugar uptake inhibition, antiviral, anti-inflammatory, and anticancer effects. Utilized as both a metabolic inhibitor and tracer, 2DG uniquely mimics D-glucose and D-mannose. The COVID-19 pandemic has revived interest in 2DG's antiviral potential. However, current synthetic routes are tedious, expensive, and low-yielding. Developing an economical, milder process for high-yield, pure 2DG synthesis could enable new antiviral drugs and treatments for hyperglycemia. Overcoming synthetic hurdles could unlock 2DG's full therapeutic value across viral infections, cancer, and metabolic disorders.

LIST OF ABBREVIATIONS

2DG   2-Deoxy-D-Glucose

DMF   N,N-Dimethylformamide

RAMA   D-Fructose-1,6-diphosphate Aldolase

ACKNOWLEDGEMENTS

The authors express their sincere gratitude to the management of Amity University, Gwalior, Madhya Pradesh, India, for providing the facilities to write and submit the book chapter for publication.

REFERENCES

[1]   Singh, R.; Gupta, V.; Singh, K. A review on synthetic methods for 2-deoxy-D-glucose. *ARKIVOC,* **2023**, *2022*(6), 199-219.
        [http://dx.doi.org/10.24820/ark.5550190.p011.946]

[2]   Singh, R.; Gupta, V.; Kumar, A.; Singh, K. 2-Deoxy-D-Glucose: A novel pharmacological agent for killing hypoxic tumor cells, oxygen dependence-lowering in Covid-19, and other pharmacological activities. *Adv. Pharmacol. Pharm. Sci.,* **2023**, *2023*, 1-15.
        [http://dx.doi.org/10.1155/2023/9993386] [PMID: 36911357]

[3]   Pająk, B.; Zieliński, R.; Manning, J.T.; Matejin, S.; Paessler, S.; Fokt, I.; Emmett, M.R.; Priebe, W. The antiviral effects of 2-Deoxy-D-glucose (2-DG), a dual D-glucose and D-mannose mimetic, against SARS-CoV-2 and other highly pathogenic viruses. *Molecules,* **2022**, *27*(18), 5928.
        [http://dx.doi.org/10.3390/molecules27185928] [PMID: 36144664]

[4]   Priebe, W.; Grynkiewicz, G. Formation and reactions of glycal derivatives. In: *Glycoscience: Chemistry and Chemical Biology I–III*; Springer Berlin Heidelberg: Berlin, Heidelberg, **2001**; pp. 749-783.
        [http://dx.doi.org/10.1007/978-3-642-56874-9_23]

[5]   Binkley, R.W.; Bankaitis, D. Photochemically based synthesis of deoxy sugars. Synthesis of 2-Deox-
        -D- Arabino-Hexopyranose (2-Deoxy-D-Glucose) and several of its derivatives from 3,4,6-Tri-
        O-Acetyl-D-Glucal. *J. Carbohydr. Chem.,* **1982**, *1*(1), 1-8.
        [http://dx.doi.org/10.1080/07328308208085074]

[6]   Monneret, C.; Choay, P. A convenient synthesis of 2-deoxy-d-arabino-hexose and of its methyl and benzyl glycosides. *Carbohydr. Res.,* **1981**, *96*(2), 299-305.
        [http://dx.doi.org/10.1016/S0008-6215(00)81880 7]

[7]   Mereyala, H. B.; Mamidyala, S. K. Process for the Synthesis of 2-Deoxy-D-Glucose. IN193296B **2004**.

[8]   Liu, F.-W.; Xu, W.; Yang, H.; Liu, Y.; Hua, Y.; He, B.; Ning, X.; Qin, Z.; Liu, H.M. Facile approaches to 2-Deoxy-d-glucose and 2-Deoxy-α-d-glucopyranonucleosides from d-Glucal. *Synthesis,* **2017**, *49*(16), 3686-3691.
        [http://dx.doi.org/10.1055/s-0036-1589501]

[9]   Hakamata, W.; Nishio, T.; Oku, T. Hydrolytic activity of α-galactosidases against deoxy derivatives of p-nitrophenyl α-d-galactopyranoside. *Carbohydr. Res.,* **2000**, *324*(2), 107-115.
        [http://dx.doi.org/10.1016/S0008-6215(99)00281-5] [PMID: 10702877]

[10]   Liu, K.K.C.; Wong, C.H. Enzymic halohydration of glycals. *J. Org. Chem.,* **1992**, *57*(13), 3748-3750.
        [http://dx.doi.org/10.1021/jo00039a050]

[11]   Fokt, I.; Skora, S.; Conrad, C.; Madden, T.; Emmett, M.; Priebe, W. d-Glucose and d-mannose-based metabolic probes. Part 3: Synthesis of specifically deuterated d-glucose, d-mannose, and 2-deoxy-d-glucose. *Carbohydr. Res.,* **2013**, *368*, 111-119.
        [http://dx.doi.org/10.1016/j.carres.2012.11.021] [PMID: 23376241]

[12]   Yadav, J.S.; Reddy, B.V.S.; Reddy, K.B.; Satyanarayana, M. CeCl3·7H2O: a novel reagent for the synthesis of 2-deoxysugars from d-glycals. *Tetrahedron Lett.,* **2002**, *43*(39), 7009-7012.
        [http://dx.doi.org/10.1016/S0040-4039(02)01584-8]

[13]   Chen, H.; Zhao, Z.; Hallis, T.M.; Guo, Z.; Liu, H. Insights into the Branched-Chain Formation of Mycarose: Methylation Catalyzed by an (S)-Adenosylmethionine-Dependent Methyltransferase. *Angew. Chem. Int. Ed.,* **2001**, *40*(3), 607-610.
[http://dx.doi.org/10.1002/1521-3773(20010202)40:3<607::AID-ANIE607>3.0.CO;2-8]

[14]   Lipshutz, B.H.; Pegram, J.J.; Morey, M.C. Chemistry of β-trimethylsilylethanol. II. A new method for protection of an anomeric center in pyranosides. *Tetrahedron Lett.,* **1981**, *22*(46), 4603-4606.
[http://dx.doi.org/10.1016/S0040-4039(01)82992-0]

[15]   Zhang, J.; Fu, J.; Si, W.; Wang, X.; Wang, Z.; Tang, J. A highly efficient deprotection of the 2,2,2-trichloroethyl group at the anomeric oxygen of carbohydrates. *Carbohydr. Res.,* **2011**, *346*(14), 2290-2293.
[http://dx.doi.org/10.1016/j.carres.2011.08.007] [PMID: 21889124]

[16]   Sridhar, P.R.; Anjaneyulu, B.; Rao, B.U. Regioselective Anomeric *O* -Benzyl Deprotection in Carbohydrates. *Eur. J. Org. Chem.,* **2021**, *2021*(41), 5665-5668.
[http://dx.doi.org/10.1002/ejoc.202101033]

[17]   Costantino, V.; Imperatore, C.; Fattorusso, E.; Mangoni, A. A mild and easy one-pot procedure for the synthesis of 2-deoxysugars from glycals. *Tetrahedron Lett.,* **2000**, *41*(47), 9177-9180.
[http://dx.doi.org/10.1016/S0040-4039(00)01643-9]

[18]   Watanabe, S.; Hirokawa, R.; Iwamura, M. Caged compounds of a 2-deoxyglucose: Facile synthesis and their photoreactivity. *Bioorg. Med. Chem. Lett.,* **1998**, *8*(23), 3375-3378.
[http://dx.doi.org/10.1016/S0960-894X(98)00623-4] [PMID: 9873737]

[19]   Masuda, Y.; Tsuda, H.; Murakami, M. C1 Oxidation/C2 reduction isomerization of unprotected aldoses induced by light/ketone. *Angew. Chem. Int. Ed.,* **2020**, *59*(7), 2755-2759.
[http://dx.doi.org/10.1002/anie.201914242] [PMID: 31823472]

[20]   Cramer, F.B.; Woodward, G.E. 2-Desoxy-D-glucose as an antagonist of glucose in yeast fermentation. *J. Franklin Inst.,* **1952**, *253*(4), 354-360.
[http://dx.doi.org/10.1016/0016-0032(52)90852-1]

[21]   Cramer, F.B. The alpha form of 2-desoxy-d-glucose. *J. Franklin Inst.,* **1954**, *257*(1), 69-70.
[http://dx.doi.org/10.1016/0016-0032(54)91056-X]

[22]   Jørgensen, C.; Pedersen, C. Preparation of 2-deoxyaldoses from aldose phenylhydrazones. *Carbohydr. Res.,* **1997**, *299*(4), 307-310.
[http://dx.doi.org/10.1016/S0008-6215(97)00022-0]

[23]   Sowden, J.C.; Fischer, H.O.L. Carbohydrate C-nitroalcohols: the acetylated nitroölefins. *J. Am. Chem. Soc.,* **1947**, *69*(5), 1048-1050.
[http://dx.doi.org/10.1021/ja01197a022] [PMID: 20240494]

[24]   Koóš, M. An alternative route to 2-deoxysugar and 2,3-unsaturated sugar derivatives *via* the corresponding 1-nitro-1-alkenes. *Tetrahedron Lett.,* **2000**, *41*(28), 5403-5406.
[http://dx.doi.org/10.1016/S0040-4039(00)00863-7]

[25]   Roush, W.R.; Straub, J.A.; VanNieuwenhze, M.S. A stereochemically general synthesis of 2-deoxyhexoses *via* the asymmetric allylboration of 2,3-epoxy aldehydes. *J. Org. Chem.,* **1991**, *56*(4), 1636-1648.
[http://dx.doi.org/10.1021/jo00004a053]

[26]   Regeling, H.; Chittenden, G.J.F. The chemistry of D-gluconic acid derivatives. Part IV Synthesis and reactions of some 2-deoxy-D-hexonic acid derivatives, a new synthesis of 2-deoxy-D- *arabino* -hexose and some related compounds. *Recl. Trav. Chim. Pays Bas,* **1989**, *108*(10), 330-334.
[http://dx.doi.org/10.1002/recl.19891081003]

[27]   van Haver, D.; Rabi, N.A.; Vandewalle, M.; Goethals, P.; Vandecasteele, C. Routine production of 2-deoxy-D-[1-^{11} C]glucose : An alternative. *J. Labelled Comp. Radiopharm.,* **1985**, *22*(7), 657-666.
[http://dx.doi.org/10.1002/jlcr.2580220704]

[28]   Yorimitsu, H.; Murakami, Y.; Takamatsu, H.; Nishimura, S.; Nakamura, E. Ultra-rapid synthesis of 15O-labeled 2-deoxy-D-glucose for positron emission tomography (PET). *Angew. Chem. Int. Ed.,* **2005**, *44*(18), 2708-2711.
[http://dx.doi.org/10.1002/anie.200500044] [PMID: 15828042]

[29]   Mi, Q.; Ma, Y.; Gao, X.; Liu, R.; Liu, P.; Mi, Y.; Fu, X.; Gao, Q. 2-Deoxyglucose conjugated platinum (II) complexes for targeted therapy: design, synthesis, and antitumor activity. *J. Biomol. Struct. Dyn.,* **2016**, *34*(11), 2339-2350.
[http://dx.doi.org/10.1080/07391102.2015.1114972] [PMID: 26524393]

[30]   Keiichi, K.; Seiji, O.; Masakazu, K.; Miki, M.; Yumiko, M.; Asuka, M.; Yoshie, Y. Radiodiagnostic agent for bacterial infections. JP2019137686A, **2019**.

[31]   Sala, L.F.; Fernández Cirelli, A.; de Lederkremer, R.M. β-elimination in aldonolactones. Synthesis of 2-deoxy-D-lyxo-hexose and 2-deoxy-D-arabino-hexose. *Carbohydr. Res.,* **1980**, *78*(1), 61-66.
[http://dx.doi.org/10.1016/S0008-6215(00)83660-5]

[32]   Murray, T.P.; Singh, U.P.; Brown, R.K. Total synthesis of several monodeoxy and dideoxy-D--hexopyranoses from 6,8-Dioxabicyclo[3.2.1]oct-2-ene and 6,8-Dioxabicyclo[3.2.1]oct-3-ene. *Can. J. Chem.,* **1971**, *49*(12), 2132-2138.
[http://dx.doi.org/10.1139/v71-345]

[33]   Berberich, S.M.; Cherney, R.J.; Colucci, J.; Courillon, C.; Geraci, L.S.; Kirkland, T.A.; Marx, M.A.; Schneider, M.F.; Martin, S.F. Total synthesis of (+)-ambruticin S. *Tetrahedron,* **2003**, *59*(35), 6819-6832.
[http://dx.doi.org/10.1016/S0040-4020(03)00370-3]

[34]   Lee, B.H.; Koh, D.W.; Territo, P.R.; Park, C.S.; Hamaker, B.R.; Yoo, S.H. Enzymatic synthesis of 2-deoxyglucose-containing maltooligosaccharides for tracing the location of glucose absorption from starch digestion. *Carbohydr. Polym.,* **2015**, *132*, 41-49.
[http://dx.doi.org/10.1016/j.carbpol.2015.06.012] [PMID: 26256322]

[35]   Percival, M.D.; Withers, S.G. Applications of enzymes in the synthesis and hydrolytic study of 2-deoxy-α-D-glucopyranosyl phosphate. *Can. J. Chem.,* **1988**, *66*(8), 1970-1972.
[http://dx.doi.org/10.1139/v88-317]

[36]   Kim, Y.M.; Okuyama, M.; Mori, H.; Nakai, H.; Saburi, W.; Chiba, S.; Kimura, A. Enzymatic synthesis of alkyl α-2-deoxyglucosides by alkyl alcohol resistant α-glucosidase from Aspergillus niger. *Tetrahedron Asymmetry,* **2005**, *16*(2), 403-409.
[http://dx.doi.org/10.1016/j.tetasy.2004.11.046]

[37]   Borysenko, C.W.; Spaltenstein, A.; Straub, J.A.; Whitesides, G.M. The synthesis of aldose sugars from half-protected dialdehydes using rabbit muscle aldolase. *J. Am. Chem. Soc.,* **1989**, *111*(26), 9275-9276.
[http://dx.doi.org/10.1021/ja00208a046]

CHAPTER 3

Characterization of 2-Deoxy-D-glucose

Ramji Lal Yadav[1,*], Neeru Singh[1], S. N. Karaiya[1], Rahul Dev[1] and Anil Kumar[1]

[1] *Analytical Research & Development, Mankind Research Centre, IMT Manesar, Gurugram, Haryana-122052, India*

Abstract: 2-Deoxy-D-glucose is an important pharmaceutical intermediate, and its analytical characterization is critical for establishing its purity and quality. This chapter summarizes spectroscopic techniques, including UV, IR, NMR, and mass spectrometry, along with HPLC and GC studies used for the complete structural elucidation and purity analysis of 2-Deoxy-D-glucose. The UV spectrum of 2-Deoxy-D-Glucose showed no distinct peaks. The IR spectrum displayed characteristic bands for the O-H and C-H functional groups. ^{1}H, ^{13}C, APT, DEPT NMR, HSQC, and HMBC experiments confirmed the nominally proposed structure. ESI-MS revealed an $[M+Na]^+$ ion at m/z 187. Specific optical rotation was measured in water. HPLC studies estimated the related substances and assay to be 1.2% and 99.8%, on an anhydrous basis, respectively. The residual solvents, such as methanol, isopropyl alcohol, ethyl acetate, and toluene, were determined by GC headspace and found to be within the limits. The collective analytical evidence confirmed that the test sample met the quality specifications for 2-Deoxy-D-glucose.

Keywords: Assay, Chromatography, Characterization, Karl fisher, Related substances, Spectroscopy, Specific optical rotation, 2-deoxy-D-glucose.

1. INTRODUCTION

2-Deoxy-D-Glucose can be described as a synthesized glucose analog that acts as an antagonist of D-glucose. It is synthesized from D-Glucal; therefore, both compounds may be present during the synthesis. Compared with glucose, the hydroxyl group at position 2 is replaced with hydrogen [1].

This chapter describes the techniques used for the characterization of 2-Deoxy-D-Glucose and the determination of its purity by high-performance liquid chromatographic (HPLC). Glucose and glucose analogs present a very unique set

---

* **Corresponding author Ramji Lal Yadav:** Analytical Research & Development, Mankind Research Centre, IMT Manesar, Gurugram, Haryana-122052, India; E-mail: rlyadav2k@gmail.com

Raman Singh, Antresh Kumar & Kuldeep Singh (Eds.)

of difficulties in HPLC analysis, which is due to the lack of chromophores on the sugar molecules, leading to poor sensitivity and specificity for ultraviolet absorption detection; therefore, HPLC with RI detection is used [2].

2. EXPERIMENTAL

2.1. Chemicals and Reagents

The synthesis of 2-DG has been reported previously [1]. 2-Deoxy-D-Glucose was manufactured by Mankind Pharma Limited. Honeywell Hydranal™ Karl Fisher reagent was used. Gradient-grade methanol and acetonitrile were purchased from Merck (Darmstadt, Germany). N, N-Dimethylacetamide, isopropanol, ethyl acetate, and toluene (AR grade) were purchased from Sigma-Aldrich (Merck, Darmstadt, Germany). Potassium bromide was obtained from Merck (Darmstadt, Germany). DMSO-d6 was procured from Eurisotop (Cambridge Isotope Laboratories, Inc.). Distilled water was obtained using a Milli-Q water purifier system (Milli-Q IX-7015; Millipore, Milford, MA, USA).

2.2. Instrumentation and Methodology

2.2.1. Sulphated ash Content

The sulfated ash content of 2-Deoxy-D-Glucose was determined by ignition of 1 g of the sample at 600°C for 3 h, along with sulfuric acid treatment of the residue and reignition until a constant weight was achieved.

2.2.2. Water Content

The moisture content of 2-Deoxy-D-Glucose was determined by Karl Fisher titration using a T5 Excellence Titrator (Mettler Toledo). The moisture content of the samples was determined using methanol of known weight (50 mg).

2.2.3. Specific Optical Rotation

Polarimetric measurements were performed using an AUTOPOL® V PLUS scientific polarimeter. The sample cell length was 1 dm and the output LED light source had a wavelength of 589 nm. A 1% w/w solution in water was used for measurements at 25 ± 0.5°C. The Rudolph Research software allows for easy determination of the angle of polarization of the solution.

2.2.4. UV-VIS Spectroscopy

The ultraviolet absorption spectrum of an approximately 10 ppm 2-Deoxy-D-Glucose solution in distilled water was recorded to determine λmax using a

PerkinElmer Lambda 365 UV-Vis spectrophotometer equipped with a quartz cell with a 1 cm path length. The obtained spectrum was processed using the UV WINLAB ES software.

2.2.5. FTIR

The samples were prepared as a potassium bromide dispersion with 0.5%w/w concentration of the test sample or standard by applying a pressure of approximately 8 tons/cm2 (800MPa) using a dye press. The IR absorption spectrum of 2-Deoxy-D-Glucose was obtained using a PerkinElmer Spectrum Two FT-IR spectrometer in the wavelength range(s) of 4000 cm-1 - 400 cm-1, with a calculated resolution of 4 cm^{-1}. Sixteen scans were obtained and processed using the Spectrum ES software.

2.2.6. Nuclear Magnetic Resonance

Nuclear magnetic resonance spectra were recorded on a Bruker Ascend 400 MHz spectrometer with DMSO-d$_6$ as the solvent, tetramethylsilane (TMS) as the internal standard, and a 5 mm PABBO BB probe. ^{1}H NMR spectra were recorded at a base frequency of 500 MHz at 24° with 10 scans, relaxation delay of 2s, and pulse angle of 90°. ^{13}C NMR had a base frequency of 100 MHz at 24°, with 3000 scans, a relaxation delay of 2s, and a pulse angle of 90°. Heteronuclear single quantum coherence spectroscopy (HSQC) and heteronuclear multiple bond correlation spectroscopy (HMBC) experiments were performed using the same instrument and in the same solvent to assign the correlation. The ^{1}H chemical shift values are reported with respect to that of the TMS peak [δ_H(TMS)= 0.00 ppm], and the ^{13}C chemical shift values are reported with respect to that of the solvent residual peak [δ_C(DMSO-d$_6$) = 39.52 ppm].

2.2.7. Mass Spectrometry

Mass Spectrometry was conducted on a Waters Xevo TQS-Micro (Waters Corp., Milford, MA, USA) mass spectrometer attached to a Waters Acquity TM Ultra Performance Liquid Chromatography (UPLC) system (Waters, Milford, MA). The analytes were identified using positive electrospray ionization mass spectrometry (ESI). The capillary voltage and collision energy were maintained at 3.5 kV and 20 eV, respectively. Nitrogen was used as desolvation gas at a flow rate of 650 L/h at 350°C. The spectra were recorded in the range of m/z 100-1000 for full scan analysis. The sample was prepared by dissolving approximately 1 mg of the sample in methanol.

2.2.8. Related Substances and Assay (By HPLC)

2.2.8.1. Instruments

The Waters 2695 HPLC system was used in this study. The HPLC system was coupled with a Waters 2414 refractive index detector. Empower 2 software was used to process HPLC data. The samples were weighed on the weighing balance of the Mettler Toledo XSE205 Dual Range model, and a pH meter (Mettler Toledo Seven Excellence S400 Bio) was used for buffer preparation.

2.2.8.2. Preparation of Solutions

2.2.8.2.1. Mobile Phase

The buffer solution was prepared by mixing 1.0 mL of ammonia solution (25%) in 1000 mL of HPLC grade water and filtering out the solution through a 0.45µm membrane filter. The mobile phase was prepared by mixing the buffer solution and acetonitrile at a ratio of 12:88 (v/v). It was then degassed by sonication. A homogenous mixture of HPLC-grade acetonitrile and water in a ratio of 70:30 v/v was used as the diluent for sample preparation and as a blank solution.

2.2.8.2.2. Standard and Sample Solutions for Related Substances

A standard stock solution (750 ppm) was obtained by transferring an accurate amount of 150 mg of 2-Deoxy-D-Glucose Reference standard into a 10 mL volumetric flask containing 5 mL of diluent, shaken well, sonicated, made up to a volume of 10 mL with diluent, and further diluting 1 mL of this solution to 20mL with diluent. To obtain a standard solution (45 ppm), 3 mL of the standard stock solution was further diluted in a 50mL volumetric flask using the diluent. The sensitivity solution (300 ppm) was prepared by diluting 1 mL of the standard stock solution with 50 mL of the diluent. 2-Deoxy-D-Glucose test samples (15000 ppm) were prepared by weighing and transferring 150 mg of the 2-Deoxy-D-Glucose sample into a 10 mL volumetric flask, adding 5mL of diluent, sonicating to dissolve the content, and diluting it to the volume using the diluent.

2.2.8.2.3. Standard and Sample Solutions for the Assay

A standard solution (7500 ppm) was obtained by transferring an accurate amount of 300 mg of 2-Deoxy-D-Glucose Reference standard into a 20 mL volumetric flask containing 5 mL of diluent, shaken well, sonicated, made up to a volume of 20 mL with diluent, and further diluting 10 mL of this solution to 20mL with diluent. 2-Deoxy-D-Glucose test samples (7500ppm) were prepared by weighing and transferring 300 mg of the 2-Deoxy-D-Glucose sample into a 20 mL volumetric flask, adding 5mL of diluent, sonicating to dissolve the content, diluting to make up the volume with diluent, and further diluting 10 mL of this solution to 20mL with diluent.

2.2.8.2.4. Forced Degradation Study

The aim of this study was to ensure the effective separation of 2-Deoxy-D-Glucose and its degradation spike at the retention time of 2-Deoxy-D-Glucose. Forced degradation studies were performed to evaluate the stability, properties, and specificity of this method. All the solutions used in the stress studies were prepared at an initial concentration of 750 ppm of 2-Deoxy-D-Glucose. All the samples were filtered before injection.

Acid degradation was carried out in 1N HCl and alkaline degradation was conducted using 1N NaOH with a 0.5mL volume individually and refluxed for 60 min at 60°C. After cooling, the solutions were neutralized to equal volumes and diluted with the mobile phase. Solutions for oxidative stress studies were prepared using 30% H_2O_2 (1.0 mL) at a concentration of 750 ppm of 2-Deoxy-D-Glucose and after reflux for 3 h at 60°C in a hot air oven. The sample solution was then cooled to room temperature and diluted with the mobile phase. For thermal stress testing, the drug solution (750ppm) was heated in a thermostat at 105°C for 24 h, cooled down, and then used. For photostability testing, the drug solution(750ppm) for photostability testing was exposed to 1.2 million lux hours and analyzed. The sample was also exposed to a higher humidity condition of 90% RH for seven days and analyzed.

2.2.8.3. Chromatographic Conditions

X-Bridge amide (Waters, 4.6 mm x 250 mm, 3.5 μm) autosampler and analytical column were kept at a constant temperature of 25°C. The detector sensitivity was set to 512 and the temperature was set to 35°C. The positive mode was selected for polarity. A water/acetonitrile (10:90, v/v) solution was used to clean the needles. The injection volume was 20 μL and the flow rate was adjusted to 0.8 mL/min. For the related chemicals, the run duration was 45 minutes, whereas for the overall assay, it was 25 minutes.

For 120 minutes, the liquid chromatographic system with the RID was allowed to acclimate to experimental conditions. A blank (diluent) was injected prior to sample sequence injections once the system reached equilibrium. The system was checked for signal response by injecting a sensitivity solution, followed by six replicates of the standard solution to determine the system suitability parameters. The sample solution was then injected into a single sample.

2.2.9. Gas Chromatography

The experiments were carried out on a Shimadzu GC-2010 Plus gas chromatograph (Shimadzu, Japan) equipped with a flame ionization detector and split/splitless injector. SKY liner, Rtx-624, 60.0m length, 0.25 mm internal diameter, and film thickness 1.4 micron (Restek, USA) were used for Shimadzu GC. The PE Split/Splitless injector (Supleco, USA) uses 4 mm split inlet sleeves. Glass wool treated with silane (Supelco, USA), fused silica wool deactivated by a base (Restek, USA), or deactivated glass wool (Restek, USA) was utilized to fill the liners. A Chromeleon 7.2, SR4 chromatography data system was used to control the gas chromatographs and collect and process the data. The compounds were separated using an Rtx-624 capillary column (Restek, USA) measuring 60.0 m in length, 0.25 mm in internal diameter, and 1.4 μm film thickness. The phase composition of the column was determined by cross-bonding 6% cyanopropylphenyl and 94% dimethylpolysiloxane. The GC system was supplied with hydrogen (99.9999%), helium (99.9999%), and air (99.9990%).

2.2.9.1. HS-GC–FID Instrumental Conditions

HS sampling was performed by using an HS20 headspace sampler. A 1mL sample loop was employed. The headspace autosampler conditions were set as follows:

Oven temperature, 80°C; sample line temperature 90°C, transfer line temperature, 100°C; shaking level 5, multi-injection time: 1; equilibrating time: 30 min, pressurize time: 2 min, pressurized equilibrating time; 0.5 min, load time: 0.5 min, load equilibration time: 0.1 min, injection time: 0.5 min, needle flush time: 15 min, GC cycle time: 40 min.

A 60m × 0.25 mm i.d. Rtx-624 column with 1.4μm film thickness (Restek, USA) was utilized for chromatographic separation of the OVIs. The carrier gas was nitrogen at a linear velocity of 27.7 cm/s (1.5mL/min). The flow was 30mL/min, the filter time constant was 200ms, and the split ratio was 1:15. The FID system was set at 300°C, and nitrogen was used as the makeup gas. The column oven temperature program involved an initial temperature of 40°C for 5 min, which increased at a rate of 10°C/min to 230°C, and held for 6 min for a total run time of 30 min.

2.2.9.2. Standard Preparation

N, N-dimethylacetamide was used to generate a standard stock solution of OVIs at the amounts listed in Table 1. N, N-dimethylacetamide was used to dilute a 1.0 mL standard stock solution to 50 mL to create a working standard. Immediately after adding 1 mL of the working standard solution to a 20 mL headspace vial, the vial was sealed with an aluminum crimp and rubber septum.

Table 1. Preparation of Standard and Stock solutions of OVIs.

OVI	Stock Standard Solution (ppm)	Working Standard (ppm)	Equivalent Concentration in Sample (ppm or µg/g)
Methanol	7500	150	3000
Isopropanol	12500	250	5000
Ethyl acetate	12500	250	5000
Toluene	2240	44.8	896

2.2.9.3. Sample Preparation

A 20 mL headspace container was filled with 50 mg of the material. After adding 1.0 mL N-dimethylacetamide, the vial was quickly sealed with an aluminum crimp cap and a rubber septum.

Before injecting the sample sequence, two blanks of N-N dimethylacetamide were injected into the HSGC system to bring it into equilibrium in the experimental setup. After preparing the samples in triplicate, the working standard was individually injected into six replicates to assess the specificity of the procedure and the sensitivity of the signal.

3. RESULTS AND DISCUSSION

3.1. UV-VIS Spectroscopy

The ultraviolet absorption spectrum of 2-Deoxy-D-Glucose does not show a clear λ_{max} but an absorbance of 0.032672 AU at 210.12 nm (Fig. **1**), which is supported by the fact that the majority of the sugars have no charge, with the exception of those having negatively charged and ionizable acid groups, and most of them do not contain chromophores and fluorophores, which leads to low absorption at UV and visible wavelengths [3, 4].

3.2. IR spectroscopic Analysis

The IR spectra of many complexes of 2-Deoxy-D-Glucose have been previously discussed [5, 6]. There has been a mention of IR analysis of 2-Deoxy-D-Glucose using ATR but there is no brief discussion of the IR bands and their comparison with theoretical values [7]. We have briefly discussed the IR absorption bands and a list of assignments for the characteristic IR bands is presented in Table **2**. The

O-H stretching mode of alcohol appeared at 3412.61 cm^{-1} and 3353.02 cm^{-1} in comparison to the theoretical range of 3650 cm^{-1} to 3200 cm^{-1} [8]. The aliphatic C-H stretching vibration, which is usually observed in the range of 3000 cm^{-1} to 2850 cm^{-1}, was observed at 2956.08 cm^{-1}, 2905.86 cm^{-1} and 2875.12 cm^{-1}. The O-H bending of deoxyglucose was observed at 1265 cm^{-1} and the C-O stretching of deoxyglucose (Figs. **2A** and **2B**).

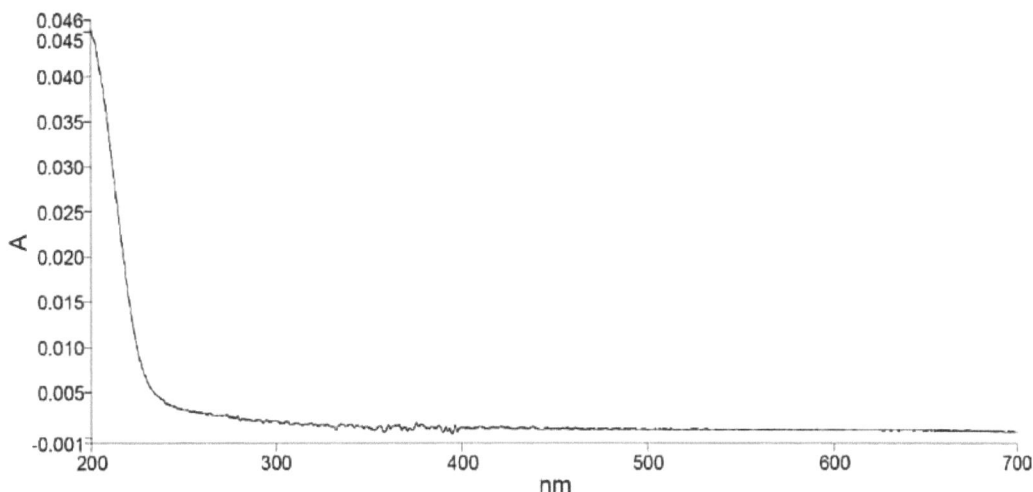

Fig. (1). UV-Visible Spectrum of 2-Deoxy-D-Glucose.

Table 2. Characteristic absorption bands observed in the FTIR spectrum of 2-Deoxy-D-Glucose.

Type of Vibration	Theoretical Value (cm^{-1})	Observed Absorption Band (cm^{-1})	Intensity
νO-H (alcohol)	3650-3200	3412.61, 3353.02	m
νC-H (aliphatic)	3000-2850	2956.08, 2905.86, 2875.12	s
O-H bending of deoxyglucose	1250-1270	1265	s
C-O stretching of deoxyglucose	1300-1000	1149.85,1065.65	s

3.3. Confirmation of Structure by NMR

2-Deoxy-D-Glucose was subjected to 1D NMR (^{1}H, ^{13}C, APT, DEPT-135, and DEPT-90) and 2D NMR (HSQC and HMBC).

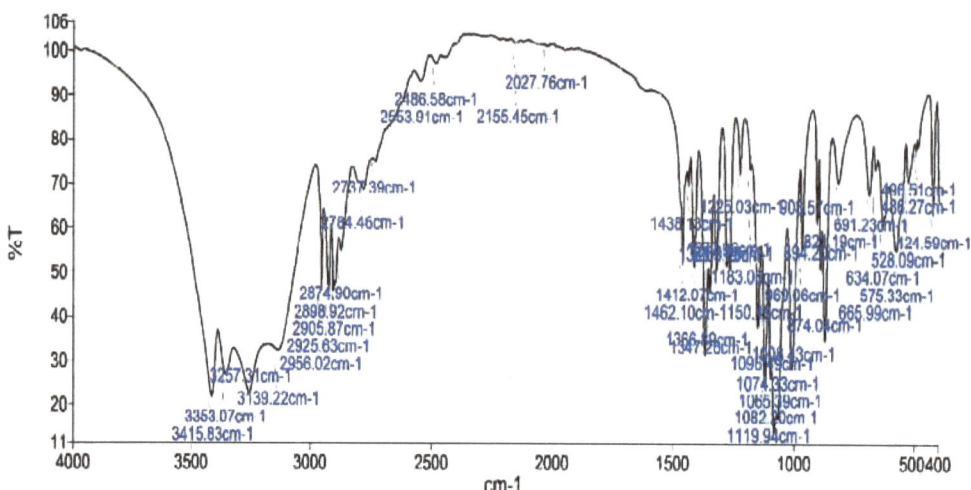

Fig. (2A). FTIR Spectrum of 2-Deoxy-D-Glucose.

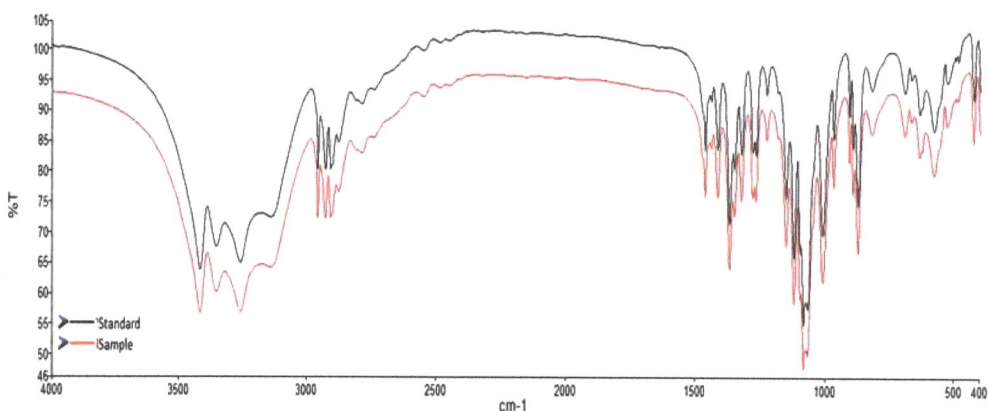

Fig. (2B). Overlaid FTIR Spectrum of 2-Deoxy-D-Glucose with Standard.

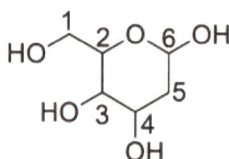

6-(hydroxymethyl)tetrahydro-2*H*-pyran-2,4,5-triol

Fig. (3). Chemical Structure of 2-Deoxy-D-Glucose.

NMR spectra of various carbohydrates and substituted deoxy sugars have been previously reported [9 - 12] and this chapter covers the first detailed discussion of the structure of 2-Deoxy-D-glucose by NMR spectroscopy. The majority of glucose in the solution was observed to be present as cyclic pyranose [13], and this was also evident when examining the 2-Deoxy-D-glucose's ^{1}H NMR spectra. The resonance of non-exchanging protons of the pyranose ring, aside from the proton connected at the anomeric carbon (C–6), is responsible for the signals detected in the range of 1.2 ppm, 2.9 ppm, and 3.3 ppm. The anomeric proton is shifted downfield from other non-exchanging protons by increased oxygen shielding, which separates the anomeric proton from other protons, as shown at 4.6 ppm. In addition, the signal observed in the region of 3.4 and 3.6 ppm corresponds to the aliphatic diastereotopic protons attached to the same carbon (C-1) with different chemical shifts in ^{1}H NMR (H-1). While the singular peak was observed at 61.40 ppm in ^{13}C NMR, similar justification can be made for the diastereotopic protons (H-5) observed at 1.2 and 1.9 ppm in ^{1}H NMR and signal at 41.38 ppm in ^{13}C NMR. The correlation of protons (H-5) with carbon (C-5) in HSQC (2D NMR) and negative phase peak ($>CH_2$) in DEPT-135 NMR confirms the evidence of the 2-Deoxy form of glucose with the support of multiple peaks of anomeric proton (H-6) due to spin-spin coupling with protons of adjacent CH_2 (C-5) and -OH protons. In addition, the signal due to the resonance of exchangeable protons (-OH) was observed downfield in the region of 4 to 6 ppm, which could be easily identified by D_2O exchange ^{1}H NMR spectra and the absence of correlation observed in HSQC NMR. All assignments given in Tables **3A** and **3B** are supported by additional experimental NMR data such as APT, DEPT-90, DEPT-135, and HMBC NMR.

Table 3A. Chemical shifts and their multiplicities with assignments (^{1}H NMR).

Chemical Shift (ppm)	Multiplicity	Number of Proton(s)	Assignment
1.232-1.317	m	1	H-5
1.877-1.925	m	1	
2.889-2.946	m	1	H-3
2.994-3.038	m	1	H-2
3.353-3.374	m	1	H-4
3.387-3.463	m	1	H-1
3.646-3.694	m	1	
4.432-4.461	t (3J= 5.6 Hz)	1	-OH(attached at C-1)
4.584-4.629	m	1	H-6
4.761-4.773	d (3J= 4.8 Hz)	1	-OH(attached at C-3 & C-4)
4.781-4.793	d (3J= 4.8 Hz)	1	
6.495-6.511	d (3J= 6.4 Hz)	1	-OH(attached at C-6)

Table 3B. Chemical shifts with assignments (^{13}C, APT, DEPT-135 and DEPT-90).

Chemical Shift (ppm)	APT	DEPT-135	DEPT-90	Assignment
41.38	>CH$_2$	>CH$_2$	-	C-5
61.40	>CH$_2$	>CH$_2$	-	C-1
70.94	>CH-	>CH-	>CH-	C-4
71.75	>CH-	>CH-	>CH-	C-3
76.91	>CH-	>CH-	>CH-	C-2
93.53	>CH-	>CH-	>CH-	C-6

The NMR (^1H, ^{13}C, APT, DEPT-135, and DEPT-90) data are presented in Tables **3A** and **3B**, the respective spectra are presented in Figs. (**4A-4G**), and HSQC and HMBC data are presented in Figs. (**4H** and **4I**), respectively.

3.4. Mass Spectrum

The ESI positive ionization mass spectrum of 2-Deoxy-D-Glucose displays that M+Na$^+$ is one of the most stable associates, with the most intense maximum at m/z = 187.00 (Fig. **5**), which is supported by the formation of a stable cyclic ion by the binding of hydroxy groups with one metal ion [14]. Additionally, glucose in the ESI source has a strong affinity towards metal ions, and there is enhanced efficiency for the formation of sodium adducts with oxygen bases [15, 16].

Fig. (4A). ^{1}H NMR Spectrum of 2-Deoxy-D-Glucose.

Fig. (4B). The ^{1}H NMR Spectrum of 2-Deoxy-D-Glucose-expanded.

Fig. (4C). The ^{1}H NMR Spectrum of 2-Deoxy-D-Glucose-expanded.

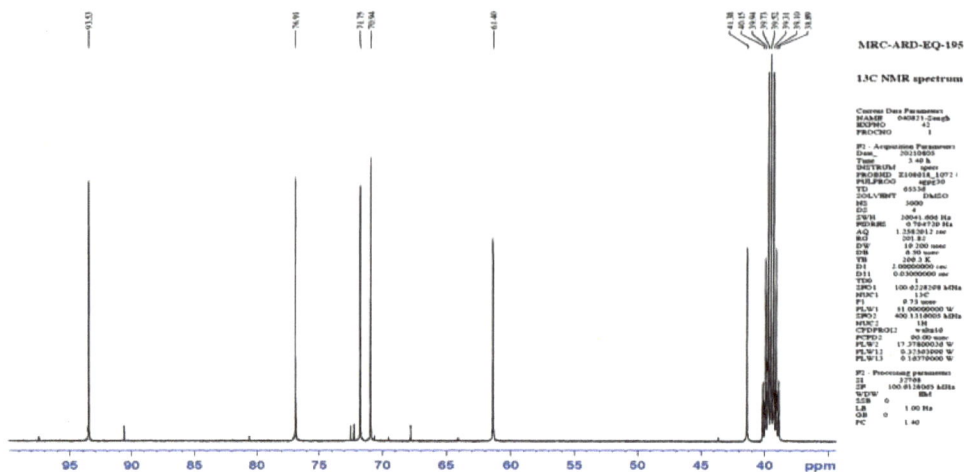

Fig. (4D). ^{13}C NMR Spectrum of 2-Deoxy-D-Glucose.

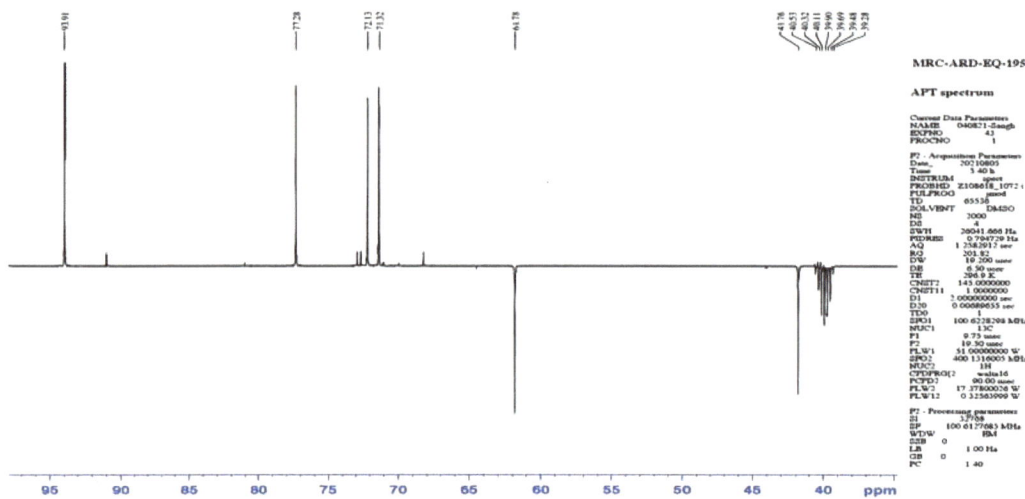

Fig. (4E). APT NMR Spectrum of 2-Deoxy-D-Glucose.

Fig. (4F). DEPT-135 NMR Spectrum of 2-Deoxy-D-Glucose.

Fig. (4G). DEPT-90 NMR Spectrum of 2-Deoxy-D-Glucose.

Fig. (4H). HSQC NMR Spectrum of 2-Deoxy-D-Glucose.

Fig. (4I). HMBC NMR Spectrum of 2-Deoxy-D-Glucose.

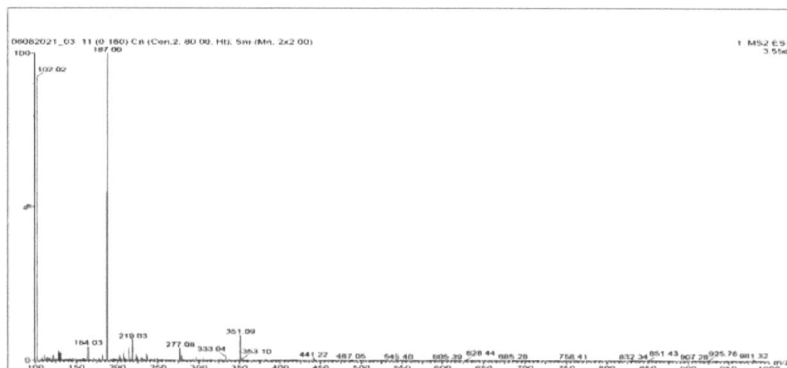

Fig. (5). Mass Spectrum of 2-Deoxy-D-Glucose.

3.5. HPLC (RS/Assay)

The purity of 2-Deoxy-D-Glucose has previously been demonstrated by gas chromatography with a derivatization method using a trimethylsilyl agent [17]. In addition, several HPLC methods have been employed to determine the purity of monosaccharides, including UV detection (a less sensitive method) [18] and derivatization methods [19 - 22]. The present study provides a newly developed and validated method for determining the purity and assay without any derivatization, which provides accurate results with a lower detection level. To establish an appropriate and reliable LC method for the better detection of 2-Deoxy-D-glucose by RI detection, various mobile phases and columns were employed to develop and optimize liquid chromatography. Ultimately, a Waters X-Bridge amide (250 x 4.6) mm, with 3.5µm column was used to measure the mobile phase, which included 0.1% ammonia solution in water and acetonitrile (12:88 v/v) at a steady flow rate of 0.8 mL/min.

3.5.1. Method Validation

To ensure accurate, dependable, and consistent results when determining the amounts of all relevant substances in all samples and 2-Deoxy-D-glucose, the HPLC methods were validated. HPLC methods were validated for accuracy, linearity, specificity, and precision [23]. A representative chromatogram obtained for 2-Deoxy-D-glucose is shown in Fig. (**6A**).

The calibration curve was linear over the concentration range of 15–68 µg/mL (Table **4A**), (Fig. **6B**), and the regression equation was y=22375 x -3017.87 with a correlation coefficient of 0.9996. The RSD in the precision studies was 2.11% (intraday) and 3.43% (interday) (Table **4B**). The % mean recovery (LOQ, 100 and 150% levels) in accuracy studies was found to be 91.36% to 100.51%. The %RSD was found to be between 2.11% and 8.69% in the robustness studies, indicating that the method was precise, accurate, and robust. The LOQ was found to be 15 µg/mL and the LOD was found to be 7.5 µg/mL.

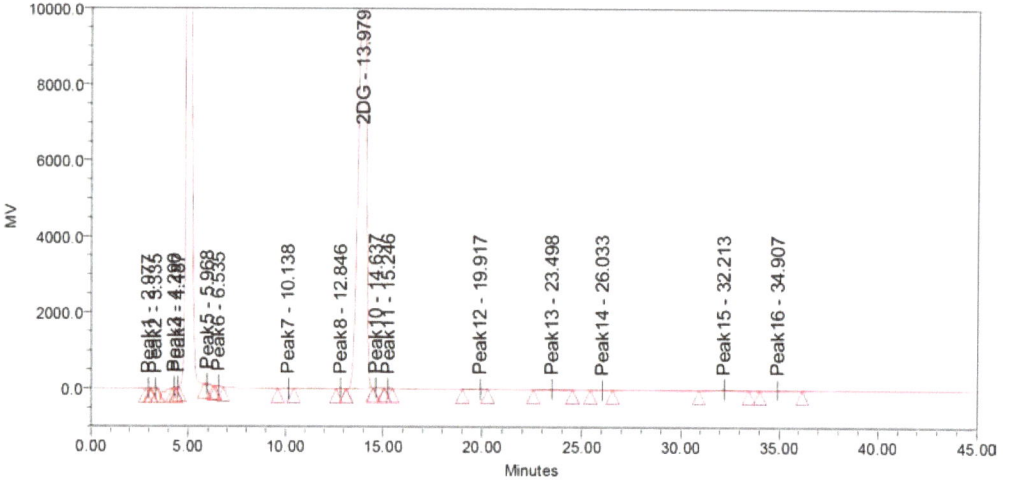

Fig. (6A). HPLC Chromatogram of 2-Deoxy-D-Glucose for Related Substances.

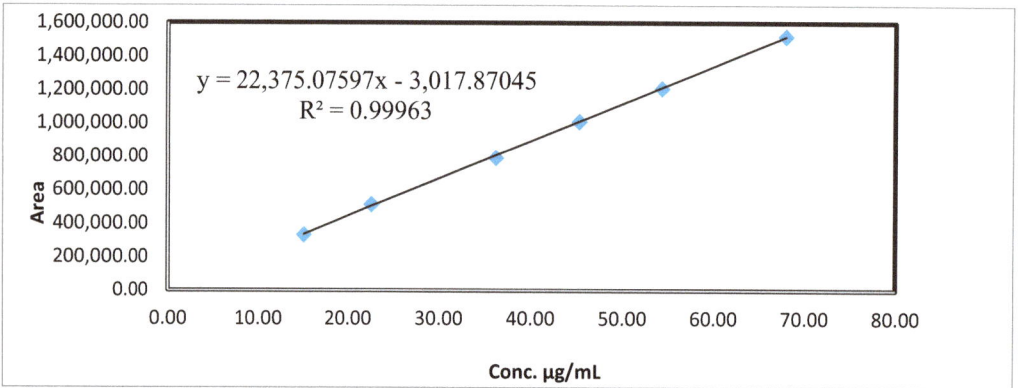

$$y = 22{,}375.07597x - 3{,}017.87045$$
$$R^2 = 0.99963$$

Fig. (6B). Linearity Curve for 2-Deoxy-D-Glucose.

Table 4A. Linearity data of 2-Deoxy-D-Glucose.

Linearity Levels	Conc. (µg/ mL)	Average Area
Linearity at LOQ	15.095	333894
Linearity at 50%	22.643	514776
Linearity at 80%	36.229	793283
Linearity at 100%	45.286	1011312
Linearity at 120%	54.343	1210672
Linearity at 150%	67.929	1522098

(Table 4A) cont.....

Linearity Levels	Conc. (µg/ mL)	Average Area
Square correlation		0.99963
Slope		22375.07597
Y-intercept		-3017.87045
Y-intercept at 100%		-0.30

Table 4B. Precision data for 2-Deoxy-D-Glucose.

Preparation	Area of 2-Deoxy-D-glucose Peak	Preparation	Area of 2-Deoxy-D-glucose Peak
Method precision-1	1050022	Intermediate precision-1	984720
Method precision-2	1049817	Intermediate precision -2	978387
Method precision-3	1044604	Intermediate precision -3	1056681
Method precision-4	1005580	Intermediate precision -4	1054764
Method precision-5	1070000	Intermediate precision -5	1017500
Method precision-6	1028792	Intermediate precision -6	992968
Average	1041469.167	Average	1014170
STD DEV	21979	STD DEV	34824
%RSD	2.11	%RSD	3.43

The results of the assay, which used the suggested method to measure 2-Deoxy-D-glucose, ranged from 98% to 102%, with a 2.0% relative standard deviation. For the 2-Deoxy-D-glucose peak, the theoretical plates were 7892 (more than 3000) and the tailing factor was 0.89 (less than 2). The assay had a 98.1 to 99.2 percent RSD value, and the accuracy at 80% to 120% was 0.34. The developed method was robust, as evidenced by the % RSD assay value of less than 2.0% under both the original and robust conditions.

3.5.2. Degradation Study

During acidic degradation, 15.2% of the drug was decomposed with 7.9% of the single highest degradant observed at 35.23 minutes. During alkaline degradation, a major degradant was observed at 5.77 min without interfering with the elution of the drug peak at 14.75 min and the percentage of drug decomposition was found to be 1.26%. No significant degradation was observed in the thermal-, photolytic-, oxidative-, and humidity-treated test samples of 2-Deoxy-D-Glucose [24].

3.6. GC-HS

In this study, a novel gas chromatography technique was employed to determine bulk residual solvents. Previously, a gas chromatography method was developed for the determination of residual solvents in 2-deoxy-2-[^{18}F] fluoro-D-glucose, but a gas chromatographic technique was used for establishing residual solvents in 2-Deoxy-D-glucose [25]. The main objective of this study was to develop a sensitive and simple gas chromatography technique to ascertain all residual solvents found in the active analyte. Trials were conducted during the development of the analytical method, and after the procedure was refined and determined to be workable, it could be implemented.

The retention times of the solvent peaks of the standard solutions matched those of the spiked test sample solutions. No interference was observed in the retention time of the solvent peak from the blank and standard/test samples (Fig. 7), which clearly resembled the specificity of the proposed method. The retention times for Methanol, Isopropanol, Ethyl acetate, and toluene were 4.8, 8.4, 11.3, and 15.6 minutes, respectively. All results obtained from the validation parameters met the ICH acceptance criteria [26]. Finally, the anticipated method was found to be suitable for routine analysis in research laboratories and quality control.

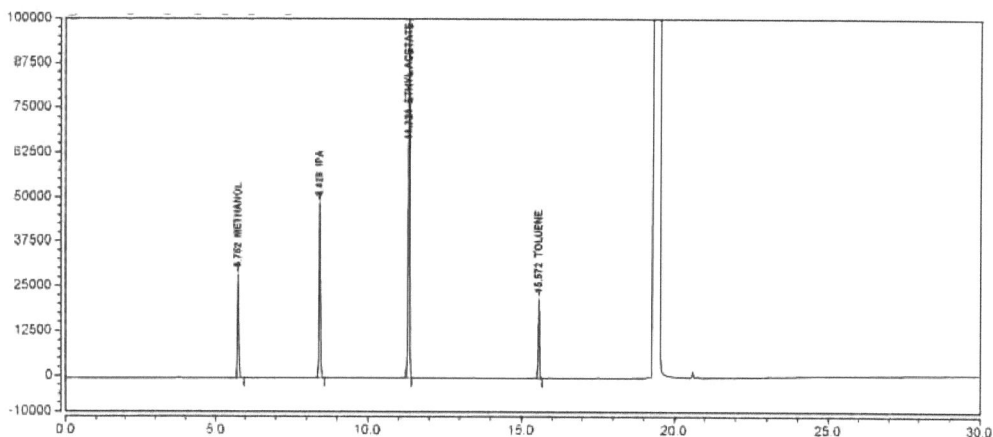

Fig. (7). GC chromatograms of standard solutions of Methanol, Isopropanol, Ethyl acetate, and toluene.

CONCLUSION

A variety of analytical methods, such as UV-VIS, FTIR, mass spectrometry, and NMR spectroscopy, have been used to characterize 2-Deoxy-D-Glucose and are in agreement with the suggested structure (Fig. **3**). Using the Waters X-Bridge amide column and RI detector, a sensitive and selective HPLC method was created to measure 2-Deoxy-D-Glucose simultaneously. The method was validated in accordance with the regulatory guidelines. The procedure was linear, exact, accurate, and appropriate for regular analysis. With excellent resolution and brief retention periods, the developed method for estimating residual solvents in 2-Deoxy-D-glucose included methanol, isopropanol, ethyl acetate, and toluene. It is also economical and precise. In the near future, this approach could be successfully applied in industry in quality control departments, testing laboratories, biopharmaceutical and bioequivalence studies, and pharmacokinetic studies.

LIST OF ABBREVIATIONS

APT	Attached Proton Test
DEPT	Distortionless Enhancement by Polarization Transfer
DMSO-d6	Dimethyl sulfoxide-d_6
ESI	Electrospray Ionization
FTIR	Fourier transform infrared.
GC	Gas Chromatography
HMBC	Heteronuclear Multiple Bond Correlation
HPLC	High-Performance Liquid Chromatography
HS	Headspace
HS	Headspace
HS-GC–FID	Headspace gas chromatography with flame ionization detection
HSQC	Heteronuclear Single Quantum Coherence
IR	Infra Red
LC	Liquid chromatographic
Min	Minute(s)
NMR	Nuclear magnetic resonance
OVIs	Organic Volatile Impurities
RI	Refractive Index
RID	Refractive Index Detection
RS	Related Substances
TMS	Tetramethylsilane
UPLC	Ultra Performance Liquid Chromatography
UV-VIS	Ultraviolet- Visible

ACKNOWLEDGEMENTS

The authors express their sincere gratitude to the scientists and colleagues of the Mankind Research Centre for providing sincere support throughout the process.

REFERENCES

[1]   Singh, K.; Singh, R.; Gupta, V. A review on synthetic methods for 2-Deoxy-D-Glucose. , **2023**, *2022*(6), 199-219.
        [http://dx.doi.org/10.24820/ark.5550190.p011.946]

[2]   Jalaludin, I.; Kim, J. Comparison of ultraviolet and refractive index detections in the HPLC analysis of sugars. *Food Chem.,* **2021**, *365*, 130514.
        [http://dx.doi.org/10.1016/j.foodchem.2021.130514] [PMID: 34247043]

[3]   Rovio, S.; Yli-Kauhaluoma, J.; Sirén, H. Determination of neutral carbohydrates by CZE with direct UV detection. *Electrophoresis,* **2007**, *28*(17), 3129-3135.
        [http://dx.doi.org/10.1002/elps.200600783] [PMID: 17661315]

[4]   Kurzyna-Szklarek, M.; Cybulska, J.; Zdunek, A. Analysis of the chemical composition of natural carbohydrates – An overview of methods. *Food Chem.,* **2022**, *394*, 133466.
        [http://dx.doi.org/10.1016/j.foodchem.2022.133466] [PMID: 35716502]

[5]   Xiong, F.; Zhu, Z.; Xiong, C.; Hua, X.; Shan, X.; Zhang, Y.; Gu, N. Preparation, characterization of 2-deoxy-D-glucose functionalized dimercaptosuccinic acid-coated maghemite nanoparticles for targeting tumor cells. *Pharm. Res.,* **2012**, *29*(4), 1087-1097.
        [http://dx.doi.org/10.1007/s11095-011-0653-9] [PMID: 22173782]

[6]   Akan, Z.; Demiroğlu, H.; Avcıbaşı, U.; Oto, G.; Ozdemir, H.; Deniz, S.; Basak, A.S. Complexion of Boric Acid with 2-Deoxy-D-glucose (DG) as a novel boron carrier for BNCT. *Medical Science and Discovery,* **2014**, *1*(3), 65-65.
        [http://dx.doi.org/10.17546/msd.74442]

[7]   Parker, F.S.; Ans, R. Infrared Spectra of Carbohydrates (700–250 cm $^{-1}$) Determined by both Attenuated Total Reflectance and Transmission Techniques. *Appl. Spectrosc.,* **1966**, *20*(6), 384-388.
        [http://dx.doi.org/10.1366/000370266774386542]

[8]   Introduction to Spectroscopy; Donald L. Pavia ... *et al.*; Stamford Cengage Learning, **2015**.

[9]   Subotkowski, W.; Friedrich, D.; Weiberth, F.J. Syntheses and NMR characterizations of epimeric 4-deoxy-4-fluoro carbohydrates. *Carbohydr. Res.,* **2011**, *346*(15), 2323-2326.
        [http://dx.doi.org/10.1016/j.carres.2011.07.019] [PMID: 21906726]

[10]   Jones, N.A.; Jenkinson, S.F.; Soengas, R.; Fanefjord, M.; Wormald, M.R.; Dwek, R.A.; Kiran, G.P.; Devendar, R.; Takata, G.; Morimoto, K.; Izumori, K.; Fleet, G.W.J. Synthesis of and NMR studies on the four diastereomeric 1-deoxy-d-ketohexoses. *Tetrahedron Asymmetry,* **2007**, *18*(6), 774-786.
        [http://dx.doi.org/10.1016/j.tetasy.2007.02.028]

[11]   Roslund, M. U. Petri Tähtinen; Matthias Niemitz; Rainer Sjöholm. Complete assignments of the 1h and 13c chemical shifts and JH,H coupling constants in NMR Spectra of D-Glucopyranose and All D-Glucopyranosyl-d-Glucopyranosides , **2008**, *343*(1), 101-112.
        [http://dx.doi.org/10.1016/j.carres.2007.10.008]

[12]   Trocka, A.; Szwarc-Karabyka, K.; Makowiec, S.; Laskowski, T. Application of the 2-deoxyglucose scaffold as a new chiral probe for elucidation of the absolute configuration of secondary alcohols. *Sci. Rep.,* **2022**, *12*(1), 16838.
        [http://dx.doi.org/10.1038/s41598-022-21174-8] [PMID: 36207399]

[13]   Kaufmann, M.; Mügge, C.; Kroh, L.W. NMR analyses of complex d -glucose anomerization. *Food Chem.,* **2018**, *265*, 222-226.
        [http://dx.doi.org/10.1016/j.foodchem.2018.05.100] [PMID: 29884376]

[14]   Aw, W.; Muoio, D.M.; Zhang, G. A Fast and sensitive method combining reversed-phase chromatography with high resolution mass spectrometry to quantify 2-Fluoro-2-Deoxyglucose and its phosphorylated metabolite for determining glucose uptake. **2019**.
        [http://dx.doi.org/10.26434/chemrxiv.7771142]

[15]   Kruve, A.; Kaupmees, K.; Liigand, J.; Oss, M.; Leito, I. Sodium adduct formation efficiency in ESI source. *J. Mass Spectrom.,* **2013**, *48*(6), 695-702.
[http://dx.doi.org/10.1002/jms.3218] [PMID: 23722960]

[16]   McIntosh, T.S.; Davis, H.M.; Matthews, D.E. A liquid chromatography-mass spectrometry method to measure stable isotopic tracer enrichments of glycerol and glucose in human serum. *Anal. Biochem.,* **2002**, *300*(2), 163-169.
[http://dx.doi.org/10.1006/abio.2001.5455] [PMID: 11779107]

[17]   Blough, H.A.; Giuntoli, R.L. Successful treatment of human genital herpes infections with 2-deoxy-D-glucose. *JAMA,* **1979**, *241*(26), 2798-2801.
[http://dx.doi.org/10.1001/jama.1979.03290520022018] [PMID: 221691]

[18]   Hughes, D.E. Determination of α-2-deoxy-d-glucose in topical formulations by high-performance liquid chromatography with ultraviolet detection. *J. Chromatogr. A,* **1985**, *331*(1), 183-186.
[http://dx.doi.org/10.1016/0021-9673(85)80020-0] [PMID: 4044738]

[19]   Anumula, K.R. Advances in fluorescence derivatization methods for high-performance liquid chromatographic analysis of glycoprotein carbohydrates. *Anal. Biochem.,* **2006**, *350*(1), 1-23.
[http://dx.doi.org/10.1016/j.ab.2005.09.037] [PMID: 16271261]

[20]   Kakita, H.; Kamishima, H.; Komiya, K.; Kato, Y. Simultaneous analysis of monosaccharides and oligosaccharides by high-performance liquid chromatography with postcolumn fluorescence derivatization. *J. Chromatogr. A,* **2002**, *961*(1), 77-82.
[http://dx.doi.org/10.1016/S0021-9673(02)00655-6] [PMID: 12186393]

[21]   Umegae, Y.; Nohta, H.; Ohkura, Y. Simultaneous determination of 2-deoxy-D-glucose and D-glucose in rat serum by high-performance liquid chromatography with post-column fluorescence derivatization. *Chem. Pharm. Bull. (Tokyo),* **1990**, *38*(4), 963-965.
[http://dx.doi.org/10.1248/cpb.38.963] [PMID: 2379291]

[22]   Gounder, M.K.; Lin, H.; Stein, M.; Goodin, S.; Bertino, J.R.; Kong, A.N.T.; DiPaola, R.S. A validated bioanalytical HPLC method for pharmacokinetic evaluation of 2-deoxyglucose in human plasma. *Biomed. Chromatogr.,* **2012**, *26*(5), 650-654.
[http://dx.doi.org/10.1002/bmc.1710] [PMID: 21932382]

[23]   *Proceedings of International Conference on Harmonization,* **2022**.

[24]   ICH Stability Testing of New Drug Substances and Products Q1A (R2), in: Proceedings of International Conference on Harmonization, **2003**.

[25]   Channing, M.A.; Huang, B.X.; Eckelman, W.C. Analysis of residual solvents in 2-[18F]FDG by GC. *Nucl. Med. Biol.,* **2001**, *28*(4), 469-471.
[http://dx.doi.org/10.1016/S0969-8051(00)00213-4] [PMID: 11395321]

[26]   Guideline for residual solvents Q3C(R8. *Proceedings of International Conference on Harmonization,* **2021**.

CHAPTER 4

[^{18}F]Fluoro Analogue of D-Glucose: A Chemistry Perspective

Mohd Faheem[1], **Vaibhav Pandey**[1] and **Manish Dixit**[1,*]

[1] *Department of Nuclear Medicine, Sanjay Gandhi Postgraduate Institute of Medical Sciences, Lucknow, Uttar Pradesh, India*

Abstract: 2-[^{18}F]fluoro-D-glucose ([^{18}F]FDG) is a versatile molecule in nuclear medicine that has evolved into a vital radiotracer in medical imaging applications *via* positron emission tomography (PET) [^{18}F]FDG is derived from its derivative, 2-deoxy-D-glucose (2-DG), where the triflate group is attached to carbon-2 [^{18}F]FDG serves as a crucial non-invasive diagnostic tool and is prominently utilized in non-invasive imaging of various metastatic diseases, particularly cancer imaging. Its importance as a tracer has been further enhanced by its unexpected attribute of generating a low body background through excretion, leading to its effective application in PET/CT for highly-sensitive and specific tumor detection. This chapter provides insight into the synthesis of [^{18}F]FDG, employing various reaction protocols such as electrophilic and nucleophilic processes. This chapter also summarized the purification and their quality assurance methods and highlighted the distinct challenges associated with each. The nucleophilic technique produces [^{18}F]FDG with a higher yield and purity than the electrophilic method for routine manufacture. Commercially devoted automated modules for FDG production use this method, demonstrating its widespread use in clinical imaging. Nucleophilic reactions of [^{18}F]fluoride ions attacking the C-2 position of mannose triflate to produce FDG are routine in clinical imaging. The final [^{18}F]FDG product satisfies safety, purity, and efficacy standards through rigorous quality control and assurance. The trajectory from glucose discovery to the development of [^{18}F]FDG exemplifies the continuing advancement of medical imaging methods. FDG's accomplishment shows how biology, chemistry, and medical technology are interrelated, providing a better understanding and treatment of complicated diseases like cancer.

Keywords: Cancer, Imaging, Nuclear medicine, PET/CT, [^{18}F]FDG.

---

* **Corresponding author Manish Dixit:** Department of Nuclear Medicine, Sanjay Gandhi Postgraduate Institute of Medical Sciences, Lucknow, Uttar Pradesh, India; E-mail: dixitm@sgpgi.ac.in

Raman Singh, Antresh Kumar & Kuldeep Singh (Eds.)
All rights reserved-© 2024 Bentham Science Publishers

1. INTRODUCTION

1.1. Definition and Background of 2-Fluoro-D-Glucose (2-FDG)

Glucose was first identified by Jean Baptiste Andre Dumas, a French chemist, in 1838 [1]. He coined the term glucose for sugars obtained from honey, grapes, starch, and cellulose. The molecular formula of glucose was established 20 years later [1 - 3]. Glucose is a simple sugar that consists of six carbon atoms. It has an open-chain structure, with aldehyde and alcohol functional groups. However, in aqueous solutions, only a negligible amount of the open-chain form of glucose remains. Glucose undergoes a ring formation reaction, forming two isomers, α-*D*-glucopyranose and β-*D*-glucopyranose. These isomers differ in the orientation of the -OH functional groups on carbon-1 [4] (Fig. **1**). Glucose has been extensively studied for its medicinal activities, particularly in anticancer treatment. The 2-deoxy-D-Glucose (2-DG) is an additive of glucose that has been investigated for its potential as an anticancer drug [5].When the -H group at the second position of the derivative of glucose (2-DG) is replaced by a [^{18}F]fluorine ion, termed as [^{18}F]FDG, which is extensively used as a non-invasive biomarker *via* positron emission tomography (PET) [6].

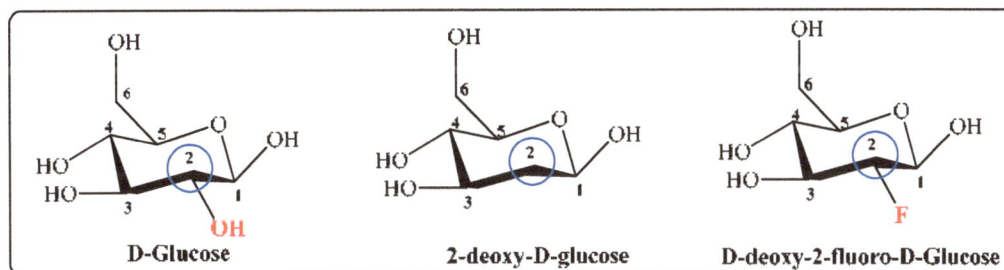

Fig. (1). The chemical skeleton of FDG, 2-DG, and glucose displaying changes at carbon-2.

1.2. Biological Importance of [^{18}F]FDG

FDG was designed based on 2-Deoxy Glucose, a derivative of glucose, wherein the hydroxyl group (-OH) on C-2 was substituted with a hydrogen atom, as shown in Fig. (**1**) [7].

Many researchers have claimed that the biological behaviour of 2-DG closely mirrors that of glucose. In view of cell uptake, the glucose, 2-DG is phosphorylated by hexokinase. The hydroxyl group on C-2 is not a critical factor for this process; however, glucose metabolism stops functioning after phosphorylation because of the essential role of the hydroxyl group on C-2 in the subsequent step involving phosphohexoseisomerase (Fig. **2**) [6 - 8]. Consequently, 2-DG6P was trapped in the cells as a metabolic record. Essentially, the elimination of the hydroxyl group from C-2 isolates is a hexokinase reaction. This unique property of 2-DG was observed by Sols and Crane in 1954, who noted this characteristic [9]. ¹⁸F-FDG is transported into the brain tissue by GLUTs and phosphorylated to ¹⁸F-FDG-6-phosphate ([¹⁸F]FDG6P) in the presence of hexokinase (HK). [¹⁸F]FDG is not further metabolized but remains trapped and can be detected in cells to evaluate brain glucose uptake. These investigations have laid the foundation for the utility of [¹⁸F]FDG, which is crucial for exploring human glucose metabolism [8, 9]. Initially, [¹⁸F]fluorine radionuclide was chosen because of its high C-F bond energy and adequate half-life of 110 min. The ¹⁸F-labeled variant of 2-DG synthesis is centered on substituting ¹⁸F at the carbon-2 atom while maintaining the characteristics of the original molecule. The logical choice for [¹⁸F]fluorine substitution at C-2 is that modifying this carbon atom would not disrupt the facilitated transport needed to penetrate the blood-brain barrier or the hexokinase reaction. The development of [¹⁸F]FDG was further supported by the successful synthesis of unlabeled FDG, which proved its efficacy as a hexokinase substrate. The significance of fluorine substitution on C-2 was evident from the considerable decrease in hexokinase affinity observed for both 3-deoxy-3-fluoro-*D*-glucose and 4-deoxy-4-fluoro-*D*-glucose simultaneously.

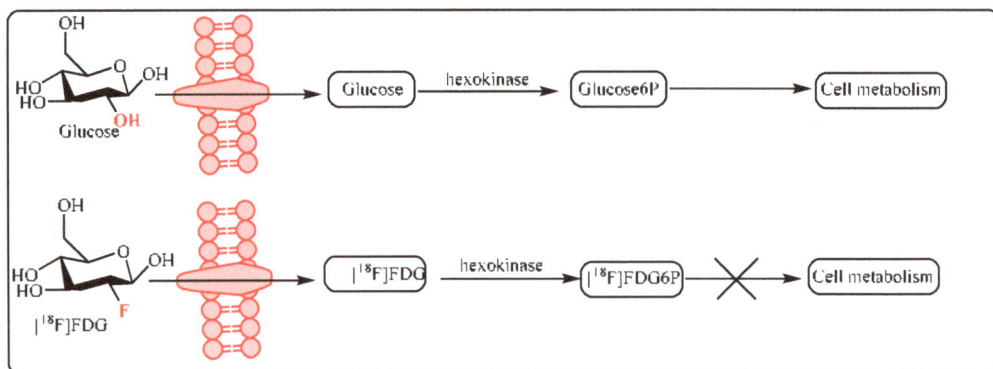

Fig. (2). Reaction pathway for [¹⁸F]FDG.

The distinctive feature of [¹⁸F]FDG, its heightened absorption in rapidly proliferating tumors owing to enhanced tumor glycolysis and its minimal background in the body, yield an exceptional signal-to-noise ratio for tumor detection (Fig. **3**). The low body background of [¹⁸F]FDG is attributed, in part, to its excretion, unlike glucose, which undergoes resorption from the urine to plasma *via* active transport across the renal tubule. Unlike glucose, the absence of a hydroxyl group on C-2 in [¹⁸F]FDG prevents active transport, contributing to its low background [7 - 10]. This unexpected property of a low body background resulting from [^{18}F]FDG excretion, not initially anticipated in its design for brain studies, has propelled it to the forefront as a tracer for managing cancer patients. The literature reports sensitivity toward different cancers, as mentioned in Table **1**.

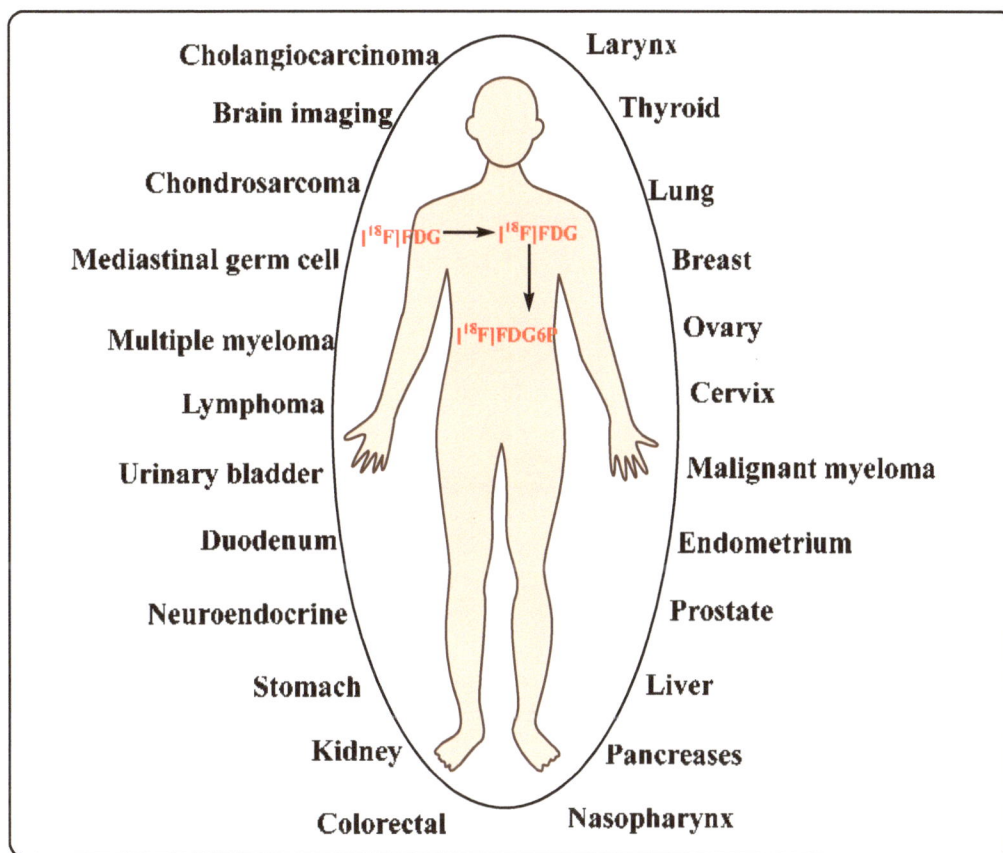

Fig. (3). The [^{18}F] used as a biomarker for different tumor detection *via* PET/CT scanner [11].

Table 1. Sensitivity, specificity, and accuracy of [^{18}F]-FDG PET/CT in different tumour types [12].

-	Sensitivity (%)	Accuracy (%)
Breast cancer	89	87
Colorectal cancer	89	90
Oesophageal cancer	94	87
Head and neck cancer	94	90
Lung cancer	81	96
Lymphoma	86	-

2. HISTORY OF [¹⁸F]FDG

The synthesis of [¹⁸F]FDG was initially designed in 1968 by Dr. Josef Pacák, ZdeněkTočík, and Miloslav Černý at the Department of Organic Chemistry, Charles University, Czechoslovakia. In the 1970s, the synthesis of fluorine-18-labeled FDG *via* an electrophilic reaction was primarily described by Wolf *et al.* at the Brookhaven National Laboratory [7, 13]. The fluorination of a glucose analog describes FDG synthesis and proceeds *via* electrophilic and nucleophilic substitution or addition reactions. This chapter describes a protocol for synthesizing [¹⁸F]FDG based on the reaction mechanism of a single roof. Fluorination can be divided into two categories (Table **2**).

Table 2. Categorization of chemical reactions for [¹⁸F]FDG production.

-	Substrate	[¹⁸F]Labeled Precursor	Refs.
Electrophilic Reaction	(structure: CH₂OAc, AcO, AcO)	$[^{18}F]F_2$	[14]
	(structure: CH₂OAc, AcO, AcO)	$CH_3CO_2{}^{18}F$	[15]
	(structure: CH₂OH, HO, HO)	$CH_3CO_2{}^{18}F$	[16]
	(structure: CH₂OAc, AcO, AcO)	$[^{18}F]XeF_2$	[17]
Nucleophilic Reaction	(structure: Ph, OTf, H₃CO, OCH₃)	$Cs[^{18}F]$	[18]
	(structure: Ph, OCH₃, O-S-O)	$Et_4N[^{18}F]$	[19]
	1,2-anhydro-3,4:5,6-di-isopropylidene-l-C-nitro- 60,61---mannitol	$KH[^{18}F]F_2$	[20]
	(structure: AcO, OTf, AcO, OAc, AcO)	$[(Krypt.222)K^+]F^-$	[21]

3. ELECTROPHILIC FLUORINATION

The electrophilic reaction occurs at an electron-rich position to produce [^{18}F]FDG and other ^{18}F-labeled products. Many studies have reported using different precursors as electrophiles, but the radiolabeled product yield is poor in real scenarios. Some modified methods further developed to improve the yield are discussed in this section (below) (Scheme **1**), but the production of ^{18}F-electrophile precursors, such as acetylhypofloride, shows multistep synthesis [14 - 17].

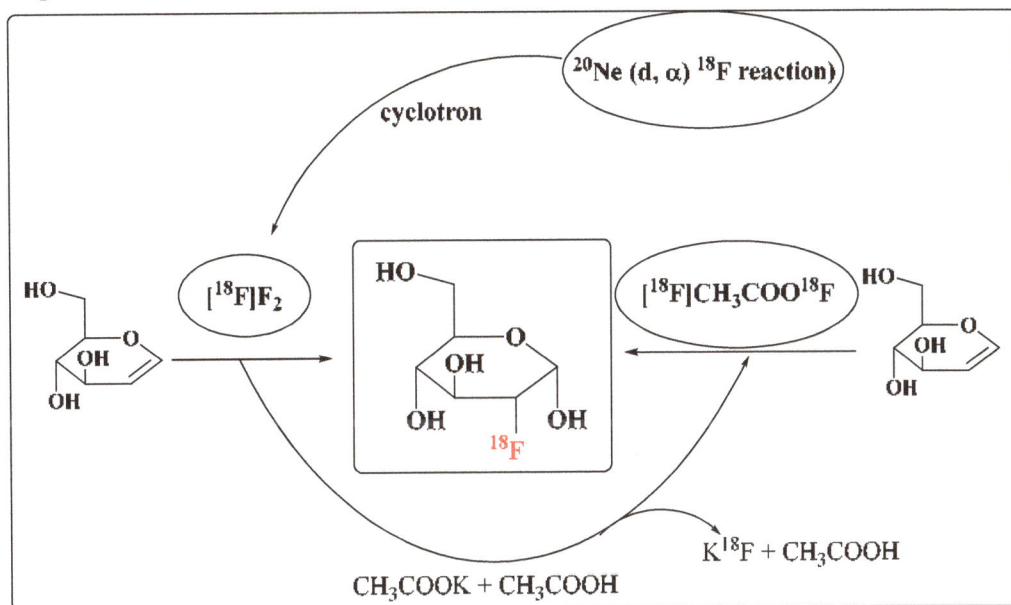

Scheme (1). Summary of the electrophilic reaction used to produce [^{18}F]FDG.

3.1. Fluorination of Carbohydrate by Electrophile

Adding fluorine atoms across a double bond, known as electrophilic fluorination, creates a difluoro six-membered derivative of the parent molecule. The 3,4,6-tri-*O*-acetyl-*D*-glucal was used as a precursor in the electrophilic fluorination reported by Wolf *et al.* A 3:1 mixture of ^{18}F-labeled derivatives of difluoro-glucose and difluoro-mannose was produced after treatment of glucal with [^{18}F]F$_2$. To obtain 2-fluoro-2-deoxyglucose, a difluoro-glucose derivative was isolated and subjected to hydrochloric acid treatment (Scheme **2**). This procedure took two hours to synthesize, yielding approximately 8%. Acetyl hypofluorite (AcO^{18}F) can be synthesized using the gas-solid-phase microchemical method described in [17b] practically and efficiently. This is particularly useful for producing ^{18}F-labeled-2-deoxy-2-fluoro-D-glucose ([^{18}F]FDG), which is used as a

PET imaging biomarker. The method allows the production of CH3COO18F with sufficient yield and purity by passing $[^{18}F]F_2$ gas at 100 mL/min through a stainless-steel tube (4 mm × 100 mm) packed with $CH_3COOK.CH_3COOH$. The synthesis reaction maintained a higher yield (Scheme **3**).

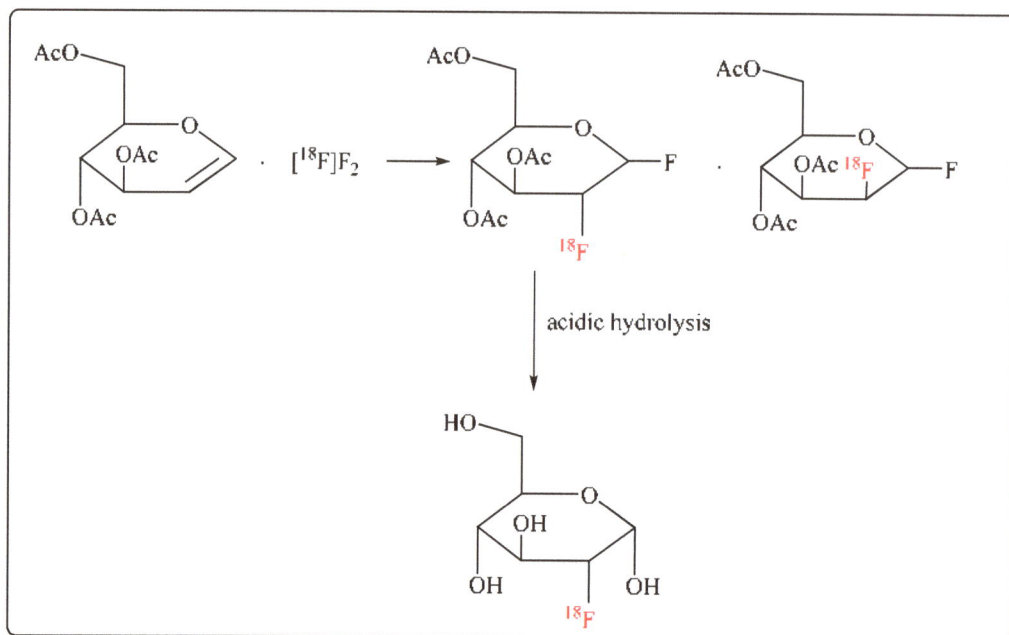

Scheme (2). Electrophilic addition reaction of ^{18}F-F_2 [14].

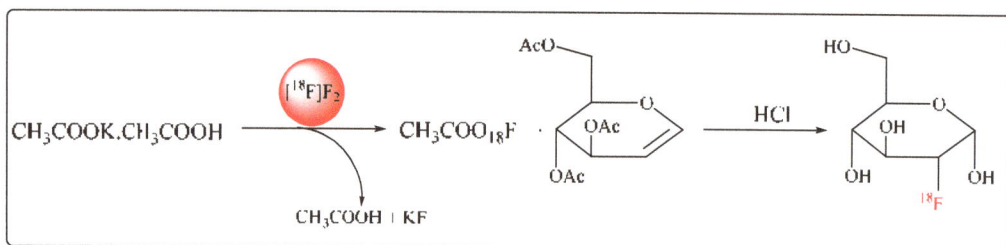

Scheme (3). Electrophilic reaction using acetylhypofluride [15, 16].

4. NUCLEOPHILIC FLUORINATION

Nucleophilic reactions are popular in organic synthesis because of their high yield. Numerous strategies have been proposed to get around the drawbacks of electrophilic *versus* nucleophile addition and substitution processes. In ^{18}F-radiolabeling, the nucleophile reaction plays a significant role in high specific activity. The nucleophile is an electron-rich species, such as $[^{18}F]$ caesium fluoride, $[^{18}F]$potassium fluoride, $[(Krypt.222)K^+]F^-$, $[^{18}F]TBAF$, and $[^{18}F]TMAF$, involving the addition of electron-deficient carbon and releasing unstable species (leaving group) by forming a new covalent bond with the inversion of the configuration of the core moiety [18 - 21] (Fig. **4**).

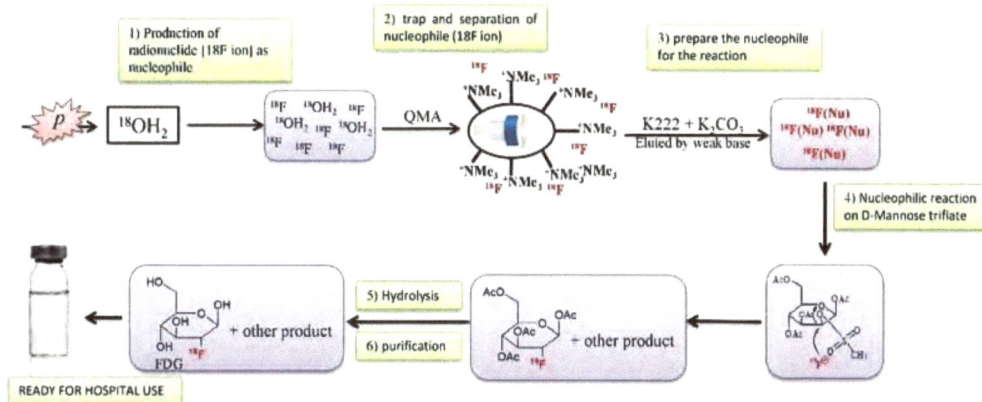

Fig. (4). Schematic overall pictorial presentation of Nucleophilic fluorination reaction.

In summary, ^{18}F-ions act as the nucleophile in the synthesis of [^{18}F]FDG by attacking the FDG precursors known as TATM at the C-2 position, the triflate group detached from the protected mannose skeleton to form acylated fluoro glucose. An acid or base then hydrolyzes this glucose to produce [^{18}F]FDG (Scheme **4**).

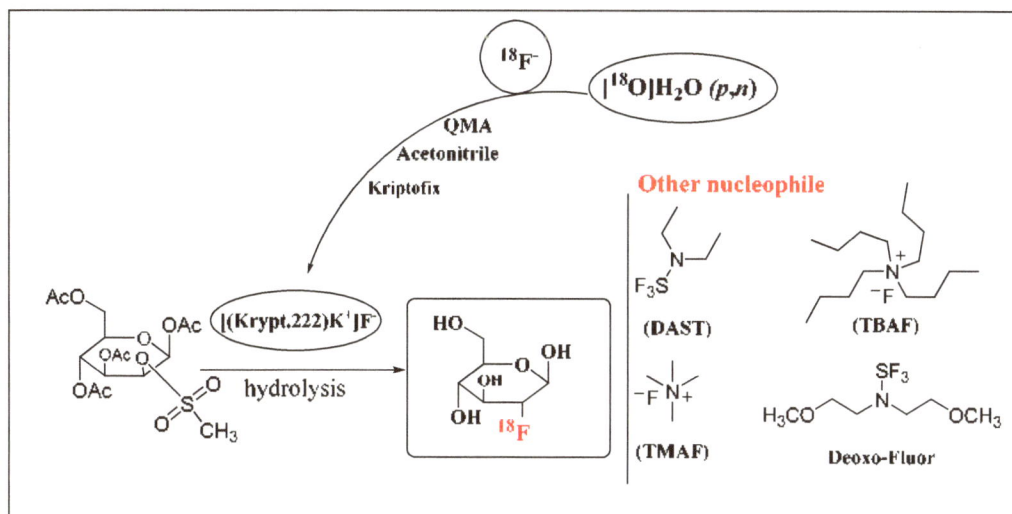

Scheme (4). Summarized scheme of nucleophile reaction for FDG production.

The nucleophilic reaction for producing [¹⁸F]FDG was standardized concerning the yield and minimized by-product. The product was subjected to quality assurance according to the recommended guidelines for clinical application. The [¹⁸F]FDG synthetic procedures and their associated quality control/assurance are discussed.

In the synthesis of [¹⁸F]FDG, seven steps were involved:

1. Production of radionuclide [¹⁸F-ion] as a nucleophile.
2. Trapping and separation of the nucleophile (¹⁸F-ion).
3. Synthesis of nucleophiles for the reaction.
4. Nucleophilic reaction over *D*-Mannose triflate.
5. Hydrolysis.
6. Purification.
7. Quality assurance.

4.1. Production of Radionuclide [¹⁸F-ion] as Nucleophile

The synthesis of [¹⁸F]FDG commences with [¹⁸O]water, an enriched variant of natural water containing the stable isotope, Oxygen-18 (O-18). In the bombardment of protons on [¹⁸O]water in a cyclotron, the O-18 isotope undergoes a proton-neutron nuclear reaction (p, n reaction), transforming into O-18 atoms to produce the F-18 isotope. The generation of F-18 nuclei occurs through a nuclear reaction, where the O-18 nucleus captures a proton and releases an energetic neutron. It is important to note that only a small fraction of the protons in the beam leads to F-18 production, with the majority of protons being lost as heat in the target. Consequently, the target was effectively engineered to handle the substantial heat generated during the bombardment. This is challenging because of the minute volume of [¹⁸O]water involved, which typically ranges from 1 to 3 ml, depending on the designed target cavity of the cyclotron (Scheme **5**) [23, 24].

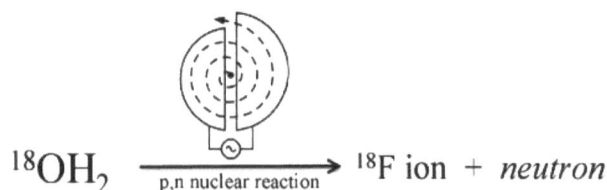

$$^{18}OH_2 \xrightarrow[\text{p,n nuclear reaction}]{} {}^{18}F \text{ ion } + neutron$$

Scheme (5). nuclear reaction (p, n) for conversion of [¹⁸O]H₂O to [¹⁸F]F-ion.

The produced F-18 atoms are in the chemical form of the [¹⁸F]fluoride ion. Subsequently, [¹⁸F]fluoride ions were collected in a single vial containing [¹⁸O]water [23].

4.2. Trapping and Separation of Nucleophiles (^{18}F-ion)

After a successful bombardment, the target's radioactive solution containing the [^{18}F]fluoride ion is moved to the automatic synthesizer or chemistry processing module placed inside the lead line closed fume hood (hot cell). The solid phase anion-exchange resin cartridge trapped [^{18}F]fluoride ion (Scheme 6). This phase transverses an ion exchange resin using Quaternary Ammonium Anion Exchange (QMA) Sep-Pak column (Waters Corporation, Accell Plus QMA Sep-Pak™), separating the [^{18}F]fluoride ion from the solution and collecting [^{18}O]water containing other impurities, for example, trace metals, into a O-18 water recovery vial.

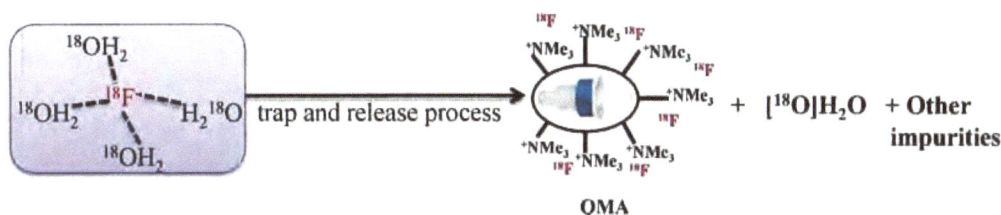

Scheme (6).   Trap of [^{18}F]F-ion from [^{18}O]H$_2$O water.

4.3. Generation of Nucleophile for the Reaction

The extraction of [^{18}F]fluorine ions from [^{18}O]water is commonly known as the "trap and release process, "which is rooted in the solid-phase ion exchange method that utilizes charges for separation. In the cartridge, anion exchange resins containing positively charged amines in QMA facilitate the exchange of negatively charged anions such as [^{18}F]fluoride ions. Subsequently, the trapped [^{18}F]fluoride ions are eluted using an acetonitrile solution containing Kryptofix®222 (4,7,13,16,21,24-Hexaoxa-1,10-diazabicyclo[8.8.8]hexacosane), and potassium carbonate as a mild base. The anhydrous conditions for the nucleophilic reaction play a favourable role. Water is evaporated using an azeotropic drying technique, and acetonitrile is mixed with the aqueous solution (with a low boiling point).

The [^{18}F]fluoride ion has a high hydration energy, and water is unsuitable for nucleophilic reactions, necessitating a polar aprotic solvent such as acetonitrile for SN^2 reactions. Acetonitrile is used as a solvent to form an azeotropic mixture with water evaporating in a supporting gas, such as N$_2$, at 80°C to achieve complete evaporation or dryness. In the FDG automatic synthesizer, the system performed this step multiple times to ensure the successful removal of all residual water and the formation of effective nucleophiles. The completely anhydrous state of the [^{18}F]fluoride ions yields a high-yield product during the nucleophilic reaction in an aprotic solvent.

At the molecular level, the process involves utilizing a group of compounds called "cryptands." Compounds such as the one known as Kryptofix®[2.2.2] (abbreviated as "K222") possess distinctive molecular properties. They effectively encrypt cations and tightly bind them to hinder the formation of solid ion pairs with anions. The chemical structure of K222, illustrated in Scheme (**7**), shows a three-dimensional cage that precisely encases potassium cations, preventing the establishment of a robust ion pair with [¹⁸F]fluoride ion [22, 23].

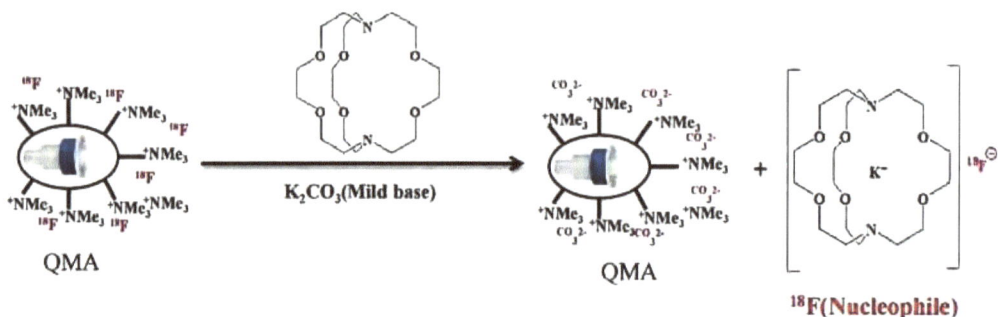

Scheme (7). Preparation of [¹⁸F]F-Kryptofix complex.

4.4. Nucleophilic Reaction on *D*-Mannose Triflate

The selection of functional groups substituted with [¹⁸F]fluoride in the precursor ion is influenced by factors such as the ease of preparation, efficiency, and high yield in the final production. The precursor molecule 1,3,4,6-*O*-Acetyl-2-*O*-trifluoromethanesulfonyl-D-mannopyranose (TATM) also known in the short term as mannose triflate is frequently used in the synthesis of [¹⁸F]FDG. The acetyl groups at the 1, 3, 4, and 6 positions of carbons through ester bonds, which are stereochemically transformed into [¹⁸F]FDG molecule and the chemical structure shown in Fig. (**5**) is similar to that of mannose triflate except at C-2 position.

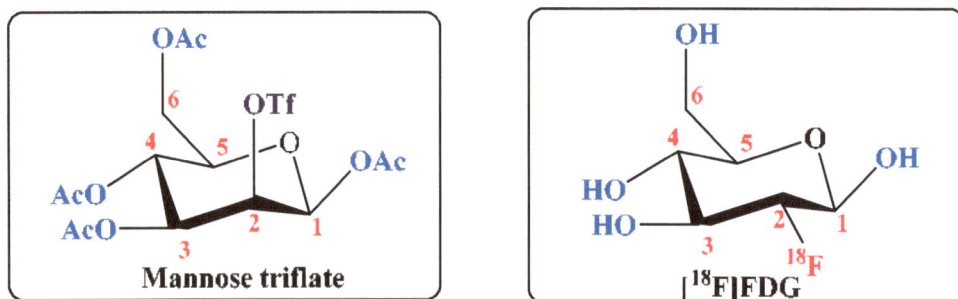

Fig. (5). The chemical skeleton of the core mannose triflate (TATM) and [¹⁸F]FDG.

The organic skeleton's core hydroxyl groups make hydrogen bonds with free fluoride ions. These acetyl groups at 1, 3, 4 and 6 positions block hydrogen bonding during fluorination. In the mannose triflate skeleton, the [^{18}F]fluoride ion attacks on carbon-2 position and the triflate group from the acetylated mannose skeleton is inversely replaced, forming [^{18}F]FDG (Scheme **8**). Acetyl groups can be efficiently removed through hydrolysis using acid or base at respective temperature conditions, producing [^{18}F]FDG.

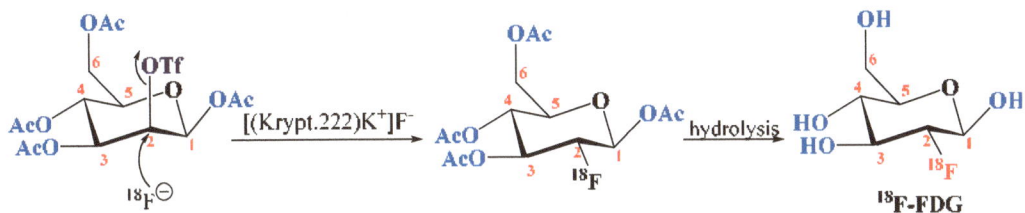

Scheme (8). Reaction scheme of [^{18}F]FDG [21].

In radiochemistry, the functional groups for the nucleophilic reaction play a very important role in yield. The selection of the leaving groups is significant for easy separation from the parent molecule. Once detached, this leaving group stabilizes its negative charge through delocalization, thereby preventing its reintegration into the parent molecule.

The common leaving groups of the nucleophiles, including triflates, tosylates, mesylates, and some other halogens except fluorine gave the best results. The choice of the leaving group is influenced by factors such as the type of precursor, solvent, precursor stability, and yield. Chloride is a poor leaving group compared to those in Fig. (**6**) [25]. Triflates showed better and more reliable yields in the [^{18}F]FDG synthesis, usually between 50% to 60%.

4.5. Hydrolysis

The last step of [^{18}F]FDG production involves the deprotection of the -OH group of positions at carbons 1,3,4, and 6. There are two ways to carry out this step: sodium hydroxide (basic hydrolysis) or hydrochloric acid (acid hydrolysis). For removing protecting groups (-OAc groups), acid hydrolysis requires a longer time and higher temperatures see Table **3** [27 - 29, 32]. Basic hydrolysis is a primarily adaptive method, which is quicker and more complete at room temperature to moderate heat, subject to the molar concentration of the base used [30, 31]. An enhanced methodology of basic hydrolysis involves affixing 1,3,4,6 acetyl-protected ^{18}F-labeled 2-deoxyglucose onto solid-phase columns. Thorough rinsing with water effectively removes all other impurities. The resulting [^{18}F]FDG product can be extracted with water, while unhydrolyzed or partially hydrolyzed

1,3,4,6 acetyl-protected ¹⁸F-labeled 2-deoxyglucose remains adhered to the column [26].

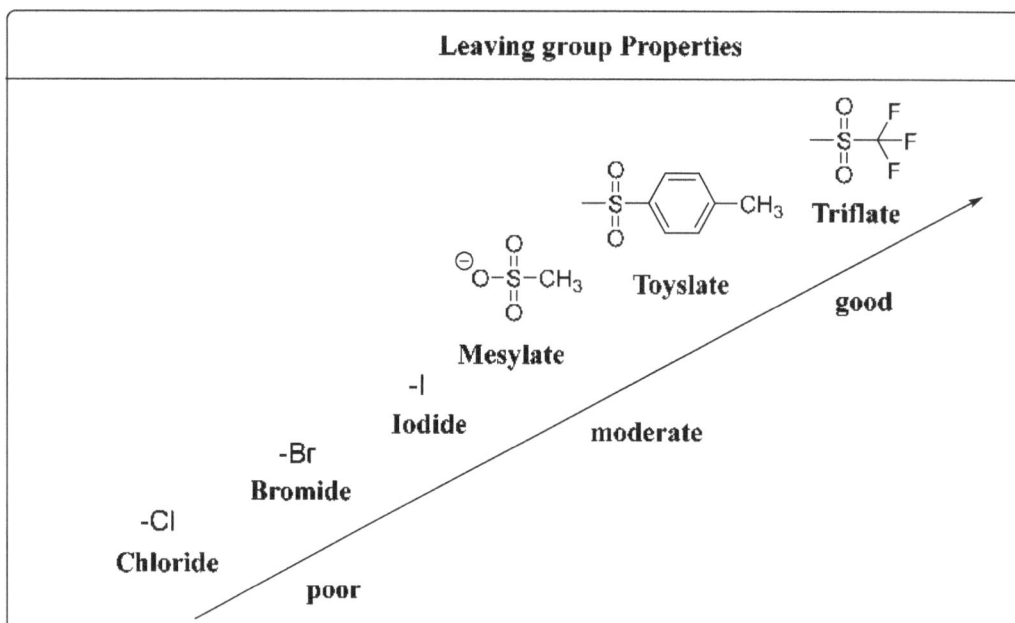

Fig. (6). Trends of leaving group by the nucleophilic reaction.

Table 3. Deprotection of –OH group under acidic and basic conditions.

Acidic Hydrolysis	Basic Hydrolysis
The reaction requires a high temperature of approx. 100-110°C.	The reaction requires a low temperature of approx. 30-35°C.
The concentration required HCl (1-2N).	The concentration required for NaOH is (0.3N-1N).
The reaction is incomplete, and [¹⁸F]fluoro-deoxy-mannose [¹⁸F]FDM may be present in the reaction mixture.	The reaction is completed within 2-3 min, and a lower amount of [¹⁸F]fluoro-deoxy-mannose [¹⁸F]FDM is present in the product.
The reaction requires a long time.	The deacetylation is rapid in a short time.

4.6. Purification

At the end of the reaction, the mixture usually contains various impurities, such as unlabeled mannose triflate, hydroxyl-protected labeled precursor, free fluoride, desired product, sodium hydroxide, and solvent.

All these by-products are removed from the desired [¹⁸F]FDG compound. Researchers have explored purification using solid-phase purification resins.

Various cation-, neutral-, and/or charge-based solid-phase cartridges were analyzed for purification. They have the unique characteristic of holding polar/nonpolar or neutral impurities. The crude [18]FDG loaded onto solid-phase cartridges and rinsed with water effectively removed all other impurities. The resulting [^{18}F]FDG product can be extracted while unhydrolyzed or partially hydrolyzed 1,3,4,6 acetyl-protected ^{18}F-labeled 2-deoxyglucose remains adhered to the column.

Various combinations of solid phase single step methods were adopted by different modules; among them, one such method utilizes purification using three different solid-phase cartridges placed in series with specific functions to remove particular impurities. This setup is more reliable and effective for completely removing all impurities. Fig. (**7**) shows three different cartridges: a cation exchange cartridge in H$^+$ form (1), a styrene-divinylbenzene-based cartridge (2), and an alumina cartridge (3). The crude products were loaded onto the columns, and all impurities remained trapped in these solid-phase resins. The final purified product was eluted in a sterile vial *via* water as eluant. In brief, cartridge 1 removes all elemental impurities, such as Na$^+$ by replacing the –H atom. After that, the Styrene-Divinylbenzene-based cartridge removes unhydrolyzed impurities, and the reaction mixture passes through the alumina cartridge (marked as 3), trapping the entire free fluoride ion from the crude compound and eluting the final pure product. For the contents of qualification, the synthesized [^{18}F]FDG product was subject to quality assurance and must comply with the regularity specifications. Table **4** shows their specifications and qualifications.

4.7. Quality Assurance

The quality standards for [^{18}F]FDG conform to various manufacturing companies in terms of efficacy, purity, and safety for clinical purposes, including the International Pharmacopoeia, United State Pharmacopeia (USP), European Pharmacopoeia (EP), and others that are used as a standard quality specification. A manufacturing, draft chemistry, and control (CMC) paper addressing [^{18}F]FDG has also been made public by regulatory bodies, explaining the different sets of standards adopted by other countries like British Pharmacopoeia (BP). The manufacturing of radiopharmaceuticals follows a regulated procedure outlined by the GMP guidelines (mentioned in IAEA Radioisotopes and Radiopharmaceutical Series No. 3, section 6.5–6.7 [33]), which are specified for radiopharmaceuticals. GMP covers various factors that influence the quality of pharmaceutical products, such as personnel, facilities, equipment, raw materials, procedures, quality control, documentation, packaging, and shipment. Establishing Standard Operating Procedures (SOPs) and validating, implementing, and monitoring the processes are crucial. Quality control involves regular daily inspection of both products and raw materials. The main goal of quality control is to assess, analyze, and appraise all materials, whether they are raw materials utilized in the manufacturing process or finalized products, and ensure that their quality meets the required standards. The release of a product for patient use depends on successful adherence to these specifications after extensive testing. By implementing a robust quality assurance program, testing a product to comply with the necessary quality specifications is transformed into a validation procedure. Quality assurance (QA) evaluates a manufacturing facility's overall PPP (processes, performance, and procedure). Within this framework, QA is the culmination of all the activities that separately or collectively affect a product's quality. In particular, radiopharmaceuticals demand short half-lives of included radionuclides, aseptic processing, parametric release of product batches, and radiation safety specifications that are required for radiopharmaceuticals.

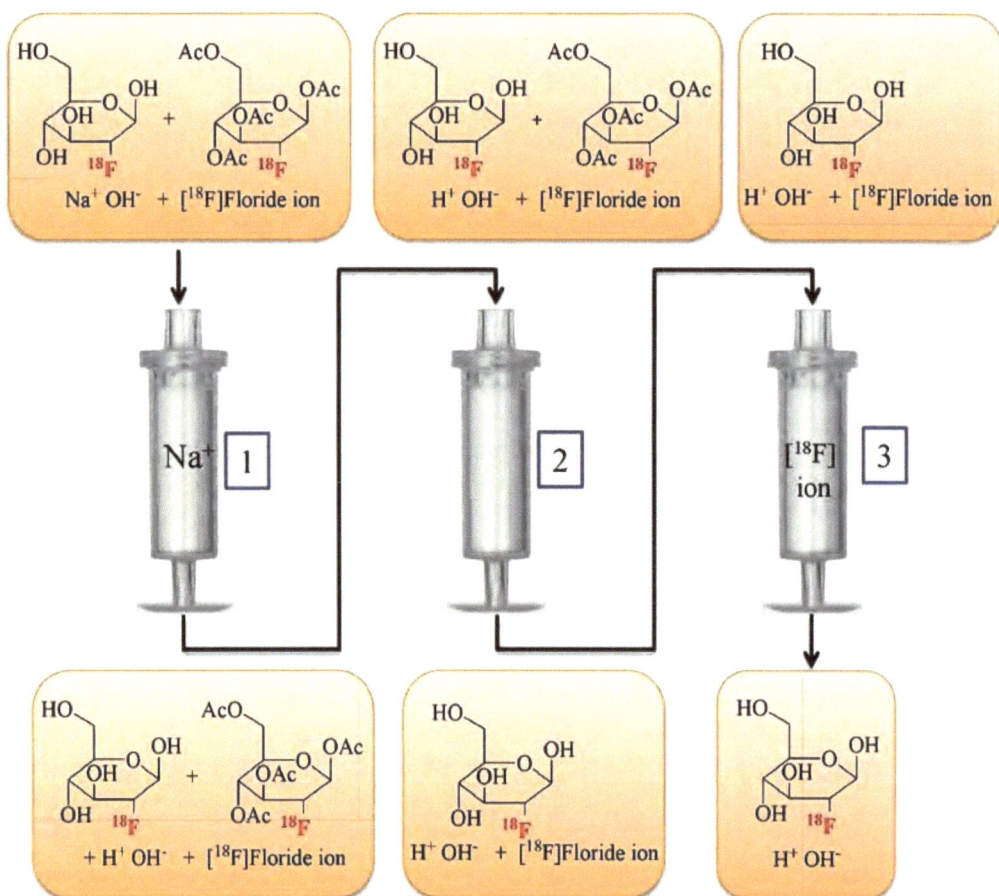

Fig. (7). Schematic diagram of the [¹⁸F]FDG purification through different solid phase cartridges.

Table 4. Quality parameter recommended by FDA.

Content/Character	Method	Accepted Criteria
Specifications	Capacity per batch	19 mL ± 2 mL
-	Radioactivity	-
-	Specific radioactivity	37 MBq/µmol
-	Half-life period	105 to 115 minutes
Characteristics	Characteristics	Transparent
-	Presence of particles	Does not recognize particles
Endotoxin test	-	0.25EU/mL or less
Sterile test	-	Does not recognize germ development
pH	-	5.0 - 8.0
Verification test	-	Recognizes a peak at 511 keV
Purity test	Radioactive heteronuclear species	Does not recognize a peak other than at 511 keV or 1,022 keV
-	Radiochemical purity	95% or higher
-	Ethanol	2,500 ppm or lower
-	Acetonitrile	200 ppm or lower
-	Aluminium ion	10 ppm or lower
-	Kryptofix222	40 ppm or lower

CONCLUSION

In conclusion, 2-[^{18}F]Fluoro-*D*-Glucose ([^{18}F]FDG) has become an important radiotracer for medical imaging of various biological processes *via* positron emission tomography (PET). [^{18}F]FDG, which is obtained from glucose and its product 2-deoxy-D-Glucose (2-DG) substituted at the triflate group on carbon-2, is an important non-invasive diagnostic tool for several diseases, most notably cancer imaging. Its use as a tracer for cancer patient management has advanced owing to the unexpected trait of low body background caused by [^{18}F]FDG excretion. This has led to its application PET/CT for tumour detection with outstanding sensitivity and specificity. This chapter describes the synthesis of [^{18}F]FDG using different reaction protocols, such as electrophilic and nucleophilic reactions. Each has its own set of difficulties, but the nucleophilic method is predominant in the routine production of this tracer with excellent yield and purity. All commercially dedicated FDG production automated modules use this nucleophilic fluorination method. Nucleophilic reactions using [^{18}F]fluoride ions to attack mannose triflate, carbon -2 of 2DG, have become routine in clinical imaging applications. This chapter also summarizes the synthesis, purification, and quality assurance variations. Quality control and assurance procedures guarantee that the final [^{18}F]FDG product satisfies safety, purity, and efficacy requirements. From the discovery of glucose to the creation of [^{18}F]FDG, the path essentially illustrates the ongoing development and improvement of medical imaging methods, providing physicians with an effective tracer for the diagnosis and surveillance of a wide range of illnesses, most notably, cancer. The success of [^{18}F]FDG highlights the relationship between biology, chemistry, and medical technology and presents a viable path for improving our comprehension and treatment of complicated disorders.

LIST OF ABBREVIATIONS

[^{18}F]FDG [^{18}F]fluorodeoxyglucose

2DG 2-deoxy-D-glucose

[^{18}F]FDM [^{18}F]fluoro-deoxy-mannose

BP British Pharmacopoeia

CMC Chemistry, Manufacturing, and Control

HK Hexokinase

IAEA International Atomic Energy Agency

K222 Kryptofix222

PET Positron Emission Tomography

TATM-1 3,4,6-*tetra-O*-acetyl-2-*O*-trifluoromethanesulfonyl-β-*D*-mannopyranose

USP United State Pharmacopeia

ACKNOWLEDGEMENTS

The authors would like to sincerely thank the HOD of the Department of Nuclear Medicine, Sanjay Gandhi Postgraduate Institute of Medical Sciences, Lucknow, for providing the facilities to write and submit the book chapter for publication.

REFERENCES

[1]   Dumas, J. B. A. *A History of Chemistry,* **1964**, 337-375.
        [http://dx.doi.org/10.1007/978-1-349-00554-3_11]

[2]   Wisniak, J. Eugène Melchior Peligot. *Educ. Quím.,* **2009**, *20*(1), 61-69.
        [http://dx.doi.org/10.1016/S0187-893X(18)30008-9]

[3]   Hudson, J. The foundation of organic chemistry. *The History of Chemistry,* **1992**, 104-121.
        [http://dx.doi.org/10.1007/978-1-349-22362-6_8]

[4]   Shendurse, A.M.; Khedkar, C.D. Glucose: properties and analysis. *Encyclopedia of food and health,* **2016**, *3*, 239-247.

[5]   Wijayasinghe, Y.S.; Bhansali, M.P.; Borkar, M.R.; Chaturbhuj, G.U.; Muntean, B.S.; Viola, R.E.; Bhansali, P.R. A comprehensive biological and synthetic perspective on 2-Deoxy- D -Glucose (2-DG), A sweet molecule with therapeutic and diagnostic potentials. *J. Med. Chem.,* **2022**, *65*(5), 3706-3728.

[http://dx.doi.org/10.1021/acs.jmedchem.1c01737] [PMID: 35192360]

[6]   Yu, S. Review of 18F-FDG synthesis and quality control. *Biij,* **2006**, *2*(4), e57.
        [http://dx.doi.org/10.2349/biij.2.4.e57] [PMID: 21614337]

[7]   Kaira, K.; Serizawa, M.; Koh, Y.; Takahashi, T.; Yamaguchi, A.; Hanaoka, H.; Oriuchi, N.; Endo, M.;
        Ohde, Y.; Nakajima, T.; Yamamoto, N. Biological significance of 18F-FDG uptake on PET in patients
        with non-small-cell lung cancer. *Lung Cancer,* **2014**, *83*(2), 197-204.
        [http://dx.doi.org/10.1016/j.lungcan.2013.11.025] [PMID: 24365102]

[8]   Groves, A.M.; Win, T.; Haim, S.B.; Ell, P.J. Non-[¹⁸F]FDG PET in clinical oncology. *Lancet Oncol.,*
        2007, *8*(9), 822-830.
        [http://dx.doi.org/10.1016/S1470-2045(07)70274-7] [PMID: 17765191]

[9]   Jadvar, H.; Alavi, A.; Gambhir, S.S. 18F-FDG uptake in lung, breast, and colon cancers: molecular
        biology correlates and disease characterization. *J. Nucl. Med.,* **2009**, *50*(11), 1820-1827.
        [http://dx.doi.org/10.2967/jnumed.108.054098] [PMID: 19837767]

[10]   Higashi, K.; Ueda, Y.; Arisaka, Y.; Sakuma, T.; Nambu, Y.; Oguchi, M.; Seki, H.; Taki, S.; Tonami,
        H.; Yamamoto, I. 18F-FDG uptake as a biologic prognostic factor for recurrence in patients with
        surgically resected non-small cell lung cancer. *J. Nucl. Med.,* **2002**, *43*(1), 39-45.
        [PMID: 11801701]

[11]   Chan, H-P.; Liu, W-S.; Liou, W-S.; Hu, C.; Chiu, Y-L.; Peng, N-J. Comparison of FDG-PET/CT for
        cancer detection in populations with different risks of underlying malignancy. *In Vivo,* **2020**, *34*(1),
        469-478.
        [http://dx.doi.org/10.21873/invivo.11797]

[12]   Almuhaideb, A.; Papathanasiou, N.; Bomanji, J. 18F-FDG PET/CT imaging in oncology. *Ann. Saudi
        Med.,* **2011**, *31*(1), 3-13.
        [http://dx.doi.org/10.4103/0256-4947.75771] [PMID: 21245592]

[13]   Fowler, J.S.; Wolf, A.P. 2-deoxy-2-[¹⁸F]fluoro-d-glucose for metabolic studies: Current status. *Int. J.
        Rad. Appl. Instrum. [A],* **1986**, *37*(8), 663-668.
        [http://dx.doi.org/10.1016/0883-2889(86)90259-5] [PMID: 3021667]

[14]   Ido, T.; Wan, C-N.; Casella, V.; Fowler, J.S.; Wolf, A.P.; Reivich, M.; Kuhl, D.E. Labeled 2-deoxy-
        D-glucose analogs. ¹⁸F-labeled 2-deoxy-2-fluoro-D-glucose, 2-deoxy-2-fluoro-D-mannose and ¹⁴C-2-
        deoxy-2-fluoro-D-glucose. *J. Labelled Comp. Radiopharm.,* **1978**, *14*(2), 175-183.
        [http://dx.doi.org/10.1002/jlcr.2580140204]

[15]   Shiue, C.Y.; Salvadori, P.A.; Wolf, A.P.; Fowler, J.S.; MacGregor, R.R. A new improved synthesis of
        2-deoxy-2-[¹⁸F]fluoro-d-glucose from 18F-labeled acetyl hypofluorite. *J. Nucl. Med.,* **1982**, *23*(10),
        899-903.
        [PMID: 7119884]

[16]   Ehrenkaufer, R.E.; Potocki, J.F.; Jewett, D.M. Simple synthesis of F-18-labeled 2-fluoro-2-deo-
        y-D-glucose: concise communication. *J. Nucl. Med.,* **1984**, *25*(3), 333-337.
        [PMID: 6699724]

[17]   (a) Shiue, C.; K.-C.; Wolf, A. P. A Rapid Synthesis of 2-deoxy-2-fluoro-d-glucose from Xenon
        Difluoride Suitable for Labelling with 18F *Journal of Labelled Compounds and
        Radiopharmaceuticals,* **1983**, *20*(2), 157-162.
        (b) Ehrenkaufer RE, Potocki JF, Jewett DM. Simple synthesis of F-18-labeled 2-fluoro-2-deo- y--
        -glucose: concise communication. *Journal of Nuclear Medicine,* **1984**, *25*(3), 333-337.
        [http://dx.doi.org/10.1002/jlcr.2580200202] [PMID: 6699724]

[18]   Levy, S.; Elmaleh, D.R.; Livni, E. A new method using anhydrous [¹⁸F]fluoride to radiolabel
        2-[¹⁸F]fluoro-2-deoxy-D-glucose. *J. Nucl. Med.,* **1982**, *23*(10), 918-922.
        [PMID: 7119887]

[19]   Tewson, T.J. Synthesis of no-carrier-added fluorine- 18 2-fluoro-2-deoxy-D-glucose. *J. Nucl. Med.,*

1983, *24*(8), 718-721.
[PMID: 6683752]

[20]   Szarek, W.A.; Hay, G.W.; Perlmutter, M.M. A rapid, stereospecific synthesis of 2-deoxy-2-fluo-o-D-glucose using the fluoride ion. *J. Chem. Soc. Chem. Commun.,* **1982**, (21), 1253.
       [http://dx.doi.org/10.1039/c39820001253]

[21]   Hamacher, K.; Coenen, H.H.; Stöcklin, G. Efficient stereospecific synthesis of no-carrier-added 2-[¹⁸F]-fluoro-2-deoxy-D-glucose using aminopolyether supported nucleophilic substitution. *J. Nucl. Med.,* **1986**, *27*(2), 235-238.
       [PMID: 3712040]

[22]   Schyler, D.J. PET tracers and radiochemistry. *Ann. Acad. Med. Singap.,* **2004**, *33*(2), 146-154.
       [http://dx.doi.org/10.47102/annals-acadmedsg.V33N2p146] [PMID: 15098627]

[23]   Kiesewetter, D.O.; Eckelman, W.C.; Cohen, R.M.; Finn, R.D.; Larson, S.M. Syntheses and D2 receptor affinities of derivatives of spiperone containing aliphatic halogens. *Int. J. Rad. Appl. Instrum. [A],* **1986**, *37*(12), 1181-1188.
       [http://dx.doi.org/10.1016/0883-2889(86)90003-1] [PMID: 3028984]

[24]   Lemaire, C.; Damhaut, P.; Lauricella, B.; Mosdzianowski, C.; Morelle, J.L.; Monclus, M.; Van Naemen, J.; Mulleneers, E.; Aerts, J.; Plenevaux, A.; Brihaye, C.; Luxen, A. Fast [¹⁸ F]FDG synthesis by alkaline hydrolysis on a low polarity solid phase support. *J. Labelled Comp. Radiopharm.,* **2002**, *45*(5), 435-447.
       [http://dx.doi.org/10.1002/jlcr.572]

[25]   Lepore, S.D.; Mondal, D. Recent advances in heterolytic nucleofugal leaving groups. *Tetrahedron,* **2007**, *63*(24), 5103-5122.
       [http://dx.doi.org/10.1016/j.tet.2007.03.049] [PMID: 19568330]

[26]   Saha, G.B. *Basics of PET imaging: physics, chemistry, and regulations*; Springer, **2015**, pp. 155-174.

[27]   Mulholland, G. K. Simple rapid hydrolysis of acetyl protecting groups in the FDG synthesis using cation exchange resins. *Nucl. Med. Biol.,* **1995**, *22*(1), 19-23.
       [PMID: 7735165]

[28]   Alexoff, D.L.; Fowler, J.S.; Gatley, S.J. Removal of the 2.2.2 cryptand (Kryptofix 2.2.2) from 18FDG by cation exchange. *Int. J. Rad. Appl. Instrum. [A],* **1991**, *42*(12), 1189-1193.
       [http://dx.doi.org/10.1016/0883-2889(91)90195-7] [PMID: 1668801]

[29]   Mock, B.H.; Vavrek, M.T.; Mulholland, G.K. Back-to-back "one-pot" [¹⁸F]FDG syntheses in a single Siemens-CTI chemistry process control unit. *Nucl. Med. Biol.,* **1996**, *23*(4), 497-501.
       [http://dx.doi.org/10.1016/0969-8051(96)00030-3] [PMID: 8832706]

[30]   Füchtner, F.; Steinbach, J.; Mäding, P.; Johannsen, B. Basic hydrolysis of in the preparation of 2-[¹⁸F]fluoro-2-deoxy-d-glucose. *Appl. Radiat. Isot.,* **1996**, *47*(1), 61-66.
       [http://dx.doi.org/10.1016/0969-8043(95)00258-8]

[31]   Meyer, G.J.; Matzke, K.H.; Hamacher, K.; Füchtner, F.; Steinbach, J.; Notohamiprodjo, G.; Zijlstra, S. The stability of 2-[¹⁸F]fluoro-deoxy-d-glucose towards epimerisation under alkaline conditions. *Appl. Radiat. Isot.,* **1999**, *51*(1), 37-41.
       [http://dx.doi.org/10.1016/S0969-8043(98)00193-6]

[32]   Singh, V.K.; Tiwari, A.K. *Faheem, Mohd. Synthetic Approach of Quinazolines Candidates*; N-Heterocycles, **2022**, pp. 313-329.
       [http://dx.doi.org/10.1007/978-981-19-0832-3_8]

[33]   https://www.iaea.org/publications/8529/cyclotron-produced-radionuclides-guidance-on-fac-lity-design-and-production-of-fluorodeoxyglucose-fdg

CHAPTER 5

Antiviral Potential of 2-DG Used in Different Viral Infections

Shaurya Prakash[1], Minakshi[1], Hemlata Kumari[1] and Antresh Kumar[1,*]

[1] Department of Biochemistry, Central University of Haryana, Mahendergarh-123031, India

Abstract: The evolution of viral infections has pushed researchers constantly to find new approaches to disseminate these infections. One such promising finding in this aspect is 2-deoxy-D-glucose (2-DG), a glucose analogue that gained attention for its potential as an antiviral agent effective against a variety of viral infections. The antiviral properties of 2-DG are due to its ability to interfere with viral replication within host cells, hence reducing the severity of infections. 2-DG is easily taken up by cells as it mimics glucose-like structure but interferes with glycolysis and other metabolic pathways. It also acts as a glycosylation inhibitor that helps in the disruption of viral assembly. Viruses are obligate and utilize the host cell machinery for proliferation. 2-DG mechanistically disrupts the energy supply by inhibiting the glycolysis cycle and providing an unfavourable environment for viral replication. 2-DG elicits broad-spectrum antiviral activity as it was found to be very effective against different families of viruses. By interfering with this process, 2-DG not only interferes with viral replication but also with the ability of the virus to enter host cells and evade the immune system. Although 2-DG has shown some promising antiviral potential, it also possesses some side effects as well. All the attributes related to the antiviral potential of 2-DG have been discussed in this chapter.

Keywords: Antiviral, Glycosylation, Viral infections, 2-deoxy-D-glucose, 2-DG analogs.

1. INTRODUCTION

Viruses are well-known opportunistic, and obligate pathogens that entirely depend on the host cell machinery for their progression and clinical implications. Their survival is accomplished by the synthesis of viral components such as nucleic acids, protein, glycans, and lipid membranes, using the host cell machinery. The progression of the viral particle entirely depends on the metabolic profile of the

* **Corresponding author Antresh Kumar:** Department of Biochemistry, Central University of Haryana, Mahendergarh-123031, India; E-mail: antreshkumar@cuh.ac.in

Raman Singh, Antresh Kumar & Kuldeep Singh (Eds.)

host cell. Thereby, viruses can modulate the metabolic profile of the host cells in multiple ways. Both retro or non-retro viruses, one way or another, regulate different metabolic pathways such as glycolysis, and pentose phosphate pathway, and induce amino acids and lipids synthesis [1]. For instance, the human cytomegalovirus (HCMV), herpesvirus-1 (HSV-1), and adenovirus upregulate the glycolysis and tricarboxylic acid (TCA) cycle and also increase nucleotide and lipid synthesis [2]. As a general notion, viral infection more often affects the glycolysis pathway. The virus-infected cells adapt metabolic alterations that aid to meet the high anabolic demand required for viral progression. Upregulation of the glycolysis cycle is the most common metabolic shift that occurs during viral infections. However, other metabolic alterations were also well reported which are often virus-specific. Previous studies reported that during viral infection, the most common enzyme induced is phosphatidylinositol-3-kinase (PI3K) or protein kinase (PKB/Akt) signaling that drives the expression glucose transporters 1 or 4 (GLUT1/ GLUT4) [3 - 5]. The expression of GLUT1/ GLUT4 glucose transporter resulted in inducing glucose uptake, which helps them to overcome the increased energy demand.

In the recent past, the entire global community faced a COVID-19 pandemic situation that affected millions of lives. This pandemic infection left no part of the world untouched and openly challenged health agencies for the development of therapeutics against the same. The COVID-19 pandemic also caused different coinfections with epidemiological impacts. Mucormycosis is a common example that rapidly emerged as a secondary infection in COVID-19 infected patients with a significant morbidity and mortality rate [6]. Different efforts have been devised to find new or repurposed existing drugs during that period and have been tested against such infections. Ivermectin, dexamethasone, ritonavir, favipiravir, remdesivir, hydroxychloroquine, *etc.* are such common examples [7]. During the same course of time, a glucose analog termed as 2-Deoxy-D-glucose (2-DG) was also employed to test the efficacy against the COVID-19 infection. 2-DG is basically, a non-metabolizing glucose analog that specifically acts up on the glycolysis cycle and blocks the functionality of enzymes involved in the glycolysis cycle along with the inhibition of viral protein glycosylation leading to the inhibition of viral replication (Fig. **1**). Apart from other inhibitory effects related to glucose metabolism, 2-DG also acts on phosphoglucoisomerase that obstructs the conversion of glucose-6-phosphaet to fructose-6-phosphate. It disturbs the metabolic ability of cells and dictates the cells toward apoptosis. 2-DG is a synthetic analog of glucose where –OH (hydroxyl group) of the second carbon position is replaced with a hydrogen atom. Similar to glucose,2-DG is taken up by the cells through glucose transporters by facilitated diffusion mainly by GLUT1 and GLUT4; and active uptake by the SGLT transporter [8, 9]. 2-DG inhibits the catalysis of hexokinase and phosphoglucoisomerase involved in the conversion of glucose to phosphoglucose, given the situation when there is a sufficient amount of 2-DG-6P generated, by the virtue of product inhibition.

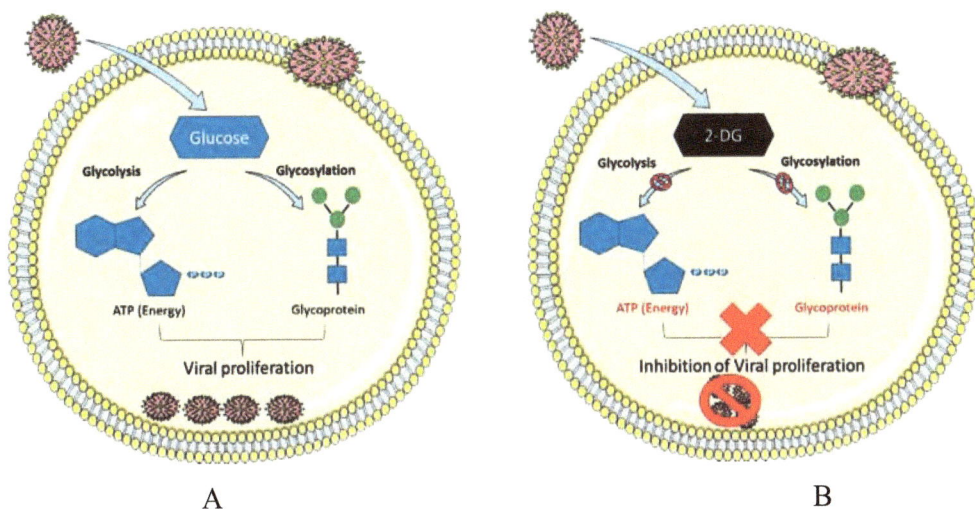

Fig. (1). (**A**) Viral proliferation in the presence of glucose, (**B**) Inhibition of viral proliferation in the presence of 2-DG.

2. HOST GLYCOSYLATION: A NECESSITY FOR VIRAL REPLICATION

Glycosylation is a process in which a carbohydrate is attached to hydroxyl or other functional groups of protein and lipids. Such modifications made macromolecules serve several cellular and physiological functions. Protein glycosylation is a process where glycan is attached to the amide nitrogen of the asparagine. This process occurs in the early stage of protein synthesis, followed by oligosaccharide trimming and remodeling during transit from ER to the Golgi apparatus. It is well established that glycosylation is primarily required for the progression of viral replication in which glycosylated viral proteins tend to promote gene expression, fusion, binding of viral particles to the cell surface receptors, and prevention of antibody neutralization. The glycosylation of the viral proteins is carried out using N-glycans synthesized in the host ER through carbohydrate metabolism [10, 11]. As virus particles invade the host cell, they tend to hijack the glycosylation pathway for modifications of their proteins. N-linked glycosylation of viral envelope or surface protein enhances its folding and subsequent trafficking. Viruses often employ calnexin and calreticulin for the facilitation of function folding of the viral proteins [12]. During the progression of viral infection, glycosylation plays a very crucial role in the modification of the proteins that help in viral particle multiplications and transmission [13]. Glycosylation patterns also tend to regulate the communication with receptors, virus entry, and escaping antibody-mediated neutralization [11, 14]. For instance, in influenza A, B, HIV, and hepatitis C, glycosylation plays a very important role in the regulation of their pathogenesis and immune invasion [15 - 17]. In the process of glycosylation, mannose is a prerequisite that enters the cells through the hexose transport channel and immediately gets phosphorylated by hexose kinase (HK) activity and then gets catabolized either by the mannose phosphate isomerase (MPI) or phosphomannomitase-2 (PMM2) [18]. The metabolic shift during viral hijack significantly upregulates HK activity and thus glycosylation for rapid production of viral particles and dissemination of infection. Keeping all the above-mentioned details in mind, inhibition of glucose centered metabolic pathways such as glycolysis, glycosylation, and others is considered to be a promising target to establish an antiviral approach for the dissemination of viral infection. In this context, one of the most widely used glycolysis inhibitors is the glucose analog, 2-deoxy-D-glucose.

3. 2-DG: BIOLOGICAL EFFECTS AND ACTION MECHANISM

2-DG is a glucose derivative that follows Lipinski's rule of five and shows various activities, as it checks hypoxic tumor cells, and lowers oxygen dependency in case of COVID-19. Till 2021, it was not approved as a drug, but after COVID-19 pandemic, it has been recognized as an anti-COVID-19 agent for its treatment as it lowers the need for oxygen supply. The action mechanism of 2-DG was debatable as a glycolysis inhibitor or an anti-viral agent. The recent studies up to some extent, have answered this question and made the picture clear. It is well established that when the virus invades the host cell, there is a sudden spike in the levels of glucose transporters in a PI3K-dependent manner [5]. Moreover, the levels of hexokinase1 (HK1) and hexokinase 2 (HK2) also increase, which augments the progression of viral particles [5, 19, 20]. However, such a metabolic shunt in the host cell is distinct from different viral infections. For instance, during lymphocytic choriomeningitis virus (LCMV) infection, expression levels of GLUT1 and GLUT3 and HK1 and HK2 were also reported to increase. Similarly, GLUT3 and HK2 induction was found during kaposi's sarcoma-associated herpes virus (KSHV) infection, and human immunodeficiency virus type 1 (HIV-1) induced GLUT1, GLUT3, GLUT 4, and GLUT6 along with HK1 [21]. During the recent SARS-CoV2 catastrophe, the metabolic profile of infected cells was found with higher levels of GLUT1, GLUT3, and GLUT4 along with HK2 [22]. The increased expression of such glucose transporters and glycolytic enzymes induces the glycolytic cycle to meet the demand for higher ATP requirements. In contrast, in LCMV infection, glucose preferentially enters in the TCA cycle, thereby overexpression of glucose transporters and glycolytic enzymes did not affect the glucose uptake [23]. Even though, depleted glucose levels did not significantly affect the rate of viral progression. However, the administration of 2-DG in such infections significantly reduced the viral load. It was due to the conversion of 2-DG into guanosine diphosphate-2-deoxy-D-glucose (GDP-2-DG). The 2-DG metabolic resultant GDP-2-DG acts as an effective competitor of GDP-mannose, which is an essential substrate for the assembly of lipid-linked oligosaccharides on the ER membrane, required for N-glycosylation of protein [24]. Reversal of 2-DG detrimental effects using mannose was also shown on LCMV and similar results have been obtained in the case of semliki forest virus, herpes simplex virus, influenza virus A, KSHV, and SARS-CoV2 [22, 24 - 26]. The restriction of protein glycosylation reduces the synthesis of glycoproteins which are an essential component of viral assembly. Deficiency in the availability of viral glycoproteins consequently affects the viral infection potential. This aberration may interfere with the cleavage, transport, and folding of proteins or the overall progression of viral infection [25, 27 - 29]. The 2-DG treatment was also reported to suppress the viral nucleoproteins and Z-protein, resulting in restricting the viral load [27]. A similar effect on the suppression of nucleoproteins and Z-protein has not been observed in LCMV treated with 2-DG treatment [4, 5, 30, 31]. The inhibition of protein glycosylation by 2-DG results in the accumulation of non-glycosylated and misfolded proteins in the ER, which induces stress to trigger the unfolded protein response (UPR) pathway. The UPR activation transmits different signalling cascades. However, some viruses can manipulate UPR response and allow selective activation of signalling for the establishment of suitable replication conditions such as AFT6 and avoid PERK and IRE1 cascade signalling [32]. Under normal conditions, the overall UPR activation is anti-viral in nature, and 2-DG mediated induction of UPR non-selectively activates UPR cascades [33, 34]. The targets of 2-DG against SARS-CoV2 have also been deduced using an *in silico* approach and determined it as a glycolysis inhibitor with anti-SARS-CoV2 activity. The 2-DG elicited minimal free energy with the glycolysis pathway enzymes rather than having a significant affinity with the 3CLp, PLp, Nsp-16p, and RdRp viral proteins [35]. The 2-DG showed a significant affinity with hexokinase but it was somewhat lesser than glucose. The difference in the binding affinities of glucose and 2-DG with hexokinase led to the speculation of competitive inhibition, hence reduction in the glycolytic flux which suppresses replication and transmission of SARS-CoV2 infections in humans [35].

4. ANTIVIRAL POTENTIAL OF 2-DG

The pathophysiological and biological effects of 2-DG on cellular metabolism made it a suitable candidate to be used as an antiviral agent or as an adjuvant agent with various approved drugs. A study on SARS-CoV2 infected Vero E6 cells showed overexpression of GLUT1, GLUT3 and, GLUT4 proteins that increased glucose influx and induced glycolysis. The 2-DG treatment of infected cells led to reduced cytopathic effect (CPE). Codo *et al.* confirmed that the 2-DG mediated glycolysis cycle restriction, resulted in inhibition of viral replication [37]. Collectively it has been deduced that the inhibition of glycolysis cycle by using 2-DG is an efficient strategy to encounter the SARS-CoV2 infection. However, viral particles carrying defective unglycosylated receptor binding domains (RBD) are reported to compromise the pathogenicity potential [22]. Similar findings were also reported when SARS-CoV2 infected the Caco-2 cell line [36].

The antiviral effect of 2-DG has also been studied against the human papillomavirus (HPV) [40 - 42]. An earlier study reported that the 2-DG treatment to HPV18-infected Hela cells reduced the viral load by inducing the expression level of tumor suppressor; p53 gene. Further findings suggested that the administration of 2-DG with TMB-8, a calcium ion (Ca^{2+}) antagonist completely abrogated viral effects *via* the involvement of 2-DG in calcium signaling [38 - 40]. However, the mechanism connecting 2-DG and calcium signaling has not been well explored. Kang *et al.* reported that HPV early gene gets downregulated by the treatment of 2-DG to the cancerous cell lines and cells undergo hypoxia conditions due to the depletion of glucose levels. They also suggested the antiviral potential of 2-DG was due to ATP limitation [41]. The regulation of HPV genes was reported to be marginally affected under such conditions. 2-DG-mediated hypoxia condition evolved in cervical carcinoma cells was the result of downregulation of the Sp1 gene through hyper-GlcNAcylation [41]. Recently, it was reported that 2-DG can sensitize the HPV-16 infected 5-fluorouracil (5-FU) resistant cervical cancer cells and restrict the cell growth. The 5-FU resistant cells elicited to upregulate the glycolysis and Aft-dependent signaling, and 2-DG treatment tends to inhibit the glycolysis pathway, thus making cells- sensitive to 5-FU [42]. Another study centered on metabolic and energy profiling of host cell upon viral infection was conducted on norovirus (NoV). The NoV-infected macrophages treated with 2-DG attenuated the pathogen by restricting replication of the viral genome, independent of type I interferon response. However, astrovirus titer remains unaffected when it was treated with 2-DG, suggesting that the metabolic shift of the hosts is virus-specific [4].

In spite of glycolysis cycle, 2-DG is also reported to target other associated pathways described earlier . For instance, rhinovirus (RV) infected HeLa cells treated with 2-DG abolished glycogenolysis with simultaneously induced the level of acylcarnitines. This acylcarnitines induction was accompanied by reducing phospholipids, sphingolipids, and ceramides levels. A similar effect of 2-DG was also assessed in the murine model that reduced lung inflammation with no evident side effects upon 2-DG treatment [20]. The 2-DG can also control the RV infection by inhibiting the RNA synthesis, resulting in reduced viral load with low RV-mediated cell death [43].

Another study of 2-DG on hepatitis B virus revealed to suppress the viral protein synthesis that inhibits DNA replication [44] and modulates the cellular AMP/ATP ratio, leading to the activation of AMP-activated protein kinase (AMPK) pathway and autophagy [45]. The current line of treatment against HBV suppresses viral replication and reduces the risk of liver cancer, but they do not ensure complete viral elimination. The inability to clear the complete viral titer may increase the risk of infection and thus, targeting the infected host cell metabolism *via* 2-DG has been proven a viable approach. Apart from these, 2-DG treatment remarkably reduces ZIKV particles in HRvEC cells and also induces the AMPK phosphorylation [46]. Similar findings on the inhibition of viral replication by 2-DG treatment were also reported in the Vero cell culture model [47].

5. SHORTCOMINGS OF 2-DG TREATMENT

However, some detrimental and adverse implications associated with the use of 2-DG have also been reported. Varanasi *et al.* warned not to use metabolic modifying drugs during HSV 1 infection. They reported that HSV 1 tends to upregulate glucose metabolism in CD4 cells. 2-DG treatment in such infections led to restrict glycolysis, resulting in suppressing immune response by inhibiting differentiation of effector T cells. Another *in vivo* study revealed that 2-DG treatment tends to diminish S-lesions because of the suppression of effector T-cell response. 2-DG-mediated inhibition of HSV 1 infection was carried out through the modulation of CD4 effector T-cells. However, some detrimental effects were also shown in the eyes of the tested mice. On the contrary, during the acute phase of ocular infection, the 2-DG treatment led to the death of the subjects from herpes encephalitis [48 - 50]. Even the 2-DG therapy was not able to restrict the growth of the HSV virus and still replicate efficiently, in fact, induction in replication was also observed, which could prove to be lethal as it leads to the proliferation of the virus in the brain. Other findings suggested viral glycoprotein's glycosylation inhibitory property of 2-DG in HSV 1 infection and this resulted in the inability for cell fusion [26]. Some studies showed the inability of 2-DG in the treatment of cutaneous HSV 1 and HSV 2 infection in mice and guinea pigs [51, 52].

6. ANTIVIRAL ACTIVITY OF 2-DG DERIVATIVES

Acetyl conjugated analogs of 2-DG were developed by Dr. Waldemar Priebe's lab and among all the tested derivatives, WP1122 (3,6-di-O-acetyl-2-deoxy- D-glucose) was found to be the most potent glycolysis inhibitor. The WP1122 derivative was synthesized in a two-step synthesis method using 3,4,6-tri-

O-acetyl-D-glucal. Initially, the substrate was deacetylated to 3,6-di-O-acetyl- D-glucal and afterward treated with an aqueous solution of hydrobromic acid. Unlike 2-DG, which is uptaken *via* glucose transporters, WP1122 is passively diffused inside the cells and gets deacetylated by the esterase to yield 2-DG. Later, 2-DG gets phosphorylated to produce 6-phospho-2-DG that competitively inhibits the HK activity leading to the inhibition of the glycolytic pathway [53]. WP1122 readily crosses the blood-brain barrier which could prove a promising strategy for glioma therapy [54] and viral encephalitis. The slower release of WP1122 makes a longer half-life than 2-DG. WP1122 also has better oral bioavailability resulting in two-fold higher plasma concentration of 2-DG when compared to the administration of 2-DG alone. WP1122 was found to be well tolerated in the orthotopic glioma mice model even after prolonged exposure [55]. Earlier studies reported that halogen derivatives of 2-DG (Fig. **2**) showed a negative relation between the size of the halogen substituent and drug activity [56]. With an increase in the size of halogen derivatives (2-FG > 2-CG > 2-BG), the HKI binding activity gradually reduced leading to a lesser yield of 6-O-phosphorylated intermediates, a glycolysis inhibitory molecule. However, the antiviral effects of these halogen derivatives need to be further explored.

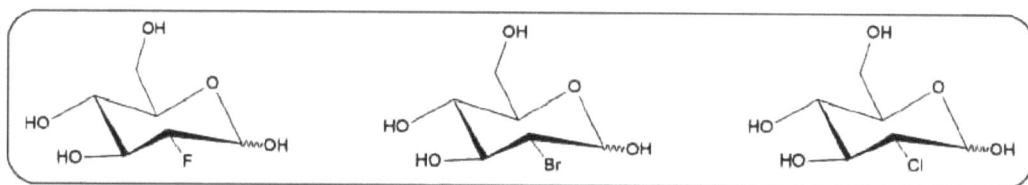

Fig. (2). Halogen derivatives of 2-DG.

CONCLUSION

The recent COVID-19 pandemic made global health agencies realize the lethal potential of viral infections. The lack of broad-spectrum antiviral therapeutics allowed the catastrophic spread of SARS-CoV2 with severely higher morbidity and mortality. Not only the SARS-CoV2, but all the other viruses discussed in this chapter can have a devastating impact on global health and the economy. There is an urgent need for the development of broad-spectrum antiviral therapy that could be potent against the majority of viral pathogens. The progression and proliferation of virus primarily alters host cell metabolism, especially targeting the glycolysis pathway. 2-DG, a derivative of D-glucose has appeared to be a promising antiviral molecule that elicited promising results to restrict the growth of viral particles by targeting various noticeable mechanisms both in host cells and viral particles. 2-DG controls the glycolysis cycle activity during viral infections in host cells resulting in ATP limitation. It also showed some promising results as discussed previously but comes with some drawbacks as well.

Drawbacks include a short half-life of 48 hours, evidence of grade 3-asymptomatic QTc prolongation, T wave flattening, and gastrointestinal bleeding. These drawbacks keep the demand for new molecules unfulfilled, which could probably serve as a potential antiviral candidate. In the course of the development of more effective drug candidates, molecules like WP1122 exhibit promising antiviral potential, however, the clinical trial findings would confirm the efficacy of the same.

LIST OF ABBREVIATIONS

2-DG	2-deoxy-D-glucose
5-FU	5-fluorouracil
AMPK	Adenosine Monophosphate Kinase
COVID-19	Coronavirus Disease 2019
CPE	Cytopathic Response
ER	Endoplasmic Reticulum
GDP-2-DG	Guanosine diphosphate-2-deoxy-D-glucose
GLUT	Glucose Transporter
GDP	Guanosine Diphosphate
HK	Hexokinase
HPV	Human Papilloma Virus
HKI	Hexokinase Isomerase
MPI	Mannose Phosphate Isomerase
PMM2	Phosphomannomitase-2
RBD	Receptor Binding Domain
SGLT	Sodium Glucose Co-transporter
TCA	Tricarboxylic Acid
UPR	Unfolded Protein Response

REFERENCES

[1]   Thaker, S.K.; Ch'ng, J.; Christofk, H.R. Viral hijacking of cellular metabolism. *BMC Biol.*, **2019**, *17*(1), 59.
[http://dx.doi.org/10.1186/s12915-019-0678-9] [PMID: 31319842]

[2]   Pająk, B.; Zieliński, R.; Manning, J.T.; Matejin, S.; Paessler, S.; Fokt, I.; Emmett, M.R.; Priebe, W. The antiviral effects of 2-Deoxy-D-glucose (2-DG), a dual D-glucose and D-mannose mimetic, against SARS-CoV-2 and other highly pathogenic viruses. *Molecules,* **2022**, *27*(18), 5928.
[http://dx.doi.org/10.3390/molecules27185928] [PMID: 36144664]

[3]   Icard, P.; Lincet, H.; Wu, Z.; Coquerel, A.; Forgez, P.; Alifano, M.; Fournel, L. The key role of warburg effect in SARS-CoV-2 replication and associated inflammatory response. *Biochimie,* **2021**, *180*, 169-177.
[http://dx.doi.org/10.1016/j.biochi.2020.11.010] [PMID: 33189832]

[4]   Passalacqua, K.D.; Lu, J.; Goodfellow, I.; Kolawole, A.O.; Arche, J.R.; Maddox, R.J.; Carnahan, K.E.; O'Riordan, M.X.D.; Wobus, C.E. Glycolysis is an intrinsic factor for optimal replication of a norovirus. *MBio,* **2019,** *10*(2), e02175-18.
[http://dx.doi.org/10.1128/mBio.02175-18] [PMID: 30862747]

[5]   Fontaine, K.A.; Sanchez, E.L.; Camarda, R.; Lagunoff, M. Dengue virus induces and requires glycolysis for optimal replication. *J. Virol.,* **2015,** *89*(4), 2358-2366.
[http://dx.doi.org/10.1128/JVI.02309-14] [PMID: 25505078]

[6]   Prakash, S.; Kumar, A. Mucormycosis threats: A systemic review. *J. Basic Microbiol.,* **2023,** *63*(2), 119-127.
[http://dx.doi.org/10.1002/jobm.202200334] [PMID: 36333107]

[7]   Chakraborty, C.; Sharma, A.R.; Bhattacharya, M.; Agoramoorthy, G.; Lee, S.S. The Drug Repurposing for COVID-19 Clinical Trials Provide Very Effective Therapeutic Combinations: Lessons Learned From Major Clinical Studies. *Front. Pharmacol.,* **2021,** *12*(November), 704205.
[http://dx.doi.org/10.3389/fphar.2021.704205] [PMID: 34867318]

[8]   Navale, A.M.; Paranjape, A.N. Glucose transporters: physiological and pathological roles. *Biophys. Rev.,* **2016,** *8*(1), 5-9.
[http://dx.doi.org/10.1007/s12551-015-0186-2] [PMID: 28510148]

[9]   Anthony, J. Cura; Carruthers, A. The role of monosaccharide transport proteins in carbohydrate assimilation, distribution, metabolism and homeostasis. *Compr. Physiol.,* **2014,** *23*(2), 1-7.
[http://dx.doi.org/10.1002/cphy.c110024.The]

[10]   Feng, T.; Zhang, J.; Chen, Z.; Pan, W.; Chen, Z.; Yan, Y.; Dai, J. Glycosylation of viral proteins: Implication in virus–host interaction and virulence. *Virulence,* **2022,** *13*(1), 670-683.
[http://dx.doi.org/10.1080/21505594.2022.2060464] [PMID: 35436420]

[11]   Mantlo, E.K.; Maruyama, J.; Manning, J.T.; Wanninger, T.G.; Huang, C.; Smith, J.N.; Patterson, M.; Paessler, S.; Koma, T. Machupo Virus with Mutations in the Transmembrane Domain and Glycosylation Sites of the Glycoprotein Is Attenuated and Immunogenic in Animal Models of Bolivian Hemorrhagic Fever. *J. Virol.,* **2022,** *96*(8), e00209-22.
[http://dx.doi.org/10.1128/jvi.00209-22] [PMID: 35343792]

[12]   Pieren, M.; Galli, C.; Denzel, A.; Molinari, M. The use of calnexin and calreticulin by cellular and viral glycoproteins. *J. Biol. Chem.,* **2005,** *280*(31), 28265-28271.
[http://dx.doi.org/10.1074/jbc.M501020200] [PMID: 15951445]

[13]   Liu, X.; Li, S.; Peng, W.; Feng, S.; Feng, J.; Mahboob, S.; Al-Ghanim, K.A.; Xu, P. Genome-wide identification, characterization and phylogenetic analysis of ATP-binding cassette (ABC) transporter genes in common carp (Cyprinus carpio). *PLoS One,* **2016,** *11*(4), e0153246.
[http://dx.doi.org/10.1371/journal.pone.0153246] [PMID: 27058731]

[14]   Koma, T.; Huang, C.; Coscia, A.; Hallam, S.; Manning, J.T.; Maruyama, J.; Walker, A.G.; Miller, M.; Smith, J.N.; Patterson, M.; Abraham, J.; Paessler, S. Glycoprotein N-linked glycans play a critical role in arenavirus pathogenicity. *PLoS Pathog.,* **2021,** *17*(3), e1009356.
[http://dx.doi.org/10.1371/journal.ppat.1009356] [PMID: 33647064]

[15]   Ramière, C.; Rodriguez, J.; Enache, L.S.; Lotteau, V.; André, P.; Diaz, O. Activity of hexokinase is increased by its interaction with hepatitis C virus protein NS5A. *J. Virol.,* **2014,** *88*(6), 3246-3254.
[http://dx.doi.org/10.1128/JVI.02862-13] [PMID: 24390321]

[16]   Kim, P.; Jang, Y.; Kwon, S.; Lee, C.; Han, G.; Seong, B. Glycosylation of hemagglutinin and neuraminidase of influenza a virus as signature for ecological spillover and adaptation among influenza reservoirs. *Viruses,* **2018,** *10*(4), 183.
[http://dx.doi.org/10.3390/v10040183] [PMID: 29642453]

[17]   Upadhyay, C.; Feyznezhad, R.; Cao, L.; Chan, K.W.; Liu, K.; Yang, W.; Zhang, H.; Yolitz, J.; Arthos, J.; Nadas, A.; Kong, X.P.; Zolla-Pazner, S.; Hioe, C.E. *Signal Peptide of HIV-1 Envelope Modulates*

Glycosylation Impacting Exposure of V1V2 and Other Epitopes; , **2020**, Vol. 16, .
[http://dx.doi.org/10.1371/journal.ppat.1009185]

[18]   Sharma, V.; Freeze, H.H. Mannose efflux from the cells: a potential source of mannose in blood. *J. Biol. Chem.,* **2011**, *286*(12), 10193-10200.
[http://dx.doi.org/10.1074/jbc.M110.194241] [PMID: 21273394]

[19]   Delgado, T.; Carroll, P.A.; Punjabi, A.S.; Margineantu, D.; Hockenbery, D.M.; Lagunoff, M. Induction of the Warburg effect by Kaposi's sarcoma herpesvirus is required for the maintenance of latently infected endothelial cells. *Proc. Natl. Acad. Sci. USA,* **2010**, *107*(23), 10696-10701.
[http://dx.doi.org/10.1073/pnas.1004882107] [PMID: 20498071]

[20]   Gualdoni, G.A.; Mayer, K.A.; Kapsch, A.M.; Kreuzberg, K.; Puck, A.; Kienzl, P.; Oberndorfer, F.; Frühwirth, K.; Winkler, S.; Blaas, D.; Zlabinger, G.J.; Stöckl, J. Rhinovirus induces an anabolic reprogramming in host cell metabolism essential for viral replication. *Proc. Natl. Acad. Sci. USA,* **2018**, *115*(30), E7158-E7165.
[http://dx.doi.org/10.1073/pnas.1800525115] [PMID: 29987044]

[21]   Kavanagh Williamson, M.; Coombes, N.; Juszczak, F.; Athanasopoulos, M.; Khan, M.; Eykyn, T.; Srenathan, U.; Taams, L.; Dias Zeidler, J.; Da Poian, A.; Huthoff, H. Upregulation of glucose uptake and hexokinase activity of primary human CD4+ T cells in response to infection with HIV-1. *Viruses,* **2018**, *10*(3), 114.
[http://dx.doi.org/10.3390/v10030114] [PMID: 29518929]

[22]   Bhatt, A.N.; Kumar, A.; Rai, Y.; Kumari, N.; Vedagiri, D.; Harshan, K.H.; Chinnadurai, V.; Chandna, S. Glycolytic inhibitor 2-deoxy-d-glucose attenuates SARS-CoV-2 multiplication in host cells and weakens the infective potential of progeny virions. *Life Sci.,* **2022**, *295*, 120411.
[http://dx.doi.org/10.1016/j.lfs.2022.120411] [PMID: 35181310]

[23]   Baďurová, L.; Polčicová, K.; Omasta, B.; Ovečková, I.; Kocianová, E.; Tomášková, J. 2-Deoxy-D-glucose inhibits lymphocytic choriomeningitis virus propagation by targeting glycoprotein N-glycosylation. *Virol. J.,* **2023**, *20*(1), 108.
[http://dx.doi.org/10.1186/s12985-023-02082-3] [PMID: 37259080]

[24]   Datema, R.; Schwarz, R.T. Interference with glycosylation of glycoproteins. Inhibition of formation of lipid-linked oligosaccharides *in vivo. Biochem. J.,* **1979**, *184*(1), 113-123.
[http://dx.doi.org/10.1042/bj1840113] [PMID: 534512]

[25]   Kaluza, G.; Schmidt, M.F.G.; Scholtissek, C. Effect of 2-deoxy-d-glucose on the multiplication of semliki forest virus and the reversal of the block by mannose. *Virology,* **1973**, *54*(1), 179-189.
[http://dx.doi.org/10.1016/0042-6822(73)90127-X] [PMID: 4736595]

[26]   Knowles, R.W.; Person, S. Effects of 2-deoxyglucose, glucosamine, and mannose on cell fusion and the glycoproteins of herpes simplex virus. *J. Virol.,* **1976**, *18*(2), 644-651.
[http://dx.doi.org/10.1128/jvi.18.2.644-651.1976] [PMID: 178901]

[27]   Wright, K.; Spiro, R.C.; Burns, J.W.; Buchmeier, M.J. Post-translational processing of the glycoproteins of lymphocytic choriomeningitis virus. *Virology,* **1990**, *177*(1), 175-183.
[http://dx.doi.org/10.1016/0042-6822(90)90471-3] [PMID: 2141203]

[28]   Leavitt, R.; Schlesinger, S.; Kornfeld, S. Tunicamycin inhibits glycosylation and multiplication of Sindbis and vesicular stomatitis viruses. *J. Virol.,* **1977**, *21*(1), 375-385.
[http://dx.doi.org/10.1128/jvi.21.1.375-385.1977] [PMID: 189071]

[29]   Padula, P.J.; de Martínez Segovia, Z.M. Replication of Junin virus in the presence of tunicamycin. *Intervirology,* **1984**, *22*(4), 227-231.
[http://dx.doi.org/10.1159/000149555] [PMID: 6096295]

[30]   Chen, B.; Boël, G.; Hashem, Y.; Ning, W.; Fei, J.; Wang, C.; Gonzalez, R.L., Jr; Hunt, J.F.; Frank, J.; Ett, A. EttA regulates translation by binding the ribosomal E site and restricting ribosome-tRNA dynamics. *Nat. Struct. Mol. Biol.,* **2014**, *21*(2), 152-159.
[http://dx.doi.org/10.1038/nsmb.2741] [PMID: 24389465]

[31] Sun, L.; Yi, L.; Zhang, C.; Liu, X.; Feng, S.; Chen, W.; Lan, J.; Zhao, L.; Tu, J.; Lin, L. Glutamine is required for snakehead fish vesiculovirus propagation *via* replenishing the tricarboxylic acid cycle. *J. Gen. Virol.,* **2016**, *97*(11), 2849-2855.
[http://dx.doi.org/10.1099/jgv.0.000597] [PMID: 27600401]

[32] Pasqual, G.; Burri, D.J.; Pasquato, A.; de la Torre, J.C.; Kunz, S. Role of the host cell's unfolded protein response in arenavirus infection. *J. Virol.,* **2011**, *85*(4), 1662-1670.
[http://dx.doi.org/10.1128/JVI.01782-10] [PMID: 21106748]

[33] Kurtoglu, M.; Maher, J.C.; Lampidis, T.J. Differential toxic mechanisms of 2-deoxy-D-glucose *versus* 2-fluorodeoxy-D-glucose in hypoxic and normoxic tumor cells. *Antioxid. Redox Signal.,* **2007**, *9*(9), 1383-1390.
[http://dx.doi.org/10.1089/ars.2007.1714] [PMID: 17627467]

[34] Leung, H.J.; Duran, E.M.; Kurtoglu, M.; Andreansky, S.; Lampidis, T.J.; Mesri, E.A. Activation of the unfolded protein response by 2-deoxy-D-glucose inhibits Kaposi's sarcoma-associated herpesvirus replication and gene expression. *Antimicrob. Agents Chemother.,* **2012**, *56*(11), 5794-5803.
[http://dx.doi.org/10.1128/AAC.01126-12] [PMID: 22926574]

[35] Ghosh, B.; Roy, S.; Singh, J.K.; Gorenstein, D.; Frolov, I.; Hilser, V.; Nikonowicz, E.; Rajarathnam, K.; Watowich, S. The mode of therapeutic action of 2-Deoxy D-Glucose: Anti-viral or glycolysis blocker? *Pers. MAPs,* **2021**, *4*(1), 66-86.
[http://dx.doi.org/10.26434/chemrxiv-2021-2z6ln]

[36] Bojkova, D.; Klann, K.; Koch, B.; Widera, M.; Krause, D.; Ciesek, S.; Cinatl, J.; Münch, C. Proteomics of SARS-CoV-2-infected host cells reveals therapy targets. *Nature,* **2020**, *583*(7816), 469-472.
[http://dx.doi.org/10.1038/s41586-020-2332-7] [PMID: 32408336]

[37] Codo, A.C.; Davanzo, G.G.; Monteiro, L.B.; de Souza, G.F.; Muraro, S.P.; Virgilio-da-Silva, J.V.; Prodonoff, J.S.; Carregari, V.C.; de Biagi Junior, C.A.O.; Crunfli, F.; Jimenez Restrepo, J.L.; Vendramini, P.H.; Reis-de-Oliveira, G.; Bispo dos Santos, K.; Toledo-Teixeira, D.A.; Parise, P.L.; Martini, M.C.; Marques, R.E.; Carmo, H.R.; Borin, A.; Coimbra, L.D.; Boldrini, V.O.; Brunetti, N.S.; Vieira, A.S.; Mansour, E.; Ulaf, R.G.; Bernardes, A.F.; Nunes, T.A.; Ribeiro, L.C.; Palma, A.C.; Agrela, M.V.; Moretti, M.L.; Sposito, A.C.; Pereira, F.B.; Velloso, L.A.; Vinolo, M.A.R.; Damasio, A.; Proença-Módena, J.L.; Carvalho, R.F.; Mori, M.A.; Martins-de-Souza, D.; Nakaya, H.I.; Farias, A.S.; Moraes-Vieira, P.M. Elevated glucose levels favor SARS-CoV-2 infection and monocyte response through a HIF-1α/Glycolysis-dependent axis. *Cell Metab.,* **2020**, *32*(3), 498-499.
[http://dx.doi.org/10.1016/j.cmet.2020.07.015] [PMID: 32877692]

[38] Sung, H.; Ferlay, J.; Siegel, R.L.; Laversanne, M.; Soerjomataram, I.; Jemal, A.; Bray, F. Global cancer statistics 2020: globocan estimates of incidence and mortality worldwide for 36 cancers in 185 countries. *CA Cancer J. Clin.,* **2021**, *71*(3), 209-249.
[http://dx.doi.org/10.3322/caac.21660] [PMID: 33538338]

[39] Läsche, M.; Urban, H.; Gallwas, J.; Gründker, C. HPV and other microbiota; who's good and who's bad: effects of the microbial environment on the development of cervical cancer—a non-systematic review. *Cells,* **2021**, *10*(3), 714.
[http://dx.doi.org/10.3390/cells10030714] [PMID: 33807087]

[40] Maehama, T.; Patzelt, A.; Lengert, M.; Hutter, K.J.; Kanazawa, K.; Zur Hausen, H.; Rösl, F. Selective down-regulation of human papillomavirus transcription by 2-deoxyglucose. *Int. J. Cancer,* **1998**, *76*(5), 639-646.
[http://dx.doi.org/10.1002/(SICI)1097-0215(19980529)76:5<639::AID-IJC5>3.0.CO;2-R] [PMID: 9610719]

[41] Kang, H.T.; Ju, J.W.; Cho, J.W.; Hwang, E.S. Down-regulation of Sp1 activity through modulation of O-glycosylation by treatment with a low glucose mimetic, 2-deoxyglucose. *J. Biol. Chem.,* **2003**, *278*(51), 51223-51231.
[http://dx.doi.org/10.1074/jbc.M307332200] [PMID: 14532290]

[42]   Ma, D.; Huang, Y.; Song, S. Inhibiting the HPV16 oncogene-mediated glycolysis sensitizes human cervical carcinoma cells to 5-fluorouracil. *OncoTargets Ther.,* **2019**, *12*, 6711-6720.
[http://dx.doi.org/10.2147/OTT.S205334] [PMID: 31695407]

[43]   Wali, L.; Karbiener, M.; Chou, S.; Kovtunyk, V.; Adonyi, A.; Gösler, I.; Contreras, X.; Stoeva, D.; Blaas, D.; Stöckl, J.; Kreil, T.R.; Gualdoni, G.A.; Gorki, A.D. Host-directed therapy with 2-deoxy-D-glucose inhibits human rhinoviruses, endemic coronaviruses, and SARS-CoV-2. *J. Virus Erad.,* **2022**, *8*(4), 100305.
[http://dx.doi.org/10.1016/j.jve.2022.100305] [PMID: 36514716]

[44]   Wu, Y.H.; Yang, Y.; Chen, C.H.; Hsiao, C.J.; Li, T.N.; Liao, K.J.; Watashi, K.; Chen, B.S.; Wang, L.H.C. Aerobic glycolysis supports hepatitis B virus protein synthesis through interaction between viral surface antigen and pyruvate kinase isoform M2. *PLoS Pathog.,* **2021**, *17*(3), e1008866.
[http://dx.doi.org/10.1371/journal.ppat.1008866] [PMID: 33720996]

[45]   Wang, X.; Lin, Y.; Kemper, T.; Chen, J.; Yuan, Z.; Liu, S.; Zhu, Y.; Broering, R.; Lu, M. AMPK and Akt/mTOR signalling pathways participate in glucose-mediated regulation of hepatitis B virus replication and cellular autophagy. *Cell. Microbiol.,* **2020**, *22*(2), e13131.
[http://dx.doi.org/10.1111/cmi.13131] [PMID: 31746509]

[46]   Patel, A.; Kaur, H.; Xess, I.; Michael, J.S.; Savio, J.; Rudramurthy, S.; Singh, R.; Shastri, P.; Umabala, P.; Sardana, R.; Kindo, A.; Capoor, M.R.; Mohan, S.; Muthu, V.; Agarwal, R.; Chakrabarti, A. A multicentre observational study on the epidemiology, risk factors, management and outcomes of mucormycosis in India. *Clin. Microbiol. Infect.,* **2020**, *26*(7), 944.e9-944.e15.
[http://dx.doi.org/10.1016/j.cmi.2019.11.021] [PMID: 31811914]

[47]   Lin, S.C.; Chen, M.C.; Liu, S.; Callahan, V.M.; Bracci, N.R.; Lehman, C.W.; Dahal, B.; de la Fuente, C.L.; Lin, C.C.; Wang, T.T.; Kehn-Hall, K. Phloretin inhibits Zika virus infection by interfering with cellular glucose utilisation. *Int. J. Antimicrob. Agents,* **2019**, *54*(1), 80-84.
[http://dx.doi.org/10.1016/j.ijantimicag.2019.03.017] [PMID: 30930299]

[48]   Subak-Sharpe, J.H.; Dargan, D.J. HSV molecular biology: general aspects of herpes simplex virus molecular biology. *Virus Genes,* **1998**, *16*(3), 239-251.
[http://dx.doi.org/10.1023/A:1008068902673] [PMID: 9654678]

[49]   Abrantes, J.L.; Alves, C.M.; Costa, J.; Almeida, F.C.L.; Sola-Penna, M.; Fontes, C.F.L.; Souza, T.M.L. Herpes simplex type 1 activates glycolysis through engagement of the enzyme 6-phosphofructo-1-kinase (PFK-1). *Biochim. Biophys. Acta Mol. Basis Dis.,* **2012**, *1822*(8), 1198-1206.
[http://dx.doi.org/10.1016/j.bbadis.2012.04.011] [PMID: 22542512]

[50]   Varanasi, S.K.; Donohoe, D.; Jaggi, U.; Rouse, B.T. Manipulating glucose metabolism during different stages of viral pathogenesis can have either detrimental or beneficial effects. *J. Immunol.,* **2017**, *199*(5), 1748-1761.
[http://dx.doi.org/10.4049/jimmunol.1700472] [PMID: 28768727]

[51]   Kern, E.R.; Glasgow, L.A.; Klein, R.J.; Friedman-Kien, A.E. Failure of 2-deoxy-D-glucose in the treatment of experimental cutaneous and genital infections due to herpes simplex virus. *J. Infect. Dis.,* **1982**, *146*(2), 159-166.
[http://dx.doi.org/10.1093/infdis/146.2.159] [PMID: 6286785]

[52]   Shannon, W.M.; Arnett, G.; Drennen, D.J. Lack of efficacy of 2-deoxy-D-glucose in the treatment of experimental herpes genitalis in guinea pigs. *Antimicrob. Agents Chemother.,* **1982**, *21*(3), 513-515.
[http://dx.doi.org/10.1128/AAC.21.3.513] [PMID: 7201777]

[53]   Raez, L.E.; Papadopoulos, K.; Ricart, A.D.; Chiorean, E.G.; DiPaola, R.S.; Stein, M.N.; Rocha Lima, C.M.; Schlesselman, J.J.; Tolba, K.; Langmuir, V.K.; Kroll, S.; Jung, D.T.; Kurtoglu, M.; Rosenblatt, J.; Lampidis, T.J. A phase I dose-escalation trial of 2-deoxy-d-glucose alone or combined with docetaxel in patients with advanced solid tumors. *Cancer Chemother. Pharmacol.,* **2013**, *71*(2), 523-530.
[http://dx.doi.org/10.1007/s00280-012-2045-1] [PMID: 23228990]

[54]   Priebe, W.; Zielinski, R.; Fokt, I.; Felix, E.; Radjendirane, V.; Arumugam, J.; Tai Khuong, M.; Krasinski, M.; Skora, S. EXTH-07. Design and evaluation of wp1122, an inhibitor of glycolysis with increased cns uptake. *Neuro-oncol.,* **2018**, *20* Suppl. 6, vi86.
       [http://dx.doi.org/10.1093/neuonc/noy148.356]

[55]   Michel, K.A.; Zieliński, R.; Walker, C.M.; Le Roux, L.; Priebe, W.; Bankson, J.A.; Schellingerhout, D. Hyperpolarized pyruvate mr spectroscopy depicts glycolytic inhibition in a mouse model of glioma. *Radiology,* **2019**, *293*(1), 168-173.
       [http://dx.doi.org/10.1148/radiol.2019182919] [PMID: 31385757]

[56]   Lampidis, T.J.; Kurtoglu, M.; Maher, J.C.; Liu, H.; Krishan, A.; Sheft, V.; Szymanski, S.; Fokt, I.; Rudnicki, W.R.; Ginalski, K.; Lesyng, B.; Priebe, W. Efficacy of 2-halogen substituted d-glucose analogs in blocking glycolysis and killing "hypoxic tumor cells". *Cancer Chemother. Pharmacol.,* **2006**, *58*(6), 725-734.
       [http://dx.doi.org/10.1007/s00280-006-0207-8] [PMID: 16555088]

CHAPTER 6

2-Deoxy-D-Glucose and its Derivatives: Dual Role in Diagnostics and Therapeutics

Anil Kumar[1,*] and **Krishnendu Barik**[1]

[1] *Department of Bioinformatics, Central University of South Bihar, Gaya-824236, India*

Abstract: This chapter delves into the multifaceted applications of 2-Deoxy-d-Glucose (2-DG) and its derivatives as versatile tools in diagnostics and therapeutics. Highlighting their dual role in the medical landscape, this chapter provides a comprehensive overview of the diverse functions and mechanisms by which these compounds contribute to both diagnostic assessments and therapeutic interventions. The first section examines the use of 2-DG and its derivatives in diagnostics, detailing their efficacy in various imaging techniques, diagnostic assays, and investigative procedures. Their unique properties and specific interactions in these contexts were explored to elucidate their significance in the accurate detection and visualization of specific physiological conditions or anomalies. The subsequent segment shifts the focus towards the therapeutic realm, where the book chapter investigates the potential and current applications of 2-DG and its derivatives in treating a spectrum of diseases and conditions. From their roles in cancer therapy to neurological disorders and severe acute respiratory syndrome-related coronavirus-2 (SARS-CoV-2) treatment, the chapter outlines the mechanisms and clinical advancements where these compounds show promise as therapeutic agents. Throughout this discussion, the chapter emphasizes the evolving landscape of 2-DG and its derivatives, touching upon ongoing research, challenges, and future prospects in harnessing their dual attributes for enhanced healthcare outcomes. The exploration of these compounds in both diagnostic and therapeutic realms not only illuminates their versatility but also underlines the potential for innovative and integrated medical approaches.

Keywords: Cancer therapy, Neurological disorders, SARS-CoV-2 treatment, Warburg effect, 2-Deoxy-D-Glucose.

1. INTRODUCTION

2-Deoxy-D-glucose (2-DG), a synthetic analog of glucose, has been captivated in the scientific field because of its various biological properties and potential therapeutic applications. 2-DG has been widely employed as a research tool in

---

* **Corresponding author Anil Kumar:** Department of Bioinformatics, Central University of South Bihar, Gaya-824236, India; E-mail: kumaranil@cub.ac.in

Raman Singh, Antresh Kumar & Kuldeep Singh (Eds.)

various biological and medical fields [1]. The lack of a hydroxyl group at the 2'-position on the pyranose ring distinguishes 2-DG from glucose and prevents it from continuing further glycolysis after being phosphorylated by hexokinase (HK), the first enzyme of the glycolytic pathway [2]. As a result, 2-DG acts as an inhibitor of pathways utilizing glucose and mannose, affecting multiple enzymes and cellular processes through various mechanisms. This multifaceted disruption interferes with the production of energy, nucleotides, and other essential macromolecules, thereby impacting cell growth and survival [1, 2]. Other cellular activities that rely on glucose, such as N-glycosylation, pentose phosphate pathway (PPP), and hexosamine biosynthesis pathway, can be influenced by 2-DG [3]. The same glucose transporters (GLUTs) mediate glucose absorption by transferring 2-DG into the cell. As a result, it preferentially accumulates in cells that consume large amounts of glucose, such as cancer cells, neurons, and immunological cells [2, 3].

Using techniques such as autoradiography, nuclear magnetic resonance, and positron emission tomography (PET), 18F-2-deoxyglucose, a derivative of 2-DG has been employed as a tracer molecule to analyze the distribution and activity of glucose metabolism in living organisms [4]. 2-DG has also been employed as a pharmaceutical agent against various illnesses such as cancer, epilepsy, neurodegeneration, and infection [5, 6]. 2-DG has shown promising results in preclinical and clinical trials as an adjuvant therapy for cancer and COVID-19 by exploiting the metabolic vulnerabilities of these diseases [6]. However, 2-DG has some limitations and challenges such as toxicity, specificity, and delivery [7]. In this chapter, we review the history, chemistry, biology, and applications of 2-DG, as well as the current status and prospects of 2-DG as a diagnostic and therapeutic tool.

Glucose serves as the predominant cellular energy source and functions as a substrate for various metabolic processes. It is primarily derived from consumed dietary carbohydrates, but it can also be produced within the body *via* gluconeogenesis [8]. Because glucose is hydrophilic, it requires specific GLUT proteins to allow cellular uptake [9]. Tumor cells require the overexpression of GLUT transporters to boost glucose uptake–20-30 times compared to normal cells [9, 10]. Glucose is the primary reservoir of energy for most cells, predominantly in the brain, muscles, and tumors. Glucose metabolism involves a series of biochemical processes that transform glucose into pyruvate or lactate, generating adenosine triphosphate (ATP) and nicotinamide adenine dinucleotide hydrogen (NADH) as energy carriers [11]. The first step of glucose metabolism is glycolysis, which occurs in the cytoplasm and does not require oxygen. Glycolysis consists of ten enzymatic reactions that split one molecule of glucose (6-carbon), yielding two pyruvate molecules (3-carbon) and producing a pair of

ATP molecules and a pair of NADH molecules [11, 12]. The fate of pyruvate relies on the availability of oxygen and the cell type. Under aerobic conditions, pyruvate is carried into the mitochondria and oxidized into acetyl-CoA, which enters the tricarboxylic acid (TCA) cycle and electron transport chain (ETC), producing more ATP and NADH [13].

Glucose metabolism in cancerous cells involves the conversion of glucose, the main source of energy for most cells, into pyruvate or lactate [12]. Cancer cells exhibit a distinct glucose metabolism compared to normal cells, characterized by increased glucose uptake and the conversion of glucose to lactate through fermentation, even when oxygen and functional mitochondria are present. This phenomenon is termed the Warburg effect, which allows cancer cells to sustain and multiply in hypoxic environments. Cancer cells rely on acquiring carbon for cell proliferation. Complete oxidation of glucose to CO_2 may hinder this process by depriving cancer cells of the necessary carbon required for producing new cells [14]. Glucose metabolism in cancer cells is regulated by multiple factors such as oncogenes, tumor suppressors, signaling pathways, and microenvironmental cues [15].

Glucose metabolism in cancer cells also affects their plasticity, which is the ability to switch between different phenotypes and behaviors such as stemness, differentiation, invasion, and metastasis [14]. Tumor cells adapt to low oxygen levels by changing gene expression and signaling pathways. In response to hypoxic stress, tumor cells undergo a series of metabolic adaptations to maintain their survival and growth. These adaptations include elevated expression of protooncogenes, such as c-Myc, the instigation of signaling pathways, such as PI3K/Akt, and the triggering of specific transcription factors, such as hypoxia-inducible factor-1α (HIF-1α) [16]. One significant alteration is the activation of HIF-1α, a transcription factor that controls the expression of many genes related to glucose metabolism. HIF-1α helps tumor cells switch from oxidative metabolism to aerobic glycolysis, which produces energy and reduces oxidative stress in the absence of oxygen. HIF-1α also regulates the intake of glucose, functioning of glycolytic enzymes, function of mitochondria, and removal of damaged mitochondria by autophagy. HIF-1α balances oxygen demand and supply as well as ATP and reactive oxygen species (ROS) production in tumor cells [17]. Shifting oxidative metabolism to aerobic glycolysis is a key strategy for tumor cells to thrive and proliferate in hypoxic environments [18].

Glycolysis occurs in the cytoplasm and does not require oxygen. Glycolysis begins when glucose enters the cell through GLUT transporters and is phosphorylated by HK to glucose 6-phosphate (G6P) (Fig. **1**) [19]. This molecule has the option to enter the PPP for NADPH and ribose-5-phosphate production or undergo conversion to fructose-6-phosphate (F-6-P) through phosphoglucose isomerase (PGI). The next step is the irreversible and ATP-dependent phosphorylation of F-6-P to fructose-1,6-biphosphate (F-1,6-BP) by phosphofructokinase (PFK), a key enzyme that controls the glycolysis rate [20]. F-1,6-BP can then be split into two three-carbon molecules: glyceraldehyde-3-P and dihydroxyacetone phosphate, which can also be used for lipid synthesis. The conversion of phosphoenol pyruvate (PEP) to pyruvate by pyruvate kinase (PK), which produces ATP and NADH, is the final step in glycolysis [19, 20]. Mammals possess four distinct PK isoforms: PKM1/PKM2, PKR, and PKL, each with its distinctive molecular structure, function, and expression in distinct tissues. The most prevalent type of PKM2 is found in fetal tissues, stem cells, and cancer cells, and allows for rapid cell development and high glucose flow [21]. PKL is also involved in gluconeogenesis, which is the reverse of glycolysis, in which glucose is synthesized from other sources such as pyruvate, lactate, and amino acids. Gluconeogenesis occurs mostly in the liver during fasting and is regulated by hormones such as glucagon, which limits PK action. Pyruvate, the last product of glycolysis, can have different fates depending on the oxygen level and cell type. In standard oxygen environments, pyruvate can enter the mitochondria and be oxidized to acetyl-CoA, which then joins the TCA cycle and ETC to produce more ATP and NADH [22]. Under low oxygen conditions or in cells that have high glycolytic rates, such as cancer cells, pyruvate can be reduced to lactate by lactate dehydrogenase (LDH), which also recycles NAD^+ for glycolysis. This is called the Warburg effect, or aerobic glycolysis, and it helps cancer cells adapt to hypoxia and avoid oxidative stress [21, 22].

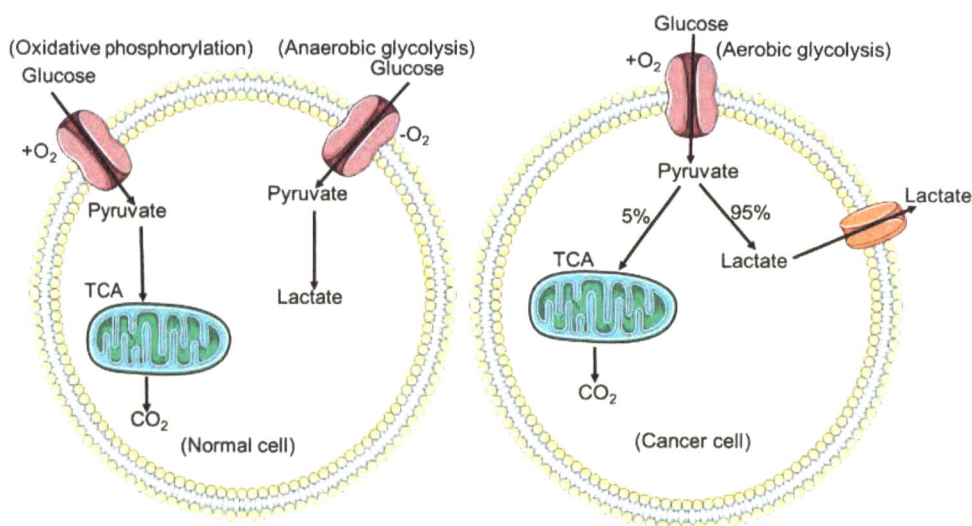

Fig. (1). Glucose metabolism in normal and cancer cells.

2. THE WARBURG EFFECT

The breakdown of glucose, allows the generation of ATP *via* carbon bond oxidation, which is required for mammalian survival. In mammals, glucose metabolism triggers the synthesis of lactate or, upon complete oxidation in the mitochondria, CO_2. In tumors and actively proliferating cells, there is a significant increase in glucose uptake, accompanied by lactate production, despite the presence of oxygen and fully functional mitochondria [23].

Aerobic glycolysis is a less efficient process for producing ATP per glucose molecule than mitochondrial respiration. However, owing to the rapid breakdown of glucose in aerobic glycolysis, lactate formation from glucose occurs 10-100 times faster than the total oxidation of glucose in the mitochondria [24]. Surprisingly, the total amount of ATP synthesized over a fixed period was equivalent between the two modes of glucose metabolism [23]. Owing to the inherent difference in kinetics, this leads to the idea that cancer uses aerobic glycolysis [24]. Theoretical estimates based on evolutionary game theory suggest that cells that produce ATP at a higher rate but with a lower yield may have a selection advantage when fighting for limited energy supplies. Tumor microenvironments, which are characterized by limited glucose availability and nutritional competition with stromal cells and the immune compartment, support this hypothesis [10].

Recent studies causing alterations in the cellular environment to greatly increase ATP demand revealed a rapid increase in aerobic glycolysis, while oxidative phosphorylation (OXPHOS) remained constant, lending credence to the Warburg Effect's involvement in rapidly responding to ATP synthesis needs. Despite the beauty of this plan, there are some obstacles. According to empirical calculations, ATP required for cell growth and division may be significantly lower than that required for normal cellular maintenance [12, 23]. As a result, ATP demand may not reach limiting levels during tumor cell growth. Moreover, the mechanisms available to other cell types for rapid ATP demand are present in tumor cells, raising the question of whether aerobic glycolysis is the only process responsible for ATP requirement. Further research is crucial to understand the impact of this pathway on the role of aerobic glycolysis [12].

The Warburg Effect has been suggested to be an adaptive mechanism to meet the metabolic needs of uncontrolled growth. In this scenario, increased glucose consumption provides a carbon source for anabolic activities necessary for cell proliferation [23, 25]. Excess carbon is utilized for the *de novo* synthesis of nucleotides, lipids, and proteins, branching into various glycolysis-derived pathways. For example, phosphoglycerate dehydrogenase (PHGDH) redirects glycolytic flow into *de novo* serine production. Proliferating cells, rather than possessing a rate-limiting requirement for ATP, require additional reducing equivalents in the form of NADPH [25]. Increased glucose absorption promotes the synthesis of these reducing equivalents in the oxidative branch of PPP, which is essential for reductive biosynthesis, particularly *de novo* lipid synthesis [26].

Another suggested explanation for the biosynthetic role of the Warburg Effect involves the regeneration of NAD^+ from NADH in the pyruvate-to-lactate phase, which completes aerobic glycolysis. To keep glycolysis functioning, NADH generated by glyceraldehyde phosphate dehydrogenase must be used in order to renew NAD^+ [25, 26]. The high rate of glycolysis keeps supply lines open, allowing metabolites, such as 3-phosphoglycerate, to be diverted to serine for one-carbon metabolism-mediated synthesis of NADPH and nucleotides. Some argue that aerobic glycolysis is a trade-off for biosynthesis, with poor ATP production at the cost of sustaining high fluxes through anabolic pathways [27]. This trade-off restricts the utilization of mitochondria to maintain a high expression of biosynthetic enzymes. In contrast to the functions within individual cells discussed earlier, the Warburg Effect may offer advantages for cell growth in a multicellular setting. Intriguing possibilities include the acidification of the microenvironment and metabolic crosstalk. Elevated glucose metabolism contributes to microenvironmental acidification through lactate secretion, leading to a decreased pH [12]. Acidosis has many possible benefits for cancer cells. According to the acid-mediated invasion hypothesis, H^+ ions generated by cancer cells permeate into the surrounding environment, changing the tumor–stroma interface and fostering increased invasiveness. Some studies have suggested that tumor-derived lactate contributes to the polarization of M2 tissue-associated macrophages [12, 23]. Additionally, the availability of glucose appears to result from competitive clashes between tumor cells and tumor-infiltrating lymphocytes (TILs). Increased glycolysis rates limit the glucose availability for TILs, which require glucose for their effector actions [23, 25].

Targeting aerobic glycolysis in tumors suppresses cancer cells and boosts glucose availability to TILs, thereby boosting their ability to destroy tumor cells. Findings from earlier studies suggest that tumor cells have the ability to interact with the immune system to promote pro-tumor immunity [28]. While the Warburg Effect most likely provides an overall benefit by promoting a tumor microenvironment favorable to cancer cell proliferation, it is regarded as an early event in oncogenesis, occurring as an immediate result of initial oncogenic mutations such as KRAS (Kirsten rat sarcoma viral oncogene homolog) in pancreatic cancer or BRAF (v-Raf murine sarcoma viral oncogene homolog B) in melanoma [23, 28]. This occurs before cell invasion, and even in benign and early stage lesions. Another consideration is that under conditions isolated from the environment, similar to the growth phase of unicellular yeast, the Warburg Effect remains the preferred choice for energy metabolism from glucose [12, 28].

The Warburg Effect provides tumor cells with direct signaling functions. This theory stands out because it establishes a direct causal role for altered glucose metabolism in cancer *via* signal transduction that affects multiple cellular processes [29]. The generation and alteration of ROS and the control of chromatin state are two areas of signaling. Additional putative signaling systems have been reported in other studies [28, 29]. Maintaining an appropriate ROS balance is critical. Excessive ROS levels can harm cell membranes and nucleic acids. Inadequate ROS impairs cell proliferation-promoting signaling mechanisms, such as the inactivation of phosphatase tensin homolog (PTEN) and tyrosine phosphatases [29]. The Warburg Effect causes changes in mitochondrial redox potential, which in turn affects ROS formation. NADH accessible to mitochondria for electron transport is an important factor in redox potential. When glycolysis rates fluctuate, cellular mechanisms that preserve redox homeostasis are activated [30]. The malate-aspartate shuttle across the mitochondria can correct the NADH imbalance up to a particular level of glycolysis. When glycolysis rates exceed the capacity of the malate-aspartate shuttle, the conversion of pyruvate to lactate *via* LDH can renew NAD^+. This process may also bring about changes in the homeostasis of ROS formation by changing the concentration of reducing equivalents in the mitochondria. This Warburg Effect may be directly related to oncogene-induced senescence (OIS) [31]. OIS has a tumor-suppressing function, and diverse studies have established that enhanced glucose oxidation *via* pyruvate dehydrogenase (PDH) can control OIS. These data show that the NADH redox balance may play a direct signaling function in the Warburg Effect [23]. Along with the Warburg Effect, metabolic pathways that promote redox equilibrium are also activated [23, 31]. NADPH and glutathione are produced by *de novo* serine metabolism, which feeds into one-carbon metabolism to control ROS levels. These findings show direct biochemical links between aerobic glycolysis and ROS availability, which might influence a range of signaling systems. In addition to ROS-mediated cell signaling, there is a well-established signaling relationship between glucose metabolism and histone acetylation. Chromatin structure governs multiple biological processes, including DNA repair and transcription [32].

Glucose flux has been shown to modulate acetyl-CoA, a substrate for histone acetylation. Studies have shown a direct link between cellular metabolism and growth gene regulation, with intracellular acetyl-CoA levels indicating a widely conserved mechanism that promotes this interaction [33]. The activity of ATP-citrate lyase, which converts citrate to acetyl-CoA, has been shown to alter histone acetylation levels [23]. Increased acetyl-CoA levels may be sufficient to induce cell proliferation through histone acetylation. When glucose is removed or

ATP-citrate lyase is reduced, the acetylation of numerous histones is lost, resulting in decreased transcription of genes involved in glucose metabolism. This points to a relationship between glucose metabolism and histone acetylation [23, 34]. Furthermore, glycolytic metabolism has been shown to influence chromatin shape. In addition to histone acetylation in response to glucose availability, food availability can influence deacetylation. Deacetylation is important in food sensing and signaling because NAD^+ levels influence the activity of several deacetylases [35]. The proportion of $NAD^+/NADH$ increases under nutrient-deprived conditions, which influences both acetylation and deacetylation. This indicates that their statuses may be consequences of the Warburg Effect [34, 35].

A pivotal difference between cancer and normal cells is the choice of energy source. Cancer cells exhibit a phenomenon called the 'Warburg effect,' which means that they prefer glycolysis over OXPHOS for energy production [23]. This metabolic trait provides the basis for targeting cancer cells with 2-DG. 2-DG is transported into the cell by the same GLUTs that mediate glucose uptake; thus, 2-DG gets phosphorylated to 2-deoxy-D-glucose-6-phosphate but cannot proceed further in glycolysis, such as cancer cells, neurons, and immune cells. 2-DG can mimic glucose and enter the glycolytic pathway, but cannot be further metabolized after phosphorylation by HK [36]. Therefore, 2-DG is trapped inside the cell as 2-deoxy-D-glucose-6-phosphate. This accumulation leads to the inhibition of glycolytic enzymes, initially targeting phosphoglucoisomerase directly. This inhibition subsequently causes product inhibition of hexokinase due to the buildup of 2-deoxy-D-glucose-6-phosphate. These upstream effects lead to a cascade that indirectly inhibits other glycolytic enzymes such as phosphofructokinase (PFK) and pyruvate kinase, reducing ATP production and increasing lactate accumulation [37]. 2-DG can also impair other glucose-dependent pathways such as N-glycosylation, which is essential for the folding and stability of proteins such as growth factor receptors and integrins. 2-DG can also affect PPP, generating NADPH and ribose-5-phosphate, which are important for the synthesis of nucleotides, fatty acids, and glutathione [36, 37]. 2-DG might intervene with the hexosamine biosynthesis pathway, which produces UDP-N-acetylglucosamine, which is associated with the modification of proteins such as transcription factors and signaling molecules. By disrupting these pathways, 2-DG can induce various cellular responses such as apoptosis, autophagy, oxidative stress, endoplasmic reticulum (ER) stress, and inflammation [1, 37].

3. 2-DG IN CANCER DIAGNOSTICS

A phase I clinical trial was initiated based on promising preclinical data. Patients were administered 2-DG orally at a dose that increased gradually, with planned evaluations including PET scans and markers of autophagy. Preliminary findings have indicated that 2-DG is generally safe, with no observed toxicity limiting the dose; however, there exists a maximum tolerable dose of 250 mg/kg body weight (BW). Interestingly, one patient with prostate cancer had stable prostate-specific antigen (PSA) levels after more than 11 treatment cycles [38]. 2-DG can be used as a tracer molecule to study the distribution and activity of glucose metabolism in living organisms using techniques such as autoradiography, nuclear magnetic resonance, and PET. PET is a non-invasive imaging technique that detects the uptake and retention of glucose or its derivatives in tumors using radioactive isotopes, such as fluorine-18, carbon-11, or oxygen-15, which emit positrons [39]. Positrons are positively charged particles that collide with electrons and produce gamma rays, which can be determined and measured by external detectors such as PET scanners. PET can offer insights into the metabolic activity and heterogeneity of tissues and tumors as well as the response to treatments that target glucose metabolism. 2-DG can be labeled with fluorine-18, a radioactive isotope with a half-life of approximately 110 min that can serve as a PET tracer [40]. 2-DG labeled with fluorine-18 is also known as 18F-2-deoxyglucose (FDG) and is the most widely used PET tracer in clinical oncology. FDG resembles glucose and enters the glycolytic pathway; however, after phosphorylation by HK, it cannot be further metabolized [6, 40]. As a result, FDG becomes trapped inside the cell and releases gamma rays that PET scanners can detect. As a result of the Warburg effect or aerobic glycolysis, FDG can represent the glucose intake and glycolytic rate of tumors, which typically surpass those of normal tissues. From the ratio of FDG to 18 F-fluoromisonidazole, a hypoxia-specific PET tracer, FDG can also detect hypoxic zones within tumors that are more resistant to radiation and chemotherapy. FDG can also be used to assess the efficacy of therapies that target glucose metabolism, such as 2-DG, by comparing FDG uptake before and after treatment [40, 41].

4. DISEASES TARGETED BY 2-DG

4.1. Cancer

Cancer significantly impacts various metabolic enzymes and pathways, altering the cellular landscape to favor growth and survival. Hexokinase, crucial for glycolysis, is often overexpressed in cancer, enhancing glucose uptake and supporting rapid cell proliferation through the Warburg effect. The Pentose Phosphate Pathway, vital for nucleotide synthesis and maintaining redox balance, is upregulated to meet the increased metabolic demands of cancer cells. Hexosamine Biosynthesis Pathway is a crucial pathway for sensing metabolic status. These enzymatic changes are pivotal in cancer pathology, offering potential targets for therapeutic intervention.

4.1.1. Inhibition of Hexokinase (HK)

The molecular targets of 2 DG are molecules or pathways that can be influenced by 2 DG, a synthetic analog of glucose, potentially disrupting glucose metabolism. 2-DG is transported into the cell by the same GLUTs that mediate glucose uptake, and as a result, it preferentially accumulates in cells with high rates of glucose consumption, such as cancer cells, neurons, and immune cells [42]. 2-DG differs from glucose in the absence of a hydroxyl group at the 2-position of the pyranose ring, which prevents it from undergoing further glycolysis after phosphorylation by HK, the first enzyme of glycolysis [43]. This enzyme catalyzes the phosphorylation of glucose to glucose-6-phosphate using ATP as a substrate and traps glucose inside the cell (Fig. **2**). 2-DG can compete with glucose for HK and form 2-DG-6-phosphate, which cannot be further metabolized by phosphoglucose isomerase (PGI), the second enzyme of glycolysis [44]. This leads to the aggregation of 2-DG-6-phosphate in the cell and the depletion of ATP and NAD^+ for glycolysis. 2-DG can also inhibit the binding of HK to the mitochondrial membrane, which can affect the coupling of glycolysis and OXPHOS and induce apoptosis [42, 44].

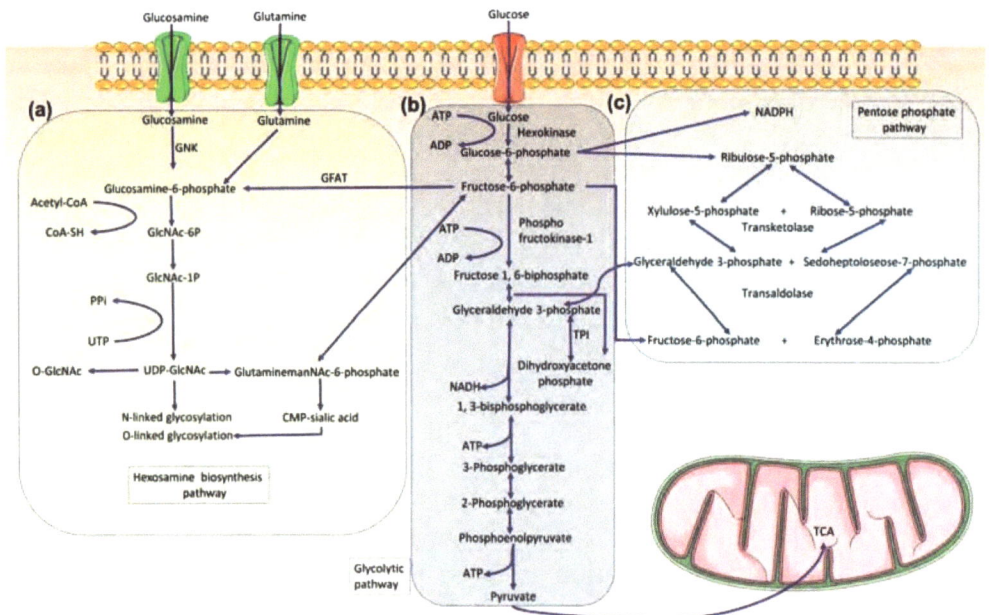

Fig. (2). Glycolysis bioenergetic and biosynthetic pathways. (**a**) Glycolysis converts glucose to pyruvate, yielding two ATP and two NADH. Intermediates serve as precursors for amino acid synthesis. (**b**) PPP, with oxidative and non-oxidative phases, produces NADPH and five-carbon sugars essential for biosynthesis and antioxidant defense. PPP links to glycolysis through TKT and TALDO. (**c**) Hexosamine biosynthesis, a glycolysis branch, starts with F-6-P, generating UDP-GlcNAc for protein glycosylation. Rate-limiting enzyme: GFAT.

4.1.2. Inhibition of Pentose Phosphate Pathway (PPP)

PPP is a metabolic process similar to glycolysis that plays a crucial role in supporting the survival and growth of cancer cells (Fig. **2**). PPP contributes to nucleic acid synthesis by producing pentose phosphate and supplying NADPH, which is required for fatty acid synthesis and cell survival under stress [45]. In cancer cells, the flux *via* PPP can be altered to improve cell survival and proliferation. Understanding the regulatory network of PPP flow appears to be a vital part of metabolic adaptation in many environmental situations in human malignancies, including cancer [46]. PPP is a critical cytosolic metabolic pathway with two branches: oxidative and non-oxidative. The oxidative branch transforms G6P into ribulose-5-phosphate (Ru5P), CO_2, and NADPH, all of which are required for cellular redox equilibrium and fast growth [47]. The non-oxidative branch generates glycolytic intermediates and sugar phosphate precursors, which are vital for the synthesis of amino acids and nucleic acids. G6PD (glucose 6-phosphate dehydrogenase) is an important regulator of PPP and acts as a 'gatekeeper' and rate-limiting enzyme. Its overexpression in cancer cells, particularly in the active dimer form, is linked to poor prognosis [46, 47].

The tumor suppressor p53 inhibits G6PD, while Polo-like kinase 1 (Plk1) promotes PPP flux, linking G6PD to cancer cell cycle progression. G6PD is also influenced by glycosylation and regulatory proteins, such as the mammalian target of rapamycin complex 1 [48]. The enzyme 6-phosphogluconate dehydrogenase (6PGD) participates in the oxidative phase of PPP and is up-regulated in various cancers. Lysine acetylation activates 6PGD, contributing to nucleotide and RNA biosynthesis, which are crucial for cancer cell growth [49]. Ribose-5-phosphate isomerase (RPI) and ribulose-5-phosphate epimerase (RPE) convert Ru5P into ribose-5-phosphate (R5P) and xylulose-5-phosphate (Xu5P), respectively [45]. Ribose-5-phosphate isomerase overexpression is associated with cancer growth, especially in colorectal cancer and hepatocellular carcinoma (HCC). It also activates β-catenin, which influences cell proliferation. Transketolase (TKT) and transaldolase (TALDO) are enzymes in non-oxidative PPP that are responsible for complicated interconversion processes [45, 49, 50].

TKT is upregulated *via* NRF2 pathway in lung, breast, and prostate malignancies. TKTL1 is believed to be a tumor marker. TALDO is overexpressed in gastric adenocarcinomas and has been linked to HCC metastasis [51]. The combination of arginine and ascorbic acid reduces TALDO activity in PPP, thereby influencing intracellular NADPH levels. The interaction between PPP and glycolysis is critical for tumor cell activity. Increased glycolysis during reperfusion reduces the PPP rate owing to their metabolic connection *via* the shared intermediate G6P [52].

Glycolysis is a two-stage conversion of glucose to pyruvate, in which HK, PFK1, and PK play important roles. HK catalyzes glucose phosphorylation, a glycolysis-regulating step. Elevated levels of HK2 in cancer cells lead to enhanced glycolysis and the inhibition of mitochondria-mediated apoptosis. Various factors, including oncogenic Ras, Bcl-2-associated athanogene-3, HIF-1α, and human papillomaviruses E6 and E7, contribute to the induction of HK2 expression. Inhibition of HK2 shows promise in suppressing tumor growth [53]. PFK1, a crucial rate-limiting enzyme, irreversibly phosphorylates F-6-P to F-1,6-BP. Its enhanced activity is observed in cancer cell lines, with increased expression documented in breast and liver malignancies. PFK1 activity is influenced by a number of regulatory mechanisms, including O-GlcNAcylation, p53 inhibitor of TIGAR activation (PITA), and cyclin D3-dependent kinase 6 (CDK6) phosphorylation [54]. Dynamic control of PFK1 improves cancer cell survival and metastasis under metabolic stress. In the final glycolytic step, PK transforms phosphoenolpyruvate into pyruvate. In cancer cells, the balance between active and inactive forms of PK determines whether glucose is directed towards OXPHOS or PPP, influencing cellular development. PKM2, which is preferentially expressed in cancer cells, is subject to intricate regulation, which influences cellular metabolism. PKM2 activity is regulated by variables such as succinylaminoimidazole-carboxamide riboside, epidermal growth factor receptor (EGFR) activation, ROS levels, and HIF-1 [45, 55].

Understanding and targeting these regulatory processes in glycolysis and PPP could lead to new cancer treatment strategies. Changes in glucose metabolism play a significant role in determining the progression and features of malignant tumors such as HCC, breast cancer, and lung cancer. These three diseases share a common thread in their metabolic alterations, which contributes considerably to global cancer incidence and mortality. Understanding these changes not only reveals the underlying science of these cancers but also opens the door to targeted prevention, early diagnosis, and treatment therapies [56]. In HCC, increased G6PD expression is associated with metastasis and a poor prognosis. G6PD silencing is directly related to reduced HCC cell proliferation, migration, and invasion, emphasizing G6PD role in disease development. G6PD activation of the Signal Transduction and Activator of Transcription 3 (STAT3) pathway increases Epithelial-Mesenchymal Transition (EMT), which contributes to HCC cell migration and invasion [57]. G6PD activity is tightly modulated by a number of regulatory mechanisms, including NRF2, microRNA-1 (miR-1), and AKT coactivator T cell leukemia/lymphoma protein IA. Furthermore, PPP is activated by an Inhibitor of Differentiation and DNA Binding-1 (ID1), which promotes oxaliplatin resistance in HCC [45, 57]. G6PD plays an important role in breast cancer, is strongly related to molecular subtypes, and serves as a negative prognostic factor. G6PD silencing results in changes in glycolytic flux, lipid synthesis, and glutamine uptake in breast cancer cells, highlighting its role in metabolic reprogramming. NSD2 overexpression in breast cancer promotes tamoxifen resistance by upregulating G6PD and HK2, thereby increasing the PPP flux. Moreover, dysregulated G6PD expression and activity contribute to the dysregulation of 5' AMP-activated protein kinase (AMPK) signaling, disrupting lipid biosynthesis, and impeding breast cancer cell growth [58].

Tetrahydrobiopterin (TKT) enzyme, which is linked to tumor growth, has emerged as a prognostic marker in breast cancer, impacting survival outcomes. Altered metabolism in lung cancer is highlighted by G6PD overexpression in Non-Small Cell Lung Carcinoma (NSCLC), where elevated G6PD levels correlate with markedly lower survival rates. G6PD inhibition increases the susceptibility of lung cancer cells to cisplatin, implying its role in therapeutic treatment [59]. Furthermore, 6PGD contributes to cisplatin resistance in lung cancer by downregulating microRNAs, highlighting its potential as a therapeutic target [60]. HK2 is essential for lung cancer cell growth both *in vitro* and *in vivo*, and its levels are influenced by the Epidermal Growth Factor Receptor (EGFR) signaling pathway. The modification of glycolytic enzymes prompted by intracellular ROS, such as PFK2/Fructose-2,6-Bisphosphatase 3 (PFKFB3), demonstrates the intricate link between metabolism and redox homeostasis in lung cancer [61]. In the metabolic environment of malignant tumors, PPP is central, orchestrating intricate networks that contribute to the progression and features of HCC, breast cancer, and lung cancer. Targeting major PPP enzymes, such as G6PD, offers a viable path for developing novel diagnostic and therapeutic techniques suited to the different metabolic profiles of various cancers [45, 59, 60].

PPP is a metabolic process that diverges from glycolysis to produce NADPH and ribose-5-phosphate, both of which are required for biosynthesis and redox equilibrium [45]. G6PD, the initial enzyme of the pathway, activates PPP by converting G6P to 6-phosphogluconate, which produces NADPH. 2-DG can inhibit PPP by competing with glucose-6-phosphate for G6PD and by lowering NADPH and ribose-5-phosphate synthesis. This can impair nucleotide, fatty acid, and glutathione synthesis and enhance cellular oxidative stress [45, 60].

4.1.3. Inhibition of Hexosamine Biosynthesis Pathway (HBP)

HBP is a crucial pathway for sensing metabolic status, involving molecules such as glucose, glutamine, uridine triphosphate (UTP), and acetate (Fig. **2**). The final product of HBP is Uridine Diphosphate N-Acetylglucosamine (UDP-GlcNAc), a high-energy sugar donor used in subsequent pathways, particularly in O-GlcNAc transferase (OGT)-catalyzed glycosylation [62]. Targeting different enzymes associated with HBP through inhibitors has been suggested as a promising strategy for cancer treatment while sparing normal cells. Glutamine-fructose-6-phosphatase aminotransferase (GFPT1), which catalyzes the conversion of F-6-P to glucosamine-6-phosphate, is a master regulator of glucose influx into HBP [63]. Its heightened expression is associated with improved overall survival in pancreatic cancer, HCC, and triple-negative breast cancer. In breast cancer, GFPT1 serves as a potential predictive marker for relapse, correlating with tumor size and predicting poor disease-free survival in aggressive subtypes [64]. Additionally, genetic fusion analysis of medullary thyroid cancer revealed the fusion of GFPT1- anaplastic lymphoma kinase. Downregulation of GFPT1 causes tumor shrinkage in pancreatic cancer, highlighting its importance [65].

GFPT1 promotes migration, invasion, and proliferation of glioblastoma cells. Furthermore, its expression is associated with the malignant grade of gliomas. Notably, in breast cancer, GFPT1 overexpression promotes HIF-1 signaling, affecting hyaluronan synthesis and controlling metabolic and cancer stem cell-like features. On the other hand, GFPT2 has unique connections, despite its functions similar to GFPT1 in limiting glucose influx. Elevated GFPT2 levels are associated with processes including EMT and the presence of cancer-associated fibroblasts (CAFs), implying an impact on cancer progression [66]. Compared to the more positive prognostic results associated with GFPT1, this underlines the various functions of GFPT2 in cancer biology. These findings highlight the intricate roles of GFPT1 and GFPT2 in HBP, highlighting their potential as targets for understanding and intervening in cancer progression across a broad range of malignancies. Glucosamine-6-phosphate N-acetyltransferase 1 (GNPNAT1), a key enzyme in the HBP, plays a critical role in catalyzing the conversion of G6P to N-acetylglucosamine-6-phosphate. Although limited research has explored its involvement in cancer, existing studies have suggested significant implications [67].

In castration-resistant prostate cancer (CRPC), GNPNAT1 expression is notably downregulated compared with that in localized prostate cancer. The loss of GNPNAT1 expression in CRPC-like cells is associated with an increase in both cell proliferation and aggressive phenotypes observed in both *in vitro* and *in vivo* conditions [67]. Notably, the underlying signaling pathways indicate that the PI3K-AKT pathway is activated in cells expressing the full-length androgen receptor, while cells containing the androgen receptor-V7 variant modulate signaling through specificity protein 1 (SP1)-regulated expression of carbohydrate response element-binding protein (ChREBP) [68].

Furthermore, studies using Abraxane treatment in lung cancer cells have provided new insights into the involvement of GNPNAT1. As a result, the downregulation of GNPNAT1 in this environment results in proliferative delay and cell adhesion problems, providing further evidence of its impact on cancer-related processes [69]. These findings highlight the importance of GNPNAT1 in cancer biology, particularly in prostate and lung cancers. However, more detailed research is required to fully understand GNPNAT1's multiple roles in the complex terrain of cancer formation and progression. Phosphoglucomutase 3 (PGM3) is a crucial enzyme in the HBP that converts N-acetylglucosamine-6-phosphate to N-acetylglucosamine-1-phosphate [68, 69]. The role of PGM3 in cancer has been explored in a variety of cancers, suggesting a range of consequences. PGM3 expression was found not only in malignant cervical samples but also in a subgroup of normal cervical samples in uterine cancer, suggesting its existence in both normal and cancerous tissues. PGM3 plays a role in pancreatic cancer, and its overexpression has been linked to gemcitabine resistance. PGM3 inhibition, however, not only reduced pancreatic cancer cell proliferation but also increased gemcitabine sensitivity, indicating its promise as a potential therapeutic target in pancreatic cancer treatment [70].

The final and second rate-limiting enzyme in HBP, UDP-N-acetylglucosamine pyrophosphorylase 1 (UAP1), is important in cancer, notably in prostate cancer. It is responsible for producing UDP-GlcNAc, a high-energy sugar donor required for glycosylation, namely O-GlcNAcylation of intracellular target proteins. Studies employing serum samples in prostate cancer found substantial variations in UAP1 expression between patients with prostate cancer and those who had undergone post-prostatectomy [71]. Several studies have discovered UAP1 overexpression in cancer cells. UAP1 positivity was favorably associated with high androgen receptor expression and negatively correlated with the Gleason score, indicating its potential as a disease progression marker. Prostate cancer cells with enhanced UAP1 expression had higher amounts of UDP-GlcNAc, which is related to resistance to N-linked glycosylation inhibitors but not to ER stress-inducing drugs [70, 71]. UAP1 knockdown reduces the proliferation and viability of prostate cancer cells. These findings imply that UAP1 expression protects prostate cancer cells from ER stress, thereby increasing proliferation and survival. This confirms that UAP1 is a prospective therapeutic target in prostate cancer, setting the stage for the development of cancer medicines that may impair UAP1's protective functions while also improving the efficacy of existing treatments [72].

O-GlcNAc transferase (OGT) is a crucial enzyme in HBP and is responsible for adding the GlcNAc residue to serine or threonine residues of intracellular target proteins using the donor molecule UDP-GlcNAc. OGT is located on the X chromosome and is indispensable for embryonic stem cell survival [73]. The C-terminus is required for its activity, and the N-terminal tetratricopeptide repeat domain aids in substrate recognition. OGT has been widely investigated in many malignancies, and its numerous roles have been demonstrated. OGT overexpression corresponds with aggressive phenotypes in breast cancer, whereas its downregulation lowers cell proliferation, accompanied by alterations in important regulatory variables. OGT is also involved in breast cancer metastasis *via* SIRT1 regulation of FOXM1. Triple-negative breast cancer (TNBC) cells are especially sensitive to OGT inhibition, implying that they may serve as a therapeutic target [74]. OGT has been linked to metastasis and metabolic profiles in prostate cancer. OGT overexpression is linked to negative clinical outcomes, and its inhibition affects cancer cell responses to several treatments, including OXPHOS inhibitors. Combining OGT inhibition with other metabolic pathway targets may provide novel treatment strategies [75]. OGT levels are elevated in HCC and are associated with recurrence. The interaction of OGT with ChREBP showed that downstream signaling events enhance HCC recurrence. Furthermore, OGT increased tumor growth and spread in HCC through palmitic acid synthesis and ER stress. OGT's role of OGT in proliferation, migration, invasion, and cancer stem cell function has been studied in a variety of additional cancers, including cholangiocarcinoma, esophageal squamous cell carcinoma, gastric cancer, thyroid cancer, and colon cancer [76].

The interaction of OGT with various signaling pathways and molecules highlights its complexity and therapeutic potential. Furthermore, the involvement of OGT in diffuse large B-cell lymphoma (DLBCL) and acute myeloid leukemia (AML) emphasizes its importance in haematological malignancies [77]. OGT is upregulated by viral oncogenes, such as HPV16 E6 and E7, which contribute to cervical cancer carcinogenesis. OGT has emerged as a key participant in carcinogenesis, impacting facets of cancer progression, such as cell proliferation, metastasis, and metabolic control. Its various roles make it an appealing target for developing innovative therapeutics for a variety of cancer types. O-GlcNAcase (OGA) is an enzyme that catalyzes the removal of GlcNAc residues from target proteins and is important in cancer. In contrast to OGT, the activities of OGA in cancer have been investigated in several studies, demonstrating its impact on tumor recurrence, survival outcomes, and phenotypic abnormalities [78]. Low OGA expression has been identified as an isolated prognostic factor for liver cancer recurrence. Similarly, decreased OGA expression is associated with poor survival rates in patients with breast cancer. OGA downregulation causes phenotypic alterations in colon cancer, including fibroblast-like shape and decreased cell growth [79]. Transcriptomic analysis of OGA-silenced cells revealed changes in the genes involved in cell proliferation, motility, and metabolic pathways, including lipids and carbohydrates. Inhibition of OGA has been associated with enhanced migration and invasion in malignancies such as ovarian cancer, HCC, and colorectal cancer. Notably, the downregulation of OGA in CD19+ bone marrow mononuclear cells from patients with pre-B-cell acute lymphoblastic leukaemia implies that it plays a significant role in leukemia [79, 80].

OGA inhibition, either with the OGA inhibitor thiamet-G or genetic silencing, activates wild-type p53 or increases the efficacy of chemotherapeutic drugs such as cisplatin [80]. This opens the door to the establishment of a novel and effective combination treatment for ovarian cancer. Furthermore, OGA inhibition with ketoconazole has demonstrated encouraging effects in sensitizing mantle cell lymphoma cells to apoptosis and reversing bortezomib resistance. Bortezomib plus OGA inhibition appears to be a promising treatment option for drug-resistant mantle cell lymphomas. OGA plays diverse roles in cancer biology by regulating variables such as recurrence, survival, phenotypic alterations, and treatment response. Targeting OGA is a possible strategy for creating novel therapeutic options for many forms of cancer [81].

HBP is a metabolic pathway that converts F-6-P, a glycolytic intermediate, to uridine diphosphate N-acetylglucosamine (UDP-GlcNAc), a substrate for O-GlcNAcylation, a post-translational modification of proteins. O-GlcNAcylation regulates the activity, stability, and interactions of different proteins, particularly those involved in signaling, transcription, and metabolism. 2-DG can inhibit the hexosamine biosynthesis pathway by competing with F-6-P for glutamine: F-6-P amidotransferase (GFAT), the rate-limiting enzyme of the pathway [82]. This can reduce UDP-GlcNAc and O-GlcNAcylation levels and affect cellular responses to nutrients, hormones, and stress. N-Glycosylation is the process of attaching sugar chains to proteins and lipids, which are important for protein folding, function, and stability. N-glycosylation occurs in the ER and Golgi apparatus and requires glucose as a precursor [83]. 2-DG can inhibit N-glycosylation by competing with mannose, a glucose-derived sugar, for the enzyme mannose-1-phosphate guanyltransferase, which catalyses the first step of N-glycosylation. This can lead to the accumulation of misfolded proteins and activation of the unfolded protein response (UPR), which can trigger apoptosis or autophagy [84].

4.1.4. Inhibition of Proliferation and Metastasis

The Warburg effect has received considerable attention in the complex field of cancer biology. This impact highlights the metabolic uniqueness of cancer cells, where glycolysis accounts for 60% of ATP synthesis [45]. This not only provides the essential components for rapid cellular growth but also creates an environment favorable for cancer cell survival. Thus, 2-DG has emerged as an intriguing anti-cancer treatment option. 2-DG enters cancer cells by enzymatic conversion into 2-DG-6-phosphate, which is regulated by HK [85]. This transition is critical because it strongly inhibits the glycolytic pathway. In particular, it inhibits the activity of HK and PGI. In mammals, there are four different isozymes of HK, with HK-1 exhibiting ubiquitous expression in the human body. HK-1 has been linked to cancer progression, in addition to its role in glycolysis [86]. This is performed by activating the MAPK/ERK pathway, which promotes cell proliferation, invasion, and metastasis in a variety of cancers, including lung, breast, pancreatic, and colorectal cancers [87]. Furthermore, 2-DG inhibits HK function in cancer cells *via* a dual mechanism that combines competitive and allosteric inhibition. This results in a decrease in lactate generation and ATP synthesis in the glycolytic pathway. Interestingly, research indicates that the combination of 2-DG and crizotinib inhibits HK-mediated cancer invasiveness, colony formation, and proliferation, which are coordinated *via* the PI3K/Akt/mTOR signaling pathway [87].

As ATP generation is hampered, the PI3K/Akt/mTOR pathway is halted, resulting in a decrease in the amount of critical proliferative proteins. The discovery that the antimicrobial peptide buforin-IIb, when coupled with 2-DG, resulted in a rapid reduction in cancer cell proliferation is noteworthy. This phenomenon was attributed to a substantial reduction in both ATP and lactate production. Matrix metalloproteinases (MMPs) play an instrumental role in orchestrating cancer invasion, with upregulated MMP-9 and MMP-2 levels fueling this process [86, 87]. In this study, 2-DG inhibited the NF-κB pathway and downregulated the expression of MMP-2 and MMP-9. Additionally, 2-DG induces autophagy, a self-regulatory process that is pivotal for maintaining cellular integrity and eliminating toxins and pathogens. A unique therapeutic method has evolved in recent years, involving the use of penfluridol, an antipsychotic medication that inhibits SIRT1 and PGC-1, slowing mitochondrial OXPHOS while activating glycolysis to compensate for energy shortages [88].

In conjunction with this technique, 2-DG successfully inhibited both mitochondrial ATP synthesis and glycolysis, resulting in a considerable reduction in lung cancer cell proliferation and progression. Autophagy is a complex intracellular process that plays an important role in maintaining cellular integrity during intracellular stress. Surprisingly, glucose deprivation and HK2 overexpression have been shown to activate autophagy *via* the Akt pathway [89]. However, the inhibition of HK2 inhibits this self-regulatory catabolic mechanism. Intriguingly, 2-DG induces the misfolding and unfolding of intracellular proteins, triggering endoplasmic reticulum stress. This, in turn, contributes to its anti-cancer properties in prostate cancer cells (PC3) by inhibiting cell proliferation, increasing ROS levels, and inducing autophagic flux-mediated cell death [90]. The effects of 2-DG on FLICE-like inhibitory protein (c-FLIP) and receptor-interacting protein (RIP), autophagy, and apoptosis modulation, as well as its impact on various cellular pathways, have been implicated in cancer progression [91]. Moreover, it highlights the potential synergistic effects of 2-DG when combined with other agents, such as buforin-IIb, penfluridol, and metformin. 2-DG is a versatile anti-cancer drug that inhibits cancer cell growth and development through many methods (Fig. **3**). Its potential in combination medicine suggests that it could lead to more effective cancer treatments. However, additional research and clinical trials are required to maximize its medicinal effects [88, 91].

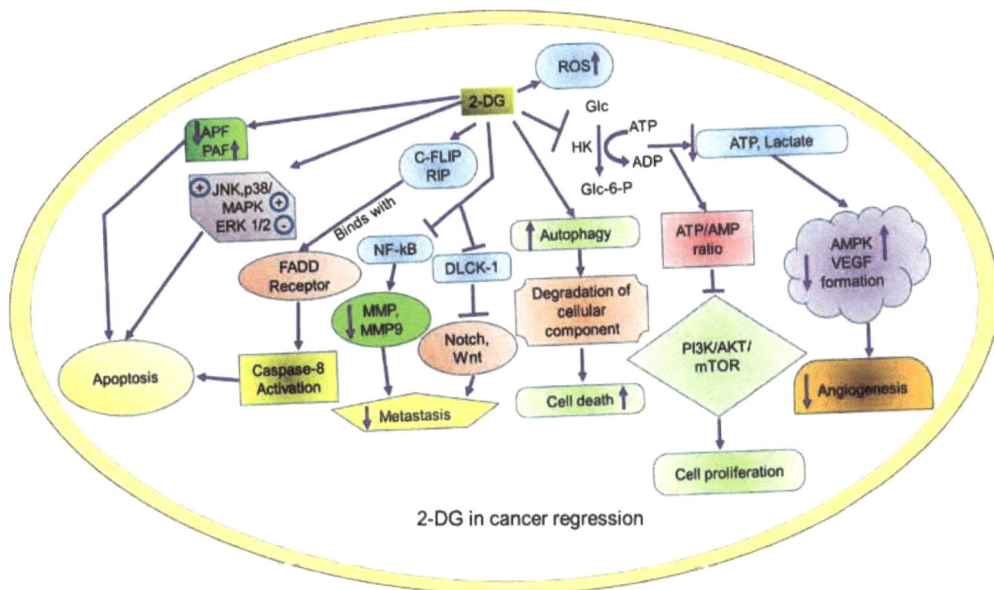

Fig. (3). Impact of 2-DG on cancer cell proliferation. 2-DG hinders glycolysis, reducing HK activity, ATP, and lactate production. This activates AMPK, suppresses VEGF, and inhibits angiogenesis. Lower ATP/AMP ratio hampers PI3K/Akt/mTOR, slowing proliferation. 2-DG impedes metastasis by suppressing NF-B, down-regulating MMP-2 and MMP-9, generating ROS, and inhibiting DCLK-1. Additionally, it inhibits c FLIP and RIP, activates JNK and p38/MAPK, hinders ERK1/2, and promotes pro-apoptotic protein production, inducing apoptosis.

4.2. Coronavirus Disease (COVID-19)

The COVID-19 pandemic, stemming from the SARS-CoV-2 virus, first emerged in Wuhan, China in November 2019 and was officially reported by the World Health Organization (WHO) on December 31, 2019. Since then, the global impact has been severe, with nearly 462 million infections and 6.06 million deaths recorded on 19th March, 2022 [92]. The pandemic has been announced as a global emergency, prompting healthcare providers to seek effective treatment regimens, especially as emerging variants challenge the efficiency of approved vaccines [93]. Despite the fast-track approval of vaccines, their effectiveness against new SARS-CoV-2 variants remains a concern. Approximately 90% of infected individuals may not require hospitalization and are manageable at home, while the remaining 10% may experience severe symptoms leading to hospitalization and potentially life-threatening conditions, such as acute respiratory distress syndrome (ARDS) and multiple organ failure. The repurposing of established drugs has gained popularity in response to the urgency to find viable treatment options [94]. This approach utilizes known compounds with established safety profiles, expediting the drug development process and potentially lowering costs. The limited availability of specific antiviral medications for COVID-19 has led to the repurposing of drugs, such as remdesivir, originally designed for hepatitis C treatment [95].

However, a comprehensive understanding of COVID-19 pathobiology is crucial for effective prophylaxis and treatment. The emergence of novel SARS-CoV-2 variants, including the delta plus variant and recently classified omicron variant, has raised concerns because of their ability to resist immunity and existing therapeutics. The delta-plus variant shows some leniency against monoclonal antibody combination therapy [96]. Additionally, recovered COVID patients exhibit rare diseases and systemic disorders, adding complexity to disease management. The connection between COVID-19 and cancer treatment lies in the shared metabolic characteristics of the virus-infected and cancer cells. Despite being distinct illnesses, both entities exhibit a rapid multiplication rate that requires substantial energy. The primary energy source, glucose, is rapidly consumed by replicating cells for survival and reproduction [97]. The pathogenicity and replication of SARS-CoV-2, the virus responsible for COVID-19, depend heavily on glycolysis and glycosylation processes. Viruses, including SARS-CoV-2, alter the metabolism of host cells to create an environment that is conducive to rapid replication. Notably, increased glucose intake supports mitochondrial signaling through aerobic glycolysis, the principal mechanism of glucose metabolism [98]. Research indicates that SARS-CoV-2 infection induces a metabolic shift in human monocytes, favoring elevated glucose cultures, promoting viral replication and cytokine formation, and impairing T cell responses. This metabolic alteration provides insights into the heightened susceptibility of diabetic patients to severe COVID-19 [97, 98].

Compound 2-DG, structurally similar to glucose, plays a pivotal role in inhibiting viral synthesis [99]. By binding to and inhibiting HK, a key enzyme in glycolysis and ATP production, 2-DG suppresses glycolysis, leading to reduced ATP production. This energy deprivation hinders viral development within host cells and deactivates the virus [100]. Furthermore, the reduced ATP concentration triggers a cascade involving AMP-mediated protein kinase, mTOR kinase, and tuberous sclerosis, ultimately inducing autophagy and cell death in virus-infected cells. This mechanism has proven effective in inhibiting the multiplication of SARS-CoV-2 in Caco-2 colon cancer cells. 2-DG is a modified glucose molecule, in which the 2-hydroxyl bonds are replaced with hydrogen, inhibiting further glycolysis [101]. It operates by impeding the synthesis of glucose-6-phosphate from glucose, which is a crucial step in glycolysis. In the liver and kidneys, 2-DG is phosphorylated by glucose HK, providing insight into tissue glucose absorption and HK activity [100, 101]. Elevated glucose uptake and HK levels are common in many cancers. This experimental drug is currently being investigated for its potential in treating both cancer and viral infections. In cancer treatment, 2-DG has been used in conjunction with chemotherapy and radiotherapy for solid tumors. However, its standalone use poses risks of toxicity, potentially affecting the nervous, cardiovascular, respiratory, and immunological systems as well as normal tissues. 2-DG depletes cellular energy and hinders cell growth by inhibiting glycolysis [6].

Structurally resembling mannose, 2-DG prevents N-glycosylation and induces endoplasmic reticulum stress, thereby activating the unfolded protein response pathway. Its biotransformation through pentose PPP, particularly in red blood cells, is known, but its implications in other cell types, as well as cancer cells, are not yet clear [1]. The ketogenic diet, explored for epilepsy treatment, has been demonstrated to be an anti-epileptic agent, highlighting the significance of glycolysis in epilepsy. 2-DG is used for PET in cancer diagnostics. Increased metabolic activity in tumors facilitates the selective uptake of 2-DG by cancer cells, facilitating their visualization in imaging studies. Despite its potential therapeutic benefits, careful consideration of its side effects and risks is crucial for safe and effective use [102]. Molecular docking is a computer technique used to anticipate the best orientations and binding conformations of molecules, allowing researchers to better understand the interactions between small pharmacological ligands and specific binding sites or receptors. Molecular docking was used to investigate the interactions between the viral nuclease nsp15 endoribonuclease, the major protease (3CLpro), and the spike glycoprotein, as well as medicines like lopinavir, favipiravir, hydroxychloroquine, and 2-DG [2].

Notably, 2-DG had higher binding energies with 3CLpro, endonuclease, and spike glycoprotein than lopinavir, favipiravir, and hydroxychloroquine. Furthermore, a 2-DG derivative, 1, 3, 4, 6-Tetra-O-acetyl-2-deoxy-D-glucopyranose, demonstrated higher binding energies than the aforementioned medicines. Importantly, 2-DG meets Lipinski's criteria for drug-like qualities associated with bioavailability [2]. Bioactivity and toxicity investigations support the idea that 2-DG and its derivatives could provide adequate oral bioavailability without inducing adverse effects or toxicity.

Based on good preliminary clinical trial results, India's Defense Research and Development Organization (DRDO) developed a promising medication, 2-DG, which gained an emergency use license from the Drug Controller General of India (DCGI). The medicine indicated the ability to expedite the recovery of hospitalized patients and minimize their need for supplementary oxygen when administered orally in powder form dissolved in water [103]. Clinical research revealed a crucial component in 2-DG that aided patient recovery and boosted the proportion of those testing negative for COVID-19 in RT-PCR tests. Second-phase trials, conducted between May and October of the previous year, affirmed the safety of the drug and its positive impact on patient recovery. The third round of trials, as well as dose-ranging tests, have confirmed its efficacy [104]. Repurposed drugs, such as remdesivir, tocilizumab, prednisone, ivermectin, and dexamethasone were used to control symptoms when specific anti-COVID therapies were limited. However, when compared to these repurposed medicines, 2-DG therapeutic COVID medication showed more promising results [105].

Despite being a repurposed drug, extensive research has indicated its superior effectiveness compared to other medications used for COVID-19 treatment. The mechanism of action involves 2-DG, a glucose analog, which hinders viral growth upon infection. By attaching to the virus, it halts multiplication and spread in the body, thereby mitigating complications and severity. Additionally, the drug alters the body's oxygen requirements during severe infections, reducing the need for supplemental oxygen [106]. Extensive research, including laboratory-based studies and usage in hospitalized settings, has demonstrated significant improvements in recovery timelines and normalization of vital parameters when compared to standard care medicines [105, 106]. The prescribed dosage involved oral consumption of 2-DG medicine mixed in water twice daily for COVID-19 patients. The approval of this drug represents a significant step forward in India's battle against the COVID-19 pandemic [106].

4.3. Inflammation

2-DG plays a crucial role in inflammation and is an effective anti-inflammatory agent (Fig. **4**). Macrophages, recognized as professional antigen-presenting cells (APCs), play a pivotal role in orchestrating inflammatory responses [87]. The polarization of inactivated macrophages into the M1 phenotype, elicited by various agents, such as interferon-γ (IFN-γ), lipopolysaccharide (LPS), and granulocyte-macrophage colony-stimulating factor (GM-CSF), hinges on glucose entry facilitated by GLUT-1 channels [107]. This influx of glucose culminates in the formation of pyruvate *via* glycolysis, subsequently driving citrate cycle and acetyl-CoA production, which are essential for histone acetylation. Crucially, 2-DG intervenes by impeding glycolysis, inhibiting the formation of HIF-1α, and activating the AMPK pathway, thereby inhibiting the mTOR pathway [108]. This dual action disrupts the glycolytic pathway, thereby affecting histone acetylation. Additionally, elevated glucose levels spur the mTOR signaling pathway, leading to increased intercellular Ca^{2+} storage and ATP formation [109].

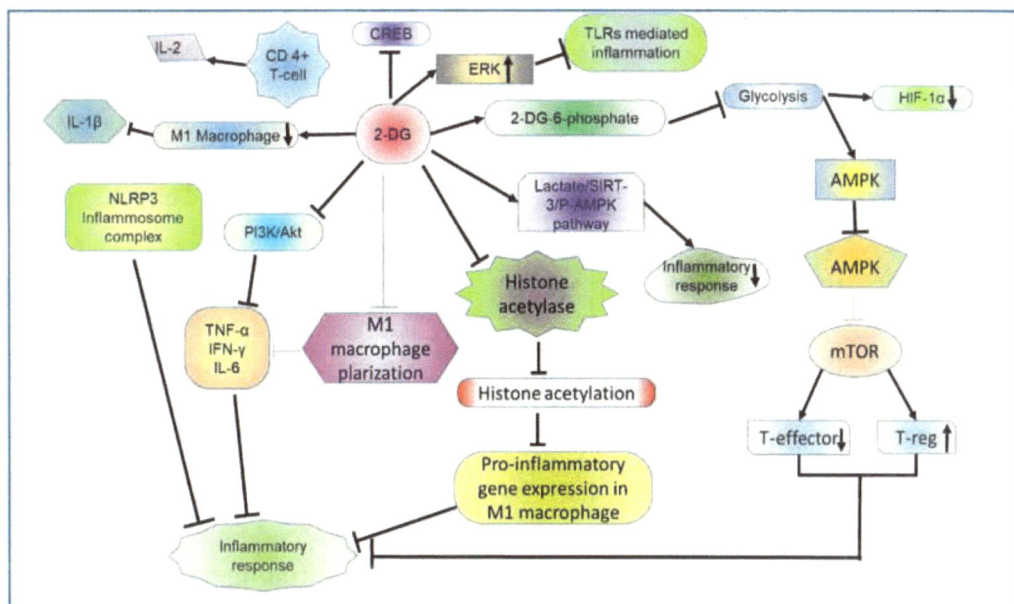

Fig. (4). Anti-inflammatory properties of 2-DG. By suppressing glycolysis, activating AMPK, and inhibiting HIF-1α, 2-DG modulates inflammation. AMPK inhibits mTOR, reduces T-effector cell development, and activates Tregs. In inflammation, 2-DG hampers human CD4+ effector T cells, activates IL-2, and suppresses TNΓ- production *via* inhibition of PI3K/Akt, M1 macrophage polarization, histone acetylation, and the NLRP3 inflammasome. It also stimulates lactate/SIRT-3/AMPK, collectively suppressing the inflammatory response.

By downregulating ATP synthesis and mTOR signaling, 2-DG suppresses effector T-cell maturation while inducing regulatory T-cell maturation, which are pivotal mechanisms in the regulation of inflammation [110]. Inflammatory responses involving IFN-γ release from Th1 cells are further influenced by 2-DG, which stimulates the secretion of anti-inflammatory cytokine (IL-2) from CD4+ cells. Regulatory T-cells (Treg cells) play a central role in cellular immune tolerance, and 2-DG enhances Treg function by inhibiting its suppressor CTLA-4 [111]. Furthermore, 2-DG exhibits the potential to suppress human CD4+ effector T cells, underscoring its potent anti-inflammatory properties through the modulation of cytokines and Treg-mediated mechanisms. The interleukin-6 (IL-6) signaling pathway, activated by binding to its receptor gp130, triggers downstream molecules (JAK1, JAK2, and TYK2) and STAT3, leading to the expression of proinflammatory genes [112]. 2-DG mitigates this response by attenuating N-linked glycosylation of IL-6 receptors, subsequently suppressing IL-6 signaling. Notably, in age-related neurodegenerative diseases, 2-DG serves as a preventive measure against IL-1β-induced neuroinflammation [113].

In the absence of infection or inflammation, most CD4+ T cells remain in a naive state, with ATP production occurring *via* mitochondrial OXPHOS. In contrast, chronic inflammation leads to the spontaneous activation of CD4+ T-cells [114]. The combination of 2-DG and metformin inhibits glycolysis and OXPHOS, effectively reducing pathological CD4+ T-cell activation and maturation, thereby exerting an anti-inflammatory effect [115]. Furthermore, studies have demonstrated that 2-DG downregulates TNF-α production during the initial stages of inflammation by inhibiting the PI3K/Akt pathway.

This action disrupts the CD33-mediated pathway, subsequently reducing the expression of adhesion molecules such as intercellular adhesion molecule (ICAM), vascular cell adhesion molecule (VCAM), and endothelial cell leukocyte adhesion molecule (ELAM), which play roles in leukocyte recruitment and inflammation promotion [116]. Toll-like receptors (TLRs) play pivotal roles in regulating inflammatory signals and responding to damage-associated molecular patterns (DAMPs) and pathogen-associated molecular patterns (PAMPs). These receptors activate pathways such as MAPK, JAK-STAT, and NF-κB, leading to glycolysis and ERK pathway activation, ultimately resulting in the production of inflammatory cytokines and adhesion molecules [115, 116].

2-DG effectively reduced TLR-induced acute and chronic inflammation by blocking glycolysis and ERK pathways. Inflammation triggered by LPS involves an upregulation of glycolysis, which 2-DG reverses, leading to a decrease in ATP production. This anti-inflammatory effect is achieved by the inhibition of proteolytic enzymes and the production of cytokines. Additionally, 2-DG downregulates phosphorylation of the transcription factor CREB, further contributing to its anti-inflammatory action [54]. Moreover, the glycolytic metabolite lactate downregulates SIRT-3 and P-AMPK expression, exacerbating inflammation and inhibiting autophagy. 2-DG counteracts this effect by blocking glycolysis and activating the lactate/SIRT-3/AMPK pathway, thereby decreasing inflammation and promoting autophagy [116, 117].

4.4. Viral Infections

2-DG exhibits potent antiviral properties against a range of viruses including HIV, SARS-CoV-2, influenza, and rhinovirus (Fig. **5**) [87]. It enters virus-infected cells through GLUTs and subsequently reduces viral infection. Additionally, 2-DG influences immune cell activation and recruitment by decreasing ATP synthesis [118]. In viral infections, it inhibits the functional activity of cytotoxic T cells (Tc cells), leading to reduced cytokine production, which is vital for glycolysis [119]. Through its action, 2-DG hinders glucose uptake inside host cells, which is a crucial step in viral replication and survival. Furthermore, 2-DG disrupts PPP and nucleotide formation, which are essential for viral replication. It also affects glutaminolysis, a process vital for viral expansion and survival [99]. By activating the AMPK pathway, 2-DG inhibits the mTOR pathway and upregulates SIRT-4 expression, effectively hindering viral replication. Furthermore, 2-DG inhibits the N-glycosylation process, blocking the attachment of sugar molecules to amino acids, and as a result, facilitating the creation of new viruses [99, 119].

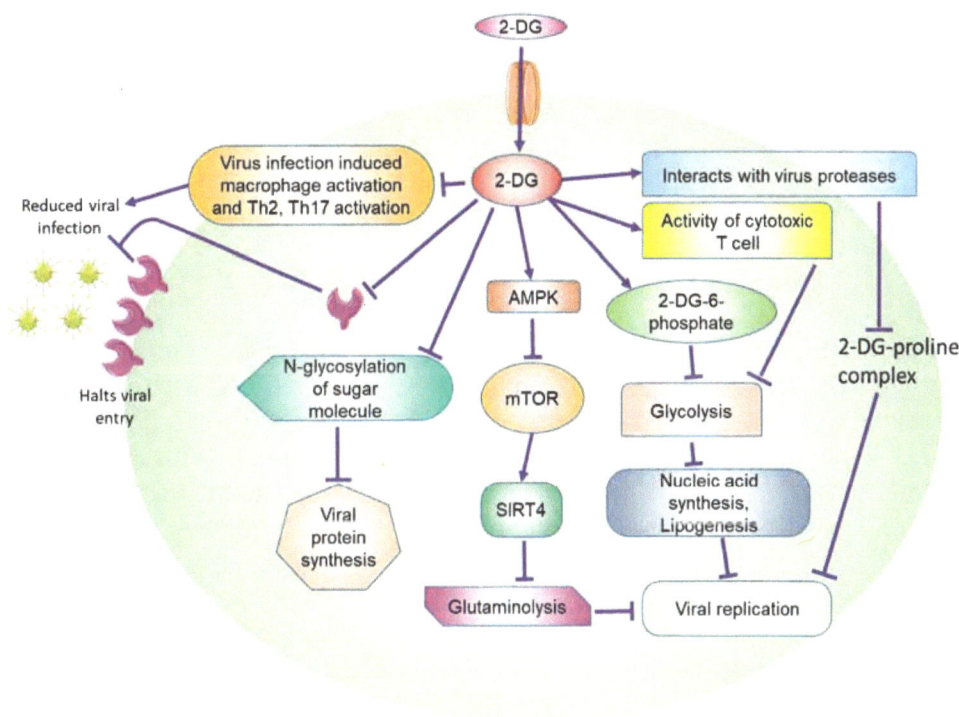

Fig. (5). Antiviral properties of 2-DG. 2-DG activates AMPK, suppressing mTOR, increasing SIRT-4 expression, and inhibiting glutaminolysis to impede viral multiplication. It inhibits viral replication through interactions with viral proteases, hindering 2-DG-proline complex formation, and disrupting glycolysis, nucleic acid synthesis, and lipogenesis. Additionally, 2-DG inhibits N-glycosylation, viral protein synthesis, macrophage activation, and Th2/Th17 responses. It also blocks the ACE2 receptor, preventing viral entry.

In case of SARS-CoV-2, 2-DG inhibits viral replication by inactivating the ACE-2 receptor. Docking research has revealed that it effectively binds to virus proteases and endoribonucleases, implying a potential inhibitory mechanism [120]. Notably, 2-DG not only reduces virus reproduction but also causes the generation of faulty virions, lowering viral infectivity to new cells. Furthermore, 2-DG inhibits macrophage, Th2, and Th17 activation, ultimately lowering viral infection and protecting virus-infected cells [121]. Several studies have shown that it is effective against influenza by preventing glycolysis and inhibiting molecule synthesis, both of which are required for viral replication and survival. 2-DG has a strong influence on non-enveloped viruses such as norovirus and Zika. It inhibits MNV infection by lowering cellular glycolysis and blocking the Akt pathway [122]. In case of the Zika virus, 2-DG reduced the severity of infection by altering AMPK phosphorylation and glycolysis levels. Overall, 2-DG has emerged as a versatile antiviral agent with diverse mechanisms for combating various viral infections. Their potential to disrupt critical pathways in virus-infected cells holds promise for developing effective antiviral treatments [122, 123].

4.5. Autosomal Dominant Polycystic Kidney Disease (ADPKD)

2-DG plays a potential therapeutic role in ADPKD owing to its influence on defective glucose metabolism [124]. A genetic mutation in ADPKD causes the development of fluid-filled cysts in the kidneys. Chiaravalli *et al.* showed that low doses of 2-DG could reduce the course of ADPKD in mouse models with inactivated Pkd1 genes [125]. This shows that 2-DG may be a potential treatment option for ADPKD. Cyst Formation Reduction: When combined with metformin, 2-DG reduces cyst formation and proliferation in human polycystic kidney cells [123, 125]. This suggests that 2-DG, especially when combined with other drugs, such as metformin, may be useful in decreasing cyst formation in ADPKD [125, 126]. Overall, the ability of 2-DG to control glucose metabolism suggests that it may be a promising choice for further research and development as a therapeutic intervention for ADPKD. However, it is crucial to emphasize that additional clinical investigations and trials are required to completely evaluate the efficacy and safety of 2-DG in the treatment of ADPKD [127].

4.6. Epilepsy

The molecular focus of epilepsy research has been on the ion channels and transporters that govern neuronal excitability at the synapse for decades [128]. Anti-seizure medicines (ASDs) have traditionally targeted synaptic components, but recent findings suggest that metabolic variables might have a significant impact on neuronal activity, impacting ion channels, such as adenosine and GABAA receptors, as well as ATP-sensitive potassium channels [127, 128]. The ketogenic diet (KD) and related variants, such as the medium-chain triglyceride (MCT) diet, modified Atkins diet (MAD), and low-glycemic-index treatment (LGIT), play critical roles in exposing the link between metabolism and epilepsy

[129]. While the precise mechanisms underlying the efficacy of these metabolic treatments in various epileptic conditions are unknown, there is growing evidence that specific metabolic substrates and enzymes may directly or indirectly induce anti-seizure and potentially neuroprotective effects [130]. In the treatment of epilepsy, not only dietary changes but also substrate or pharmacological modifications of critical metabolic processes have shown similar advantages. The KD was created to imitate the physiological consequences of fasting because it was discovered that when carbs were ingested, seizure control could be lost [131]. This gave rise to the concept that limiting carbohydrate intake alone could potentially safeguard against seizure activity and that a reduction in overall calorie intake could also decrease seizures and offer neuroprotection. As a highly energy-dependent organ, the brain relies on glucose as its obligatory energy supply [131, 132]. Seizures increase the metabolic demands of the brain owing to increased neuronal activity. The abnormal high-voltage activity found in neurons and brain networks during seizures reflects this requirement [133]. Neurometabolic coupling, which is required for neuronal excitability maintenance, involves both neuronal and astrocytic energy metabolisms. Astrocytes may supply neurons with fuel such as lactate *via* mechanisms such as the lactate shuttle. The integrity of the brain microvasculature is critical for supporting the neurometabolic fluctuations required for neuronal excitability [134]. Deficiencies in glucose availability and utilization have been associated with various neurological disorders, and increased neuronal activity during epileptic seizures considerably boosts regional blood glucose utilization. Human PET findings lend credence to the notion that metabolic therapies affecting glucose utilization could provide a rationale for seizure control [135].

KD mimics fasting by restricting carbohydrate intake, while increasing fat and protein intake to produce ketone bodies as an alternative energy source [136]. The seizure control mechanisms in KD are complex, but they avoid glycolysis, implying that glycolysis may be relevant for seizure activity [130]. This implies that blocking or reducing glycolysis may be an important strategy for KD therapy. Inhibitors of glycolysis may mimic the therapeutic effects of KD, as ketolysis decreases glycolytic flux and ketone bodies attenuate neuronal cellular excitability through this mechanism [130, 132]. With established agents known to limit glycolytic flux, this hypothesis is likely to be tested. The glucose analog 2-DG is a promising glycolytic inhibitor for seizure protection. It differs from glucose by substituting oxygen at the 2' position. 2-DG is transported into cells and phosphorylated to 2-DG-6-phosphate by HK but cannot be converted to F-6-P by PGI [132, 137]. This phosphorylated substrate is trapped in the cell, inhibiting rate-limiting enzymes, specifically PGI and HK, and therefore partially preventing glycolysis. Inhibiting PGI redirects glycolysis to PPP, resulting in the production of ribulose and glutathione [130]. Glial cells also take up 2-DG, which inhibits astrocytic glycolysis. Various studies suggest that astrocytes may transfer their glycolytic end-product, lactate, to neurons as an alternate fuel source *via* the "astrocyte-neuron lactate shuttle" (ANLS) [138]. This biochemical property has been successfully used to detect energetically active cells such as hyperexcitable brain cells or cancer cells that divide rapidly [130, 138]. 2-DG increases OXPHOS, counteracting the Warburg effect, and has been safely used as a tracer in PET for decades to indicate regional glucose utilization. 2-DG has been shown to display a diverse range of effects in *in vitro* and *in vivo* models of acute seizures. *In vitro*, 2-DG reduces high-frequency epileptiform bursting in the presence of two chemoconvulsants, 4-aminopyridine (4-AP) and bicuculline (a - aminobutyric acid (GABAA) receptor antagonist) [55]. It also worked in hippocampal brain slices, regardless of synaptic activity in CA3 pyramidal neurons. CA3 neuronal firing continues even after intracellular delivery of 2-DG, indicating that the inhibition of glycolysis in individual neurons is insufficient to cease neuronal activation [139].

In a dose-dependent manner, bath application of 2-DG in hippocampal slices prevented epileptiform bursts caused by an Mg^{2+}-free solution containing 4-AP [130]. These findings indicate that 2-DG has the potential to suppress epileptiform activity during both interictal and ictal stages. However, in rat hippocampal slices, a recent study found that 2-DG reduced Cs^{2+}- and bicuculline-induced interictal-like activity while enhancing ictal-like activity [140]. In numerous animal models of seizures, 2-DG has demonstrated antiseizure properties. It elevated the mean after-discharge threshold in the rat perforant path kindling model, suppressed seizure activity in the 6-Hz corneal stimulation paradigm, and inhibited seizures in audiogenic seizure-prone mice. Additionally, it significantly postponed seizure onset in the pilocarpine model and decreased seizure intensity and duration in the kainate (KA) model [55, 141]. However, it did not provide protection against seizures induced by pentylenetetrazol (PTZ) or maximum electroshock (MES). Despite its variable efficacy in certain experimental models, the activity profile of 2-DG was identified as distinct from that of existing anti-seizure drugs [140]. It is predominantly taken up by metabolically active cells, offering an advantage for therapeutic approaches targeting brain regions exhibiting hyperexcitable and hypersynchronous discharges, as observed in epileptic convulsions. The acute and chronic effects of 2-DG in various model systems are most likely caused by different cellular and molecular pathways [140, 141].

The processes through which 2-DG decreases seizures are complex. The mechanism by which 2-DG lowers brain-derived neurotrophic factor (BDNF) and its receptor tyrosine kinase receptor B (TrkB), both of which are essential for kindling, is intriguing [142]. 2-DG can activate KATP channels, which are specialized potassium channels that are sensitive to intracellular ATP levels. This activation causes neuronal cell membranes to hyperpolarize, lowers neuronal excitement, and prevents epilepsy [143]. In a rat model of temporal lobe epilepsy, 2-DG diminishes the synthesis of brain-derived neurotrophic factor (BDNF) and its receptor TrkB. This decline is attributed to the reduction of the transcription factor neural restrictive silencing factor (NRSF) following 2-DG treatment. Different studies have indicated that lower levels of BDNF and TrkB result in fewer seizures [144]. 2-DG stimulates NADPH generation by improving PPP metabolism. Increased NADPH levels boost neurosteroid production, which improves GABAergic inhibition, a procedure known to lower neuronal excitability [145]. Bcl-2-associated death promoter (BAD) plays a role in the regulation of both apoptosis and glucose metabolism. Changes in BAD function can affect glucose metabolism and activate ATP-sensitive KATP channels, resulting in seizure resistance [146]. High dosages of F-1,6-BP, an inhibitor of the rate-limiting enzyme PFK1 in glycolysis, have also been demonstrated to suppress seizures in animals, lending credence to glycolysis inhibition as a therapeutic option for epilepsy [144].

Evidence suggests that BDNF and TrkB inhibition slows kindling progression, potentially serving as the primary mechanism behind 2-DG's anti-epileptogenic effects (Fig. **6**). 2-DG has also been demonstrated to be neuroprotective, preventing the harmful oxidative and metabolic effects of kainic acid in rat hippocampal cell cultures by improving stress responses and lowering seizure occurrence in a mouse bilateral carotid artery ligation model [144, 146].

5. NOVEL 2-DG DERIVATIVES

Prodrugs based on the acetates of 2-deoxy monosaccharides, such as WP1122, demonstrate effective cellular entry, blood-brain barrier penetration, and glycolysis inhibition. WP1122, derived from 2-deoxyglucose (2-DG), acts as a competitive HK inhibitor [1]. It showed promising results in inhibiting glycolysis in U87 cell lines, positioning it as a prospective candidate for treating brain tumors, including glioblastoma (GBM). 2-Fluoro-d-Mannose (2-FM) competes with mannose for N-linked protein glycosylation, but not for incorporation into lipid-linked oligosaccharides (LLOs) [147]. Hence, 2-FM exhibits lower potency as an inhibitor of protein glycosylation compared to 2-DG. *In vitro* studies have suggested that 2-FM, along with 2-DG, effectively inhibits glycoprotein synthesis in breast cancer cell lines. 2-fluoro-2-deoxy-D-glucose (2-FDG), structurally similar to glucose, is particularly effective in inhibiting glycolysis [148]. Molecular modeling indicates that 2-FDG-6P acts similarly to G6P in allosteric HK inhibition. 2-FDG is a more efficient substrate for HK2 than 2-DG, leading to greater inhibition of glycolysis, especially under hypoxic conditions [99, 148]. Lampidis *et al.* synthesized and compared three 2-halogenated d-glucose analogs

(2-FDG, 2-chloro-2-deoxy-D-glucose, and 2-bromo-2-deoxy-D-glucose). These compounds compete with glucose for binding to GLUTs and HK. Studies have shown that the size of the halogen substituent at the C-2 position is negatively correlated with the drug activity [99]. Larger halogens lead to reduced binding to HK, resulting in decreased glycolysis inhibition, growth inhibition, and cytotoxicity [149].

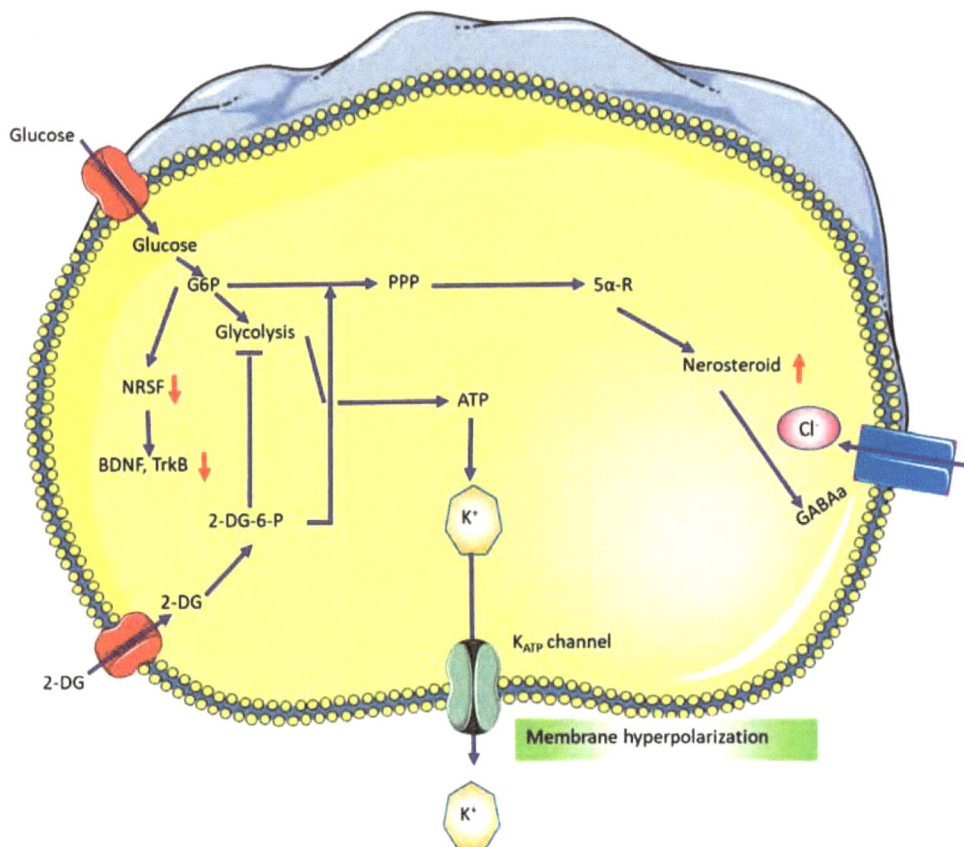

Fig. (6). 2-DG demonstrates an antiepileptic mechanism. 2-DG hinders glucose energetics, leading to a decrease in ATP levels. This reduction in glycolysis enhances PPP metabolism and augments GABAergic strength [91]. Additionally, 2-DG retards the progression of epilepsy by exerting NRSF-dependent metabolic control over BDNF and TrkB (5α-R: 5α-reductase).

CONCLUSION

An in-depth analysis of 2-DG and its wide-ranging therapeutic applications has been performed. With a distinct chemical structure that distinguishes it from glucose, 2-DG has emerged as a potent inhibitor of glucose metabolism, influencing cellular energy production and key processes. Notably, cancer cells exhibit unique metabolic behavior by favoring glycolysis even in environments abundant with oxygen, a phenomenon known as the Warburg effect. This characteristic serves as the basis for targeting cancer cells with 2-DG, which selectively accumulates in environments with high glucose consumption. By disrupting glycolytic enzymes and influencing critical pathways, such as N-glycosylation, PPP, and HBP, 2-DG induces a spectrum of cellular responses, including apoptosis, autophagy, oxidative stress, ER stress, and inflammation. Translation of preclinical data to clinical trials has yielded encouraging outcomes, with notable stability in PSA levels observed in prostate cancer cases following multiple treatment cycles. This chapter also underscores the utility of 2-DG as a tracer molecule, particularly through PET scans, for comprehensive assessments of metabolic activity and treatment responses targeting glucose metabolism. The integration of 2-DG with advanced imaging techniques holds substantial promise in advancing disease understanding and treatment modalities. Furthermore, this chapter delves into the molecular targets of 2-DG across diverse medical contexts and provides valuable insights into its potential as a versatile therapeutic agent. It emphasizes 2-DG's impact on critical metabolic pathways and discusses its potential applications in treating conditions, such as COVID-19, inflammation, ADPKD, and epilepsy. Additionally, novel derivatives of 2-DG have been introduced, which demonstrate promise in inhibiting glycolysis in various cellular contexts. This comprehensive chapter illuminates 2-DG's multifaceted properties, its influence on glucose metabolism in both normal and cancer cells, and its potential applications in cancer diagnostics and therapy.

LIST OF ABBREVIATIONS

2-DG   2-deoxy-D-Glucose

2-FDG   2-fluoro-2-Deoxy-D-Glucose

2-FM   2-Fluoro-D-Mannose

ADPKD   Autosomal Dominant Polycystic Kidney Disease

AML   Acute Myeloid Leukaemia

AMPK   AMP-Activated Protein Kinase

ASDs   Anti-Seizure Medicines

ATP   Adenosine Triphosphate

BAD   Bcl-2-Associated Death Promoter

BDNF   Brain-Derived Neurotrophic Factor

CAFs   Cancer-Associated Fibroblasts

CD33   Cluster of Differentiation 33

ChREBP   Carbohydrate Response Element-binding Protein

CREB   cAMP Response Element-Binding Protein

CRPC	Castration-Resistant Prostate Cancer
CTLA-4	Cytotoxic T-Lymphocyte-Associated Protein 4
DAMPs	Damage-Associated Molecular Patterns
DCLK-1	Doublecortin-like Kinase-1
DLBCL	Diffuse Large B-cell Lymphoma
EGFR	Epidermal Growth Factor Receptor
ELAM	Endothelial Cell Leukocyte Adhesion Molecule
EMT	Epithelial-Mesenchymal Transition
ERK	Extracellular Signal-regulated Kinase
ETC	Electron Transport Chain
F-1, 6-BP	Fructose-1,6-biphosphate
F-6-P	Fructose-6-phosphate
G6P	Glucose 6-phosphate
GABAA	Gamma-Aminobutyric Acid A
GBM	Glioblastoma
GFPT1	Glutamine-Fructose-6-Phosphatase Aminotransferase
GLUTs	Glucose Transporters
GM-CSF	Granulocyte-Macrophage Colony-Stimulating Factor
HBP	Hexosamine Biosynthetic Pathway
HCC	Hepatocellular Carcinoma
HIF-1α	Hypoxia-Inducible Factor-1α
HK	Hexokinase
ICAM	Intercellular Adhesion Molecule
IFN-γ	Interferon-gamma
IL-2	Interleukin-2
IL-6	Interleukin-6
JAK1	Janus Kinase 1
JAK2	Janus Kinase 2
KD	Ketogenic Diet
LDH	Lactate Dehydrogenase
LGIT	Low-Glycemic-Index Treatment
LLOs	Lipid-linked Oligosaccharides
LPS	Lipopolysaccharide
MAD	Modified Atkins Diet
MAPK	Mitogen-Activated Protein Kinase

MCT	Medium-Chain Triglyceride
mTOR	Mammalian Target of Rapamycin
NAD	Nicotinamide Adenine Dinucleotide
NRSF	Neural Restrictive Silencing Factor
NSCLC	Non-Small Cell Lung Carcinoma
OGT	O-GlcNAc Transferase
OIS	Oncogene-induced Senescence
OXPHOS	Oxidative Phosphorylation
P-AMPK	Phosphorylated AMP-activated Protein Kinase
PAMPs	Pathogen-Associated Molecular Patterns
PET	Positron emission tomography
PFK	Phosphofructokinase
PFKFB3	PFK2/Fructose-2, 6-Bisphosphatase 3
PGI	Phosphoglucose-Isomerase
PGM3	Phosphoglucomutase 3
PHGDH	Phosphoglycerate Dehydrogenase
PI3K/Akt	Phosphoinositide 3-kinase/protein kinase B
PK	Pyruvate Kinase
Pkd1	Polycystic Kidney Disease 1
Plk1	Polo-like Kinase 1
PPP	Pentose Phosphate Pathway
PTEN	Phosphatase Tensin Homolog
RIP	Receptor-Interacting Protein
ROS	Reactive Oxygen Species
RPI	Ribose-5-Phosphate Isomerase
Ru5P	Ribulose-5-Phosphate
SIRT-3	Sirtuin-3
STAT3	Signal Transducer and Activator of Transcription 3
STAT3	Signal Transduction and Activator of Transcription 3
TALDO	Transaldolase
TCA	Tricarboxylic Acid Cycle
TILs	Tumor-Infiltrating Lymphocytes
TKT	Tetrahydrobiopterin
TKT	Transketolase
TLRs	Toll-Like Receptors

TNBC	Triple-Negative Breast Cancer
TNF-α	Tumor necrosis Factor-alpha
Treg Cells	Regulatory T-cells
TrkB	Tyrosine Kinase Receptor B
TYK2	Tyrosine Kinase 2
UAP1	UDP-N-Acetylglucosamine Pyrophosphorylase 1
VCAM	Vascular Cell Adhesion Molecule
Xu5P	Xylulose-5-phosphate

ACKNOWLEDGEMENTS

The authors would like to express their sincere gratitude to the Central University of South Bihar for providing the facilities to write and submit the book chapter for publication.

REFERENCES

[1]   Pajak, B.; Siwiak, E.; Sołtyka, M.; Priebe, A.; Zieliński, R.; Fokt, I.; Ziemniak, M.; Jaśkiewicz, A.; Borowski, R.; Domoradzki, T.; Priebe, W. 2-Deoxy-d-glucose and its analogs: from diagnostic to therapeutic agents. *Int. J. Mol. Sci.,* **2019**, *21*(1), 234.
[http://dx.doi.org/10.3390/ijms21010234] [PMID: 31905745]

[2]   Huang, Z.; Chavda, V.P.; Vora, L.K.; Gajjar, N.; Apostolopoulos, V.; Shah, N.; Chen, Z.S. 2-Deox- -D-glucose and its derivatives for the COVID-19 treatment: an update. *Front. Pharmacol.,* **2022**, *13*, 899633.
[http://dx.doi.org/10.3389/fphar.2022.899633] [PMID: 35496298]

[3]   Stock, A.; Wang, K.; Sun, C.; Liu, C.; Gong, Y.; Liu, Y. A DNA damage response-independent mechanism for telomere shortening-elicited age-related pathologies. *Innov. Aging,* **2020**, *4* Suppl. 1, 885.
[http://dx.doi.org/10.1093/geroni/igaa057.3268]

[4]   Harris, W.J.; Asselin, M.C.; Hinz, R.; Parkes, L.M.; Allan, S.; Schiessl, I.; Boutin, H.; Dickie, B.R. *In vivo* methods for imaging blood–brain barrier function and dysfunction. *Eur. J. Nucl. Med. Mol. Imaging,* **2023**, *50*(4), 1051-1083.
[http://dx.doi.org/10.1007/s00259-022-05997-1] [PMID: 36437425]

[5]   Long, Y.; Zhuang, K.; Ji, Z.; Han, Y.; Fei, Y.; Zheng, W.; Song, Z.; Yang, H. 2-Deoxy-d-glucose exhibits anti-seizure effects by mediating the netrin-g1-katp signaling pathway in epilepsy. *Neurochem. Res.,* **2019**, *44*(4), 994-1004.
[http://dx.doi.org/10.1007/s11064-019-02734-3] [PMID: 30805800]

[6]   Singh, R.; Gupta, V.; Kumar, A.; Singh, K. A novel pharmacological agent for killing hypoxic tumor cells, oxygen dependence-lowering in covid-19, and other pharmacological activities. *Adv. Pharmacol. Pharm. Sci,* **2023**, *2023*.

[7]   Kozal, K.; Jóźwiak, P.; Krześlak, A. Contemporary perspectives on the warburg effect inhibition in cancer therapy. *Cancer Contr.,* **2021**, 28.
[http://dx.doi.org/10.1177/10732748211041243] [PMID: 34554006]

[8]   Wood, I.S.; Trayhurn, P. Glucose transporters (GLUT and SGLT): expanded families of sugar transport proteins. *Br. J. Nutr.,* **2003**, *89*(1), 3-9.
[http://dx.doi.org/10.1079/BJN2002763] [PMID: 12568659]

[9]   Herling, A.; König, M.; Bulik, S.; Holzhütter, H.G. Enzymatic features of the glucose metabolism in
        tumor cells. *FEBS J.,* **2011**, *278*(14), 2436-2459.
        [http://dx.doi.org/10.1111/j.1742-4658.2011.08174.x] [PMID: 21564549]

[10]   Ganapathy-Kanniappan, S.; Geschwind, J.F.H. Tumor glycolysis as a target for cancer therapy:
        progress and prospects. *Mol. Cancer,* **2013**, *12*(1), 152.
        [http://dx.doi.org/10.1186/1476-4598-12-152] [PMID: 24298908]

[11]   Wilson, D.F. Oxidative phosphorylation: regulation and role in cellular and tissue metabolism. *J.
        Physiol.,* **2017**, *595*(23), 7023-7038.
        [http://dx.doi.org/10.1113/JP273839] [PMID: 29023737]

[12]   Vander Heiden, M.G.; Cantley, L.C.; Thompson, C.B. Understanding the Warburg effect: the
        metabolic requirements of cell proliferation. *Science,* **2009**, *324*(5930), 1029-1033.
        [http://dx.doi.org/10.1126/science.1160809] [PMID: 19460998]

[13]   Jose, C.; Bellance, N.; Rossignol, R. Choosing between glycolysis and oxidative phosphorylation: A
        tumor's dilemma? *Biochim. Biophys. Acta Bioenerg.,* **2011**, *1807*(6), 552-561.
        [http://dx.doi.org/10.1016/j.bbabio.2010.10.012] [PMID: 20955683]

[14]   Lin, X.; Xiao, Z.; Chen, T.; Liang, S.H.; Guo, H. Glucose metabolism on tumor plasticity, diagnosis,
        and treatment. *Front. Oncol.,* **2020**, *10*, 317.
        [http://dx.doi.org/10.3389/fonc.2020.00317] [PMID: 32211335]

[15]   Marbaniang, C.; Kma, L. Dysregulation of glucose metabolism by oncogenes and tumor suppressors
        in cancer cells. *Asian Pac. J. Cancer Prev. APJCP,* **2018**, *19*(9), 2377-2390.
        [http://dx.doi.org/10.22034/APJCP.2018.19.9.2377] [PMID: 30255690]

[16]   Justus, C.; Sanderlin, E.; Yang, L. Molecular connections between cancer cell metabolism and the
        tumor microenvironment. *Int. J. Mol. Sci.,* **2015**, *16*(5), 11055-11086.
        [http://dx.doi.org/10.3390/ijms160511055] [PMID: 25988385]

[17]   Ziello, J.E.; Jovin, I.S.; Huang, Y. Hypoxia-inducible factor (HIF)-1 regulatory pathway and its
        potential for therapeutic intervention in malignancy and ischemia. *Yale J. Biol. Med.,* **2007**, *80*(2), 51-
        60.
        [PMID: 18160990]

[18]   Semenza, G.L. HIF-1: upstream and downstream of cancer metabolism. *Curr. Opin. Genet. Dev.,*
        2010, *20*(1), 51-56.
        [http://dx.doi.org/10.1016/j.gde.2009.10.009] [PMID: 19942427]

[19]   Kroemer, G.; Pouyssegur, J. Tumor cell metabolism: cancer's Achilles' heel. *Cancer Cell,* **2008**,
        13(6), 472-482.
        [http://dx.doi.org/10.1016/j.ccr.2008.05.005] [PMID: 18538731]

[20]   Christofk, H.R.; Vander Heiden, M.G.; Harris, M.H.; Ramanathan, A.; Gerszten, R.E.; Wei, R.;
        Fleming, M.D.; Schreiber, S.L.; Cantley, L.C. The M2 splice isoform of pyruvate kinase is important
        for cancer metabolism and tumour growth. *Nature,* **2008**, *452*(7184), 230-233.
        [http://dx.doi.org/10.1038/nature06734] [PMID: 18337823]

[21]   Zhang, Z.; Deng, X.; Liu, Y.; Liu, Y.; Sun, L.; Chen, F. PKM2, function and expression and
        regulation. *Cell Biosci.,* **2019**, *9*(1), 52.
        [http://dx.doi.org/10.1186/s13578-019-0317-8] [PMID: 31391918]

[22]   Gray, L.R.; Tompkins, S.C.; Taylor, E.B. Regulation of pyruvate metabolism and human disease. *Cell.
        Mol. Life Sci.,* **2014**, *71*(14), 2577-2604.
        [http://dx.doi.org/10.1007/s00018-013-1539-2] [PMID: 24363178]

[23]   Liberti, M.V.; Locasale, J.W. The warburg effect: how does it benefit cancer cells? *Trends Biochem.
        Sci.,* **2016**, *41*(3), 211-218.
        [http://dx.doi.org/10.1016/j.tibs.2015.12.001] [PMID: 26778478]

[24]   Fadaka, A.; Ajiboye, B.; Ojo, O.; Adewale, O.; Olayide, I.; Emuowhochere, R. Biology of glucose
        metabolization in cancer cells. *Journal of Oncological Sciences,* **2017**, *3*(2), 45-51.
        [http://dx.doi.org/10.1016/j.jons.2017.06.002]

[25]   Pavlova, N.N.; Zhu, J.; Thompson, C.B. The hallmarks of cancer metabolism: Still emerging. *Cell
        Metab.,* **2022**, *34*(3), 355-377.
        [http://dx.doi.org/10.1016/j.cmet.2022.01.007] [PMID: 35123658]

[26]   Lu, J.; Tan, M.; Cai, Q. The warburg effect in tumor progression: mitochondrial oxidative metabolism
        as an anti-metastasis mechanism. *Cancer Lett.,* **2015**, *356*(2), 156-164.
        [http://dx.doi.org/10.1016/j.canlet.2014.04.001] [PMID: 24732809]

[27]   Rosenzweig, A.; Blenis, J.; Gomes, A.P. Beyond the warburg effect: How dCancer cells regulate one-
        carbon metabolism? *Front. Cell Dev. Biol.,* **2018**, *6*, 90.
        [http://dx.doi.org/10.3389/fcell.2018.00090] [PMID: 30159313]

[28]   Zhou, D.; Duan, Z.; Li, Z.; Ge, F.; Wei, R.; Kong, L. The significance of glycolysis in tumor
        progression and its relationship with the tumor microenvironment. *Front. Pharmacol.,* **2022**, *13*,
        1091779.
        [http://dx.doi.org/10.3389/fphar.2022.1091779] [PMID: 36588722]

[29]   Hosios, A.M.; Manning, B.D. Cancer signaling drives cancer metabolism: akt and the warburg effect.
        Cancer Res., **2021**, *81*(19), 4896-4898.
        [http://dx.doi.org/10.1158/0008-5472.CAN-21-2647] [PMID: 34598998]

[30]   Zhao, R.Z.; Jiang, S.; Zhang, L.; Yu, Z.B. Mitochondrial electron transport chain, ROS generation and
        uncoupling (Review). *Int. J. Mol. Med.,* **2019**, *44*(1), 3-15.
        [http://dx.doi.org/10.3892/ijmm.2019.4188] [PMID: 31115493]

[31]   Lu, M.; Zhou, L.; Stanley, W.C.; Cabrera, M.E.; Saidel, G.M.; Yu, X. Role of the malate–aspartate
        shuttle on the metabolic response to myocardial ischemia. *J. Theor. Biol.,* **2008**, *254*(2), 466-475.
        [http://dx.doi.org/10.1016/j.jtbi.2008.05.033] [PMID: 18603266]

[32]   Bishayee, K.; Lee, S.H.; Park, Y.S. The illustration of altered glucose dependency in drug-resistant
        cancer cells. *Int. J. Mol. Sci.,* **2023**, *24*(18), 13928.
        [http://dx.doi.org/10.3390/ijms241813928] [PMID: 37762231]

[33]   Galdieri, L.; Zhang, T.; Rogerson, D.; Lleshi, R.; Vancura, A. Protein acetylation and acetyl coenzyme
        a metabolism in budding yeast. *Eukaryot. Cell,* **2014**, *13*(12), 1472-1483.
        [http://dx.doi.org/10.1128/EC.00189-14] [PMID: 25326522]

[34]   Wellen, K.E.; Hatzivassiliou, G.; Sachdeva, U.M.; Bui, T.V.; Cross, J.R.; Thompson, C.B. ATP-citrate
        lyase links cellular metabolism to histone acetylation. *Science,* **2009**, *324*(5930), 1076-1080.
        [http://dx.doi.org/10.1126/science.1164097] [PMID: 19461003]

[35]   Fan, J.; Krautkramer, K.A.; Feldman, J.L.; Denu, J.M. Metabolic regulation of histone post-
        translational modifications. *ACS Chem. Biol.,* **2015**, *10*(1), 95-108.
        [http://dx.doi.org/10.1021/cb500846u] [PMID: 25562692]

[36]   Barbosa, A.M.; Martel, F. Targeting glucose transporters for breast cancer therapy: the effect of
        natural and synthetic compounds. *Cancers (Basel),* **2020**, *12*(1), 154.
        [http://dx.doi.org/10.3390/cancers12010154] [PMID: 31936350]

[37]   Akella, N.M.; Ciraku, L.; Reginato, M.J. Fueling the fire: emerging role of the hexosamine
        biosynthetic pathway in cancer. *BMC Biol.,* **2019**, *17*(1), 52.
        [http://dx.doi.org/10.1186/s12915-019-0671-3] [PMID: 31272438]

[38]   DiPaola, R.S.; Stein, M.N.; Goodin, S.; Eddy, S.; Rubin, E.H.; Doyle-Lindrud, S.; Dvorzhinski, D.;
        Beers, S.; Shih, W.J.; White, E. Warburg science goes to the bedside: A phase I trial of 2-
        deoxyglucose in patients with prostate cancer and advanced malignancies. *J. Clin. Oncol.,* **2008**,
        26(15_suppl) Suppl., 16087-16087.
        [http://dx.doi.org/10.1200/jco.2008.26.15_suppl.16087]

[39]   Ali, J.S.; Ain, N.; Naz, S.; Zia, M. Biomarker selection and imaging design in cancer: A link with biochemical pathways for imminent engineering. *Heliyon,* **2020,** *6*(2), e03340.
[http://dx.doi.org/10.1016/j.heliyon.2020.e03340] [PMID: 32055737]

[40]   Pulumati, A.; Pulumati, A.; Dwarakanath, B.S.; Verma, A.; Papineni, R.V.L. Technological advancements in cancer diagnostics: Improvements and limitations. *Cancer Rep.,* **2023,** *6*(2), e1764.
[http://dx.doi.org/10.1002/cnr2.1764] [PMID: 36607830]

[41]   Alauddin, M.M. Positron emission tomography (PET) imaging with (18)F-based radiotracers. *Am. J. Nucl. Med. Mol. Imaging,* **2012,** *2*(1), 55-76.
[PMID: 23133802]

[42]   Aft, R.L.; Zhang, F.W.; Gius, D. Evaluation of 2-deoxy-D-glucose as a chemotherapeutic agent: mechanism of cell death. *Br. J. Cancer,* **2002,** *87*(7), 805-812.
[http://dx.doi.org/10.1038/sj.bjc.6600547] [PMID: 12232767]

[43]   Zhang, Y.; Huang, F.; Wang, J.; Luo, H.; Wang, Z. 2-DG-regulated rip and c-flip effect on liver cancer cell apoptosis induced by trail. *Med. Sci. Monit.,* **2015,** *21*, 3442-3448.
[http://dx.doi.org/10.12659/MSM.895034] [PMID: 26552967]

[44]   Magier, Z.; Jarzyna, R. The role of glucose transporters in human metabolic regulation. *Postepy Biochem.,* **2013,** *59*(1), 70-82.
[PMID: 23821945]

[45]   Jin, L.; Zhou, Y. Crucial role of the pentose phosphate pathway in malignant tumors (Review). *Oncol. Lett.,* **2019,** *17*(5), 4213-4221.
[http://dx.doi.org/10.3892/ol.2019.10112] [PMID: 30944616]

[46]   Vazquez, A.; Kamphorst, J.J.; Markert, E.K.; Schug, Z.T.; Tardito, S.; Gottlieb, E. Cancer metabolism at a glance. *J. Cell Sci.,* **2016,** *129*(18), 3367-3373.
[http://dx.doi.org/10.1242/jcs.181016] [PMID: 27635066]

[47]   Patra, K.C.; Hay, N. The pentose phosphate pathway and cancer. *Trends Biochem. Sci.,* **2014,** *39*(8), 347-354.
[http://dx.doi.org/10.1016/j.tibs.2014.06.005] [PMID: 25037503]

[48]   Pavlova, N.N.; Thompson, C.B. The emerging hallmarks of cancer metabolism. *Cell Metab.,* **2016,** *23*(1), 27-47.
[http://dx.doi.org/10.1016/j.cmet.2015.12.006] [PMID: 26771115]

[49]   Kathagen-Buhmann, A.; Schulte, A.; Weller, J.; Holz, M.; Herold-Mende, C.; Glass, R.; Lamszus, K. Glycolysis and the pentose phosphate pathway are differentially associated with the dichotomous regulation of glioblastoma cell migration *versus* proliferation. *Neuro-oncol.,* **2016,** *18*(9), 1219-1229.
[http://dx.doi.org/10.1093/neuonc/now024] [PMID: 26917237]

[50]   Stincone, A.; Prigione, A.; Cramer, T.; Wamelink, M.M.C.; Campbell, K.; Cheung, E.; Olin-Sandoval, V.; Grüning, N.M.; Krüger, A.; Tauqeer Alam, M.; Keller, M.A.; Breitenbach, M.; Brindle, K.M.; Rabinowitz, J.D.; Ralser, M. The return of metabolism: biochemistry and physiology of the pentose phosphate pathway. *Biol. Rev. Camb. Philos. Soc.,* **2015,** *90*(3), 927-963.
[http://dx.doi.org/10.1111/brv.12140] [PMID: 25243985]

[51]   Xu, I.M.J.; Lai, R.K.H.; Lin, S.H.; Tse, A.P.W.; Chiu, D.K.C.; Koh, H.Y.; Law, C.T.; Wong, C.M.; Cai, Z.; Wong, C.C.L.; Ng, I.O.L. Transketolase counteracts oxidative stress to drive cancer development. *Proc. Natl. Acad. Sci. USA,* **2016,** *113*(6), E725-E734.
[http://dx.doi.org/10.1073/pnas.1508779113] [PMID: 26811478]

[52]   Kamenisch, Y.; Baban, T.S.A.; Schuller, W.; von Thaler, A.K.; Sinnberg, T.; Metzler, G.; Bauer, J.; Schittek, B.; Garbe, C.; Rocken, M.; Berneburg, M. UVA-irradiation induces melanoma invasion *via* the enhanced warburg effect. *J. Invest. Dermatol.,* **2016,** *136*(9), 1866-1875.
[http://dx.doi.org/10.1016/j.jid.2016.02.815] [PMID: 27185340]

[53]   Li, X.; Gu, J.; Zhou, Q. Review of aerobic glycolysis and its key enzymes – new targets for lung

cancer therapy. *Thorac. Cancer,* **2015**, *6*(1), 17-24.
[http://dx.doi.org/10.1111/1759-7714.12148] [PMID: 26273330]

[54]   Zuo, J.; Tang, J.; Lu, M.; Zhou, Z.; Li, Y.; Tian, H.; Liu, E.; Gao, B.; Liu, T.; Shao, P. Glycolysis rate-limiting enzymes: novel potential regulators of rheumatoid arthritis pathogenesis. *Front. Immunol.,* **2021**, *12*, 779787.
[http://dx.doi.org/10.3389/fimmu.2021.779787] [PMID: 34899740]

[55]   Schiliro, C.; Firestein, B.L. Mechanisms of metabolic reprogramming in cancer cells supporting enhanced growth and proliferation. *Cells,* **2021**, *10*(5), 1056.
[http://dx.doi.org/10.3390/cells10051056] [PMID: 33946927]

[56]   Cho, E.S.; Cha, Y.H.; Kim, H.S.; Kim, N.H.; Yook, J.I. The pentose phosphate pathway as a potential target for cancer therapy. *Biomol. Ther. (Seoul),* **2018**, *26*(1), 29-38.
[http://dx.doi.org/10.4062/biomolther.2017.179] [PMID: 29212304]

[57]   Lu, M.; Lu, L.; Dong, Q.; Yu, G.; Chen, J.; Qin, L.; Wang, L.; Zhu, W.; Jia, H. Elevated G6PD expression contributes to migration and invasion of hepatocellular carcinoma cells by inducing epithelial-mesenchymal transition. *Acta Biochim. Biophys. Sin. (Shanghai),* **2018**, *50*(4), 370-380.
[http://dx.doi.org/10.1093/abbs/gmy009] [PMID: 29471502]

[58]   Yang, H.C.; Stern, A.; Chiu, D.T.Y. G6PD: A hub for metabolic reprogramming and redox signaling in cancer. *Biomed. J.,* **2021**, *44*(3), 285-292.
[http://dx.doi.org/10.1016/j.bj.2020.08.001] [PMID: 33097441]

[59]   Yang, H.C.; Wu, Y.H.; Yen, W.C.; Liu, H.Y.; Hwang, T.L.; Stern, A.; Chiu, D.T.Y. The redox role of g6pd in cell growth, cell death, and cancer. *Cells,* **2019**, *8*(9), 1055.
[http://dx.doi.org/10.3390/cells8091055] [PMID: 31500396]

[60]   Baptista, I.; Karakitsou, E.; Cazier, J.B.; Günther, U.L.; Marin, S.; Cascante, M. TKTL1 knockdown impairs hypoxia-induced glucose-6-phosphate dehydrogenase and glyceraldehyde-3-phosphate dehydrogenase overexpression. *Int. J. Mol. Sci.,* **2022**, *23*(7), 3574.
[http://dx.doi.org/10.3390/ijms23073574] [PMID: 35408935]

[61]   Patra, K.C.; Wang, Q.; Bhaskar, P.T.; Miller, L.; Wang, Z.; Wheaton, W.; Chandel, N.; Laakso, M.; Muller, W.J.; Allen, E.L.; Jha, A.K.; Smolen, G.A.; Clasquin, M.F.; Robey, R.B.; Hay, N. Hexokinase 2 is required for tumor initiation and maintenance and its systemic deletion is therapeutic in mouse models of cancer. *Cancer Cell,* **2013**, *24*(2), 213-228.
[http://dx.doi.org/10.1016/j.ccr.2013.06.014] [PMID: 23911236]

[62]   Lam, C.; Low, J.Y.; Tran, P.T.; Wang, H. The hexosamine biosynthetic pathway and cancer: Current knowledge and future therapeutic strategies. *Cancer Lett.,* **2021**, *503*, 11-18.
[http://dx.doi.org/10.1016/j.canlet.2021.01.010] [PMID: 33484754]

[63]   Marshall, S.; Bacote, V.; Traxinger, R.R. Discovery of a metabolic pathway mediating glucose-induced desensitization of the glucose transport system. Role of hexosamine biosynthesis in the induction of insulin resistance. *J. Biol. Chem.,* **1991**, *266*(8), 4706-4712.
[http://dx.doi.org/10.1016/S0021-9258(19)67706-9] [PMID: 2002019]

[64]   Bond, M.R.; Hanover, J.A. A little sugar goes a long way: The cell biology of O-GlcNAc. *J. Cell Biol.,* **2015**, *208*(7), 869-880.
[http://dx.doi.org/10.1083/jcb.201501101] [PMID: 25825515]

[65]   Munkley, J.; Mills, I.G.; Elliott, D.J. The role of glycans in the development and progression of prostate cancer. *Nat. Rev. Urol.,* **2016**, *13*(6), 324-333.
[http://dx.doi.org/10.1038/nrurol.2016.65] [PMID: 27091662]

[66]   Sethi, J.K.; Vidal-Puig, A.J. Wnt signalling at the crossroads of nutritional regulation. *Biochem. J.,* **2008**, *416*(2), e11-e13.
[http://dx.doi.org/10.1042/BJ20082074] [PMID: 18990086]

[67]   Li, L.; Shao, M.; Peng, P.; Yang, C.; Song, S.; Duan, F.; Jia, D.; Zhang, M.; Zhao, J.; Zhao, R.; Wu,

W.; Wang, L.; Li, C.; Wu, H.; Zhang, J.; Wu, X.; Ruan, Y.; Gu, J. High expression of GFAT1 predicts unfavorable prognosis in patients with hepatocellular carcinoma. *Oncotarget,* **2017**, *8*(12), 19205-19217.
[http://dx.doi.org/10.18632/oncotarget.15164] [PMID: 28186970]

[68]   Kaushik, A.K.; Shojaie, A.; Panzitt, K.; Sonavane, R.; Venghatakrishnan, H.; Manikkam, M.; Zaslavsky, A.; Putluri, V.; Vasu, V.T.; Zhang, Y.; Khan, A.S.; Lloyd, S.; Szafran, A.T.; Dasgupta, S.; Bader, D.A.; Stossi, F.; Li, H.; Samanta, S.; Cao, X.; Tsouko, E.; Huang, S.; Frigo, D.E.; Chan, L.; Edwards, D.P.; Kaipparettu, B.A.; Mitsiades, N.; Weigel, N.L.; Mancini, M.; McGuire, S.E.; Mehra, R.; Ittmann, M.M.; Chinnaiyan, A.M.; Putluri, N.; Palapattu, G.S.; Michailidis, G.; Sreekumar, A. Inhibition of the hexosamine biosynthetic pathway promotes castration-resistant prostate cancer. *Nat. Commun.,* **2016**, *7*(1), 11612.
[http://dx.doi.org/10.1038/ncomms11612] [PMID: 27194471]

[69]   Zhao, M.; Li, H.; Ma, Y.; Gong, H.; Yang, S.; Fang, Q.; Hu, Z. Nanoparticle abraxane possesses impaired proliferation in A549 cells due to the underexpression of glucosamine 6-phosphate N-acetyltransferase 1 (GNPNAT1/GNA1). *Int. J. Nanomedicine,* **2017**, *12*, 1685-1697.
[http://dx.doi.org/10.2147/IJN.S129976] [PMID: 28280335]

[70]   Zuñiga Martinez, M.L.; López Mendoza, C.M.; Tenorio Salazar, J.; García Carrancá, A.M.; Cerbón Cervantes, M.A.; Alcántara-Quintana, L.E. Establishment, authenticity, and characterization of cervical cancer cell lines. *Mol. Cell. Oncol.,* **2022**, *9*(1), 2078628.
[http://dx.doi.org/10.1080/23723556.2022.2078628] [PMID: 35692560]

[71]   Zou, Y.; Liu, Z.; Liu, W.; Liu, Z. Current knowledge and potential intervention of hexosamine biosynthesis pathway in lung cancer. *World J. Surg. Oncol.,* **2023**, *21*(1), 334.
[http://dx.doi.org/10.1186/s12957-023-03226-z] [PMID: 37880766]

[72]   Storm, M.; Sheng, X.; Arnoldussen, Y.J.; Saatcioglu, F. Prostate cancer and the unfolded protein response. *Oncotarget,* **2016**, *7*(33), 54051-54066.
[http://dx.doi.org/10.18632/oncotarget.9912] [PMID: 27303918]

[73]   Shafi, R.; Iyer, S.P.N.; Ellies, L.G.; O'Donnell, N.; Marek, K.W.; Chui, D.; Hart, G.W.; Marth, J.D. The O-GlcNAc transferase gene resides on the X chromosome and is essential for embryonic stem cell viability and mouse ontogeny. *Proc. Natl. Acad. Sci. USA,* **2000**, *97*(11), 5735-5739.
[http://dx.doi.org/10.1073/pnas.100471497] [PMID: 10801981]

[74]   Barkovskaya, A.; Seip, K.; Hilmarsdottir, B.; Maelandsmo, G.M.; Moestue, S.A.; Itkonen, H.M. O-GlcNAc transferase inhibition differentially affects breast cancer subtypes. *Sci. Rep.,* **2019**, *9*(1), 5670.
[http://dx.doi.org/10.1038/s41598-019-42153-6] [PMID: 30952976]

[75]   Guinez, C.; Filhoulaud, G.; Rayah-Benhamed, F.; Marmier, S.; Dubuquoy, C.; Dentin, R.; Moldes, M.; Burnol, A.F.; Yang, X.; Lefebvre, T.; Girard, J.; Postic, C. O-GlcNAcylation increases ChREBP protein content and transcriptional activity in the liver. *Diabetes,* **2011**, *60*(5), 1399-1413.
[http://dx.doi.org/10.2337/db10-0452] [PMID: 21471514]

[76]   Phoomak, C.; Silsirivanit, A.; Wongkham, C.; Sripa, B.; Puapairoj, A.; Wongkham, S. Overexpression of O-GlcNAc-transferase associates with aggressiveness of mass-forming cholangiocarcinoma. *Asian Pac. J. Cancer Prev.,* **2012**, *13* Suppl., 101-105.
[PMID: 23480751]

[77]   Zhe, Q.; Chengxue, D.; Bin, Z.; Shaomin, L.; Wei, Z.; Jiantao, J.; Jin, Z.; Ranran, K.; Yuefeng, M. O-linked N-acetylglucosamine transferase (OGT) is overexpressed and promotes O-linked protein glycosylation in esophageal squamous cell carcinoma. *J. Biomed. Res.,* **2012**, *26*(4), 268-273.
[http://dx.doi.org/10.7555/JBR.26.20110121] [PMID: 23554759]

[78]   Zhu, Q.; Zhou, L.; Yang, Z.; Lai, M.; Xie, H.; Wu, L.; Xing, C.; Zhang, F.; Zheng, S. O-GlcNAcylation plays a role in tumor recurrence of hepatocellular carcinoma following liver transplantation. *Med. Oncol.,* **2012**, *29*(2), 985-993.
[http://dx.doi.org/10.1007/s12032-011-9912-1] [PMID: 21461968]

[79] Zhang, B.; Zhou, P.; Li, X.; Shi, Q.; Li, D.; Ju, X. Bitterness in sugar: O-GlcNAcylation aggravates pre-B acute lymphocytic leukemia through glycolysis *via* the PI3K/Akt/c-Myc pathway. *Am. J. Cancer Res.,* **2017**, *7*(6), 1337-1349.
[PMID: 28670495]

[80] de Queiroz, R.M.; Madan, R.; Chien, J.; Dias, W.B.; Slawson, C. Changes in o-linked n-acetylglucosamine (o-glcnac) homeostasis activate the p53 pathway in ovarian cancer cells. *J. Biol. Chem.,* **2016**, *291*(36), 18897-18914.
[http://dx.doi.org/10.1074/jbc.M116.734533] [PMID: 27402830]

[81] Fardini, Y.; Dehennaut, V.; Lefebvre, T.; Issad, T. O-glcnacylation: a new cancer hallmark? *Front. Endocrinol. (Lausanne),* **2013**, *4*, 99.
[http://dx.doi.org/10.3389/fendo.2013.00099] [PMID: 23964270]

[82] Paneque, A.; Fortus, H.; Zheng, J.; Werlen, G.; Jacinto, E. The hexosamine biosynthesis pathway: regulation and function. *Genes (Basel),* **2023**, *14*(4), 933.
[http://dx.doi.org/10.3390/genes14040933] [PMID: 37107691]

[83] Yang, X.; Qian, K. Protein O-GlcNAcylation: emerging mechanisms and functions. *Nat. Rev. Mol. Cell Biol.,* **2017**, *18*(7), 452-465.
[http://dx.doi.org/10.1038/nrm.2017.22] [PMID: 28488703]

[84] Schlesinger, M.; McDonald, C.; Ahuja, A.; Alvarez Canete, C.A.; Nuñez del Prado, Z.; Naipauer, J.; Lampidis, T.; Mesri, E.A. Glucose and mannose analogs inhibit KSHV replication by blocking *N* -glycosylation and inducing the unfolded protein response. *J. Med. Virol.,* **2023**, *95*(1), e28314.
[http://dx.doi.org/10.1002/jmv.28314] [PMID: 36380418]

[85] Li, Y.; Tian, H.; Luo, H.; Fu, J.; Jiao, Y.; Li, Y. Prognostic significance and related mechanisms of hexokinase 1 in ovarian cancer. *OncoTargets Ther.,* **2020**, *13*, 11583-11594.
[http://dx.doi.org/10.2147/OTT.S270688] [PMID: 33204111]

[86] Wanyan, Y.; Xu, X.; Liu, K.; Zhang, H.; Zhen, J.; Zhang, R.; Wen, J.; Liu, P.; Chen, Y. 2-Deoxy-d-glucose promotes buforin iib-induced cytotoxicity in prostate cancer du145 cells and xenograft tumors. *Molecules,* **2020**, *25*(23), 5778.
[http://dx.doi.org/10.3390/molecules25235778] [PMID: 33297583]

[87] Dey, S.; Murmu, N.; Mondal, T.; Saha, I.; Chatterjee, S.; Manna, R.; Haldar, S.; Dash, S.K.; Sarkar, T.R.; Giri, B. Multifaceted entrancing role of glucose and its analogue, 2-deoxy-D-glucose in cancer cell proliferation, inflammation, and virus infection. *Biomed. Pharmacother.,* **2022**, *156*, 113801.
[http://dx.doi.org/10.1016/j.biopha.2022.113801] [PMID: 36228369]

[88] Lai, T.C.; Lee, Y.L.; Lee, W.J.; Hung, W.Y.; Cheng, G.Z.; Chen, J.Q.; Hsiao, M.; Chien, M.H.; Chang, J.H. Synergistic tumor inhibition *via* energy elimination by repurposing penfluridol and 2-deoxy-d-glucose in lung cancer. *Cancers (Basel),* **2022**, *14*(11), 2750.
[http://dx.doi.org/10.3390/cancers14112750] [PMID: 35681729]

[89] Pandey, A.; Yadav, P.; Shukla, S. Unfolding the role of autophagy in the cancer metabolism. *Biochem. Biophys. Rep.,* **2021**, *28*, 101158.
[http://dx.doi.org/10.1016/j.bbrep.2021.101158] [PMID: 34754952]

[90] Kunhiraman, H.; Edatt, L.; Thekkeveedu, S.; Poyyakkara, A.; Raveendran, V.; Kiran, M.S.; Sudhakaran, P.; Kumar, S.V.B. 2-Deoxy glucose modulates expression and biological activity of VEGF in a SIRT-1 dependent mechanism. *J. Cell. Biochem.,* **2017**, *118*(2), 252-262.
[http://dx.doi.org/10.1002/jcb.25629] [PMID: 27302189]

[91] Amaravadi, R.K.; Lippincott-Schwartz, J.; Yin, X.M.; Weiss, W.A.; Takebe, N.; Timmer, W.; DiPaola, R.S.; Lotze, M.T.; White, E. Principles and current strategies for targeting autophagy for cancer treatment. *Clin. Cancer Res.,* **2011**, *17*(4), 654-666.
[http://dx.doi.org/10.1158/1078-0432.CCR-10-2634] [PMID: 21325294]

[92] Hillary, V.E.; Ceasar, S.A. An update on COVID-19: SARS-CoV-2 variants, antiviral drugs, and

vaccines. *Heliyon,* **2023**, *9*(3), e13952.
[http://dx.doi.org/10.1016/j.heliyon.2023.e13952] [PMID: 36855648]

[93]   Harky, A.; Ala'Aldeen, A.; Butt, S.; Duric, B.; Roy, S.; Zeinah, M. COVID-19 and multiorgan response: the long-term impact. *Curr. Probl. Cardiol.,* **2023**, *48*(9), 101756.
[http://dx.doi.org/10.1016/j.cpcardiol.2023.101756] [PMID: 37088175]

[94]   Moghadas, S.M.; Vilches, T.N.; Zhang, K.; Wells, C.R.; Shoukat, A.; Singer, B.H.; Meyers, L.A.; Neuzil, K.M.; Langley, J.M.; Fitzpatrick, M.C.; Galvani, A.P. The impact of vaccination on COVID-19 outbreaks in the United States. *medRxiv,* **2021**, 2020.11.27.20240051.
[http://dx.doi.org/10.1101/2020.11.27.20240051]

[95]   Ng, Y.L.; Salim, C.K.; Chu, J.J.H. Drug repurposing for COVID-19: Approaches, challenges and promising candidates. *Pharmacol. Ther.,* **2021**, *228*, 107930.
[http://dx.doi.org/10.1016/j.pharmthera.2021.107930] [PMID: 34174275]

[96]   Khandia, R.; Singhal, S.; Alqahtani, T.; Kamal, M.A.; El-Shall, N.A.; Nainu, F.; Desingu, P.A.; Dhama, K. Emergence of SARS-CoV-2 Omicron (B.1.1.529) variant, salient features, high global health concerns and strategies to counter it amid ongoing COVID-19 pandemic. *Environ. Res.,* **2022**, *209*, 112816.
[http://dx.doi.org/10.1016/j.envres.2022.112816] [PMID: 35093310]

[97]   Sinha, S.; Kundu, C.N. Cancer and COVID-19: Why are cancer patients more susceptible to COVID-19? *Med. Oncol.,* **2021**, *38*(9), 101.
[http://dx.doi.org/10.1007/s12032-021-01553-3] [PMID: 34302557]

[98]   Wang, T.; Cao, Y.; Zhang, H.; Wang, Z.; Man, C.H.; Yang, Y.; Chen, L.; Xu, S.; Yan, X.; Zheng, Q.; Wang, Y.P. COVID-19 metabolism: Mechanisms and therapeutic targets. *MedComm,* **2022**, *3*(3), e157.
[http://dx.doi.org/10.1002/mCO$_2$.157] [PMID: 35958432]

[99]   Pająk, B.; Zieliński, R.; Manning, J.T.; Matejin, S.; Paessler, S.; Fokt, I.; Emmett, M.R.; Priebe, W. The antiviral effects of 2-Deoxy-D-glucose (2-DG), a Dual D-Glucose and D-Mannose Mimetic, against SARS-CoV-2 and other highly pathogenic viruses. *Molecules,* **2022**, *27*(18), 5928.
[http://dx.doi.org/10.3390/molecules27185928] [PMID: 36144664]

[100] Cao, J.; Liao, S.; Zeng, F.; Liao, Q.; Luo, G.; Zhou, Y. Effects of altered glycolysis levels on CD8$^+$ T cell activation and function. *Cell Death Dis.,* **2023**, *14*(7), 407.
[http://dx.doi.org/10.1038/s41419-023-05937-3] [PMID: 37422501]

[101] Afzal, O.; Altamimi, A.S.A.; Mubeen, B.; Alzarea, S.I.; Almalki, W.H.; Al-Qahtani, S.D.; Atiya, E.M.; Al-Abbasi, F.A.; Ali, F.; Ullah, I.; Nadeem, M.S.; Kazmi, I. mTOR as a potential target for the treatment of microbial infections, inflammatory bowel diseases, and colorectal cancer. *Int. J. Mol. Sci.,* **2022**, *23*(20), 12470.
[http://dx.doi.org/10.3390/ijms232012470] [PMID: 36293326]

[102] Barañano, K.W.; Hartman, A.L. The ketogenic diet: Uses in epilepsy and other neurologic illnesses. *Curr. Treat. Options Neurol.,* **2008**, *10*(6), 410-419.
[http://dx.doi.org/10.1007/s11940-008-0043-8] [PMID: 18990309]

[103] Sahu, K.; Kumar, R. Role of 2-Deoxy-D-Glucose (2-DG) in COVID-19 disease: A potential game-changer. *J. Family Med. Prim. Care,* **2021**, *10*(10), 3548-3552.
[http://dx.doi.org/10.4103/jfmpc.jfmpc_1338_21] [PMID: 34934645]

[104] Hu, B.; Guo, H.; Zhou, P.; Shi, Z.L. Characteristics of SARS-CoV-2 and COVID-19. *Nat. Rev. Microbiol.,* **2021**, *19*(3), 141-154.
[http://dx.doi.org/10.1038/s41579-020-00459-7] [PMID: 33024307]

[105] Salasc, F.; Lahlali, T.; Laurent, E.; Rosa-Calatrava, M.; Pizzorno, A. Treatments for COVID-19: Lessons from 2020 and new therapeutic options. *Curr. Opin. Pharmacol.,* **2022**, *62*, 43-59.
[http://dx.doi.org/10.1016/j.coph.2021.11.002] [PMID: 34915400]

[106]   Xiang, R.; Yu, Z.; Wang, Y.; Wang, L.; Huo, S.; Li, Y.; Liang, R.; Hao, Q.; Ying, T.; Gao, Y.; Yu, F.; Jiang, S. Recent advances in developing small-molecule inhibitors against SARS-CoV-2. *Acta Pharm. Sin. B,* **2022**, *12*(4), 1591-1623.
[http://dx.doi.org/10.1016/j.apsb.2021.06.016] [PMID: 34249607]

[107]   Francis, R.; Singh, P.K.; Singh, S.; Giri, S.; Kumar, A. Glycolytic inhibitor 2-deoxyglucose suppresses inflammatory response in innate immune cells and experimental staphylococcal endophthalmitis. *Exp. Eye Res.,* **2020**, *197*, 108079.
[http://dx.doi.org/10.1016/j.exer.2020.108079] [PMID: 32454039]

[108]   Maher, J.C.; Wangpaichitr, M.; Savaraj, N.; Kurtoglu, M.; Lampidis, T.J. Hypoxia-inducible factor-1 confers resistance to the glycolytic inhibitor 2-deoxy- D -glucose. *Mol. Cancer Ther.,* **2007**, *6*(2), 732-741.
[http://dx.doi.org/10.1158/1535-7163.MCT-06-0407] [PMID: 17308069]

[109]   Murray, P.J. Macrophage Polarization. *Annu. Rev. Physiol.,* **2017**, *79*(1), 541-566.
[http://dx.doi.org/10.1146/annurev-physiol-022516-034339] [PMID: 27813830]

[110]   Obaid, M.; Udden, S.M.N.; Alluri, P.; Mandal, S.S. LncRNA HOTAIR regulates glucose transporter Glut1 expression and glucose uptake in macrophages during inflammation. *Sci. Rep.,* **2021**, *11*(1), 232.
[http://dx.doi.org/10.1038/s41598-020-80291-4] [PMID: 33420270]

[111]   Ip, W.K.E.; Hoshi, N.; Shouval, D.S.; Snapper, S.; Medzhitov, R. Anti-inflammatory effect of IL-10 mediated by metabolic reprogramming of macrophages. *Science,* **2017**, *356*(6337), 513-519.
[http://dx.doi.org/10.1126/science.aal3535] [PMID: 28473584]

[112]   de Groot, A.E.; Pienta, K.J. Epigenetic control of macrophage polarization: implications for targeting tumor-associated macrophages. *Oncotarget,* **2018**, *9*(29), 20908-20927.
[http://dx.doi.org/10.18632/oncotarget.24556] [PMID: 29755698]

[113]   Tan, S.Y.; Kelkar, Y.; Hadjipanayis, A.; Shipstone, A.; Wynn, T.A.; Hall, J.P. Metformin and 2-Deoxyglucose collaboratively suppress human CD4[+] T Cell effector functions and activation-induced metabolic reprogramming. *J. Immunol.,* **2020**, *205*(4), 957-967.
[http://dx.doi.org/10.4049/jimmunol.2000137] [PMID: 32641388]

[114]   Vallee, K.A.J.; Fields, J.A. Caloric restriction mimetic 2-deoxyglucose reduces inflammatory signaling in human astrocytes: implications for therapeutic strategies targeting neurodegenerative diseases. *Brain Sci.,* **2022**, *12*(3), 308.
[http://dx.doi.org/10.3390/brainsci12030308] [PMID: 35326266]

[115]   Wilson, C.S.; Stocks, B.T.; Hoopes, E.M.; Rhoads, J.P.; McNew, K.L.; Major, A.S.; Moore, D.J. Metabolic preconditioning in CD4+ T cells restores inducible immune tolerance in lupus-prone mice. *JCI Insight,* **2021**, *6*(19), e143245.
[http://dx.doi.org/10.1172/jci.insight.143245] [PMID: 34403367]

[116]   Østerud, B.; Bjørklid, E. Role of monocytes in atherogenesis. *Physiol. Rev.,* **2003**, *83*(4), 1069-1112.
[http://dx.doi.org/10.1152/physrev.00005.2003] [PMID: 14506301]

[117]   Zhang, K.; Sowers, M.L.; Cherryhomes, E.I.; Singh, V.K.; Mishra, A.; Restrepo, B.I.; Khan, A.; Jagannath, C. Sirtuin-dependent metabolic and epigenetic regulation of macrophages during tuberculosis. *Front. Immunol.,* **2023**, *14*, 1121495.
[http://dx.doi.org/10.3389/fimmu.2023.1121495] [PMID: 36993975]

[118]   Mayer, K.A.; Stöckl, J.; Zlabinger, G.J.; Gualdoni, G.A. Hijacking the supplies: metabolism as a novel facet of virus-host interaction. *Front. Immunol.,* **2019**, *10*, 1533.
[http://dx.doi.org/10.3389/fimmu.2019.01533] [PMID: 31333664]

[119]   Sears, J.D.; Waldron, K.J.; Wei, J.; Chang, C.H. Targeting metabolism to reverse T-cell exhaustion in chronic viral infections. *Immunology,* **2021**, *162*(2), 135-144.
[http://dx.doi.org/10.1111/imm.13238] [PMID: 32681647]

[120]   Wu, C.; Liu, Y.; Yang, Y.; Zhang, P.; Zhong, W.; Wang, Y.; Wang, Q.; Xu, Y.; Li, M.; Li, X.; Zheng,

M.; Chen, L.; Li, H. Analysis of therapeutic targets for SARS-CoV-2 and discovery of potential drugs by computational methods. *Acta Pharm. Sin. B,* **2020**, *10*(5), 766-788.
[http://dx.doi.org/10.1016/j.apsb.2020.02.008] [PMID: 32292689]

[121]   Maksoud, S.; El Hokayem, J. The cytokine/chemokine response in *Leishmania*/HIV infection and co-infection. *Heliyon,* **2023**, *9*(4), e15055.
[http://dx.doi.org/10.1016/j.heliyon.2023.e15055] [PMID: 37082641]

[122]   Ren, L.; Zhang, W.; Zhang, J.; Zhang, J.; Zhang, H.; Zhu, Y.; Meng, X.; Yi, Z.; Wang, R.; Influenza, A. Influenza a virus (H1N1) infection induces glycolysis to facilitate viral replication. *Virol. Sin.,* **2021**, *36*(6), 1532-1542.
[http://dx.doi.org/10.1007/s12250-021-00433-4] [PMID: 34519916]

[123]   Lian, X.; Wu, X.; Li, Z.; Zhang, Y.; Song, K.; Cai, G.; Li, Q.; Lin, S.; Chen, X.; Bai, X.Y. The combination of metformin and 2-deoxyglucose significantly inhibits cyst formation in miniature pigs with polycystic kidney disease. *Br. J. Pharmacol.,* **2019**, *176*(5), 711-724.
[http://dx.doi.org/10.1111/bph.14558] [PMID: 30515768]

[124]   Leonhard, W.N.; Happe, H.; Peters, D.J.M. Variable cyst development in autosomal dominant polycystic kidney disease: the biologic context. *J. Am. Soc. Nephrol.,* **2016**, *27*(12), 3530-3538.
[http://dx.doi.org/10.1681/ASN.2016040425] [PMID: 27493259]

[125]   Chiaravalli, M.; Rowe, I.; Mannella, V.; Quilici, G.; Canu, T.; Bianchi, V.; Gurgone, A.; Antunes, S.; D'Adamo, P.; Esposito, A.; Musco, G.; Boletta, A. 2-Deoxy-d-Glucose ameliorates PKD progression. *J. Am. Soc. Nephrol.,* **2016**, *27*(7), 1958-1969.
[http://dx.doi.org/10.1681/ASN.2015030231] [PMID: 26534924]

[126]   Haumann, S.; Müller, R.U.; Liebau, M.C. Metabolic changes in polycystic kidney disease as a potential target for systemic treatment. *Int. J. Mol. Sci.,* **2020**, *21*(17), 6093.
[http://dx.doi.org/10.3390/ijms21176093] [PMID: 32847032]

[127]   Tsukamoto, S.; Urate, S.; Yamada, T.; Azushima, K.; Yamaji, T.; Kinguchi, S.; Uneda, K.; Kanaoka, T.; Wakui, H.; Tamura, K. Comparative Efficacy of pharmacological treatments for adults with autosomal dominant polycystic kidney disease: a systematic review and network meta-analysis of randomized controlled trials. *Front. Pharmacol.,* **2022**, *13*, 885457.
[http://dx.doi.org/10.3389/fphar.2022.885457] [PMID: 35662736]

[128]   Oyrer, J.; Maljevic, S.; Scheffer, I.E.; Berkovic, S.F.; Petrou, S.; Reid, C.A. Ion channels in genetic epilepsy: from genes and mechanisms to disease-targeted therapies. *Pharmacol. Rev.,* **2018**, *70*(1), 142-173.
[http://dx.doi.org/10.1124/pr.117.014456] [PMID: 29263209]

[129]   Zarnowska, I.M. Therapeutic use of the ketogenic diet in refractory epilepsy: what we know and what still needs to be learned. *Nutrients,* **2020**, *12*(9), 2616.
[http://dx.doi.org/10.3390/nu12092616] [PMID: 32867258]

[130]   Rho, J.M.; Shao, L.R.; Stafstrom, C.E. 2-Deoxyglucose and beta-hydroxybutyrate: metabolic agents for seizure control. *Front. Cell. Neurosci.,* **2019**, *13*, 172.
[http://dx.doi.org/10.3389/fncel.2019.00172] [PMID: 31114484]

[131]   D'Andrea Meira, I.; Romão, T.T.; Pires do Prado, H.J.; Krüger, L.T.; Pires, M.E.P.; da Conceição, P.O. Ketogenic diet and epilepsy: what we know so far. *Front. Neurosci.,* **2019**, *13*, 5.
[http://dx.doi.org/10.3389/fnins.2019.00005] [PMID: 30760973]

[132]   Shao, L.; Rho, J. M.; Stafstrom, C. E. Glycolytic inhibition: a novel approach toward controlling neuronal excitability and seizures. *Epilepsia Open,* **2018**, *3*(2), 191-197.
[http://dx.doi.org/10.1002/epi4.12251]

[133]   Sumadewi, K.T.; Harkitasari, S.; Tjandra, D.C. Biomolecular mechanisms of epileptic seizures and epilepsy: a review. *Acta Epileptologica,* **2023**, *5*(1), 28.
[http://dx.doi.org/10.1186/s42494-023-00137-0]

[134] Beard, E.; Lengacher, S.; Dias, S.; Magistretti, P.J.; Finsterwald, C. Astrocytes as key regulators of brain energy metabolism: new therapeutic perspectives. *Front. Physiol.,* **2022**, *12*, 825816.
[http://dx.doi.org/10.3389/fphys.2021.825816] [PMID: 35087428]

[135] Malkov, A.; Ivanov, A.I.; Buldakova, S.; Waseem, T.; Popova, I.; Zilberter, M.; Zilberter, Y. Seizure-induced reduction in glucose utilization promotes brain hypometabolism during epileptogenesis. *Neurobiol. Dis.,* **2018**, *116*, 28-38.
[http://dx.doi.org/10.1016/j.nbd.2018.04.016] [PMID: 29705187]

[136] Zhu, H.; Bi, D.; Zhang, Y.; Kong, C.; Du, J.; Wu, X.; Wei, Q.; Qin, H. Ketogenic diet for human diseases: the underlying mechanisms and potential for clinical implementations. *Signal Transduct. Target. Ther.,* **2022**, *7*(1), 11.
[http://dx.doi.org/10.1038/s41392-021-00831-w] [PMID: 35034957]

[137] Stafstrom, C.E.; Roopra, A.; Sutula, T.P. Seizure suppression *via* glycolysis inhibition with 2-deoxy--D-glucose (2DG). *Epilepsia,* **2008**, *49*(s8) Suppl. 8, 97-100.
[http://dx.doi.org/10.1111/j.1528-1167.2008.01848.x] [PMID: 19049601]

[138] Faria-Pereira, A.; Morais, V.A. Synapses: the brain's energy-demanding sites. *Int. J. Mol. Sci.,* **2022**, *23*(7), 3627.
[http://dx.doi.org/10.3390/ijms23073627] [PMID: 35408993]

[139] Dumas, T.C.; Uttaro, M.R.; Barriga, C.; Brinkley, T.; Halavi, M.; Wright, S.N.; Ferrante, M.; Evans, R.C.; Hawes, S.L.; Sanders, E.M. Removal of area CA3 from hippocampal slices induces postsynaptic plasticity at Schaffer collateral synapses that normalizes CA1 pyramidal cell discharge. *Neurosci. Lett.,* **2018**, *678*, 55-61.
[http://dx.doi.org/10.1016/j.neulet.2018.05.011] [PMID: 29738844]

[140] Nedergaard, S.; Andreasen, M. Opposing effects of 2-deoxy- D -glucose on interictal- and ictal-like activity when K $^+$ currents and GABA $_A$ receptors are blocked in rat hippocampus *in vitro*. *J. Neurophysiol.,* **2018**, *119*(5), 1912-1923.
[http://dx.doi.org/10.1152/jn.00732.2017] [PMID: 29412775]

[141] Ahmed Juvale, I.I.; Che Has, A.T. The evolution of the pilocarpine animal model of status epilepticus. *Heliyon,* **2020**, *6*(7), e04557.
[http://dx.doi.org/10.1016/j.heliyon.2020.e04557] [PMID: 32775726]

[142] Wang, X.; Hu, Z.; Zhong, K. The Role of brain-derived neurotrophic factor in epileptogenesis: an update. *Front. Pharmacol.,* **2021**, *12*, 758232.
[http://dx.doi.org/10.3389/fphar.2021.758232] [PMID: 34899313]

[143] Lutas, A.; Yellen, G. The ketogenic diet: metabolic influences on brain excitability and epilepsy. *Trends Neurosci.,* **2013**, *36*(1), 32-40.
[http://dx.doi.org/10.1016/j.tins.2012.11.005] [PMID: 23228828]

[144] Fei, Y.; Shi, R.; Song, Z.; Wu, J. Metabolic control of epilepsy: a promising therapeutic target for epilepsy. *Front. Neurol.,* **2020**, *11*, 592514.
[http://dx.doi.org/10.3389/fneur.2020.592514] [PMID: 33363507]

[145] Khatibi, V.A.; Rahdar, M.; Rezaei, M.; Davoudi, S.; Nazari, M.; Mohammadi, M.; Raoufy, M.R.; Mirnajafi-Zadeh, J.; Hosseinmardi, N.; Behzadi, G.; Janahmadi, M. The glycolysis inhibitor 2-deoxy--d-glucose exerts different neuronal effects at circuit and cellular levels, partially reverses behavioral alterations and does not prevent nadph diaphorase activity reduction in the intrahippocampal kainic acid model of temporal lobe epilepsy. *Neurochem. Res.,* **2023**, *48*(1), 210-228.
[http://dx.doi.org/10.1007/s11064-022-03740-8] [PMID: 36064822]

[146] Mann, J.; Githaka, J.M.; Buckland, T.W.; Yang, N.; Montpetit, R.; Patel, N.; Li, L.; Baksh, S.; Godbout, R.; Lemieux, H.; Goping, I.S. Non-canonical BAD activity regulates breast cancer cell and tumor growth *via* 14-3-3 binding and mitochondrial metabolism. *Oncogene,* **2019**, *38*(18), 3325-3339.
[http://dx.doi.org/10.1038/s41388-018-0673-6] [PMID: 30635657]

[147]   Schildhauer, P.; Selke, P.; Scheller, C.; Strauss, C.; Horstkorte, R.; Leisz, S.; Scheer, M. Glycation leads to increased invasion of glioblastoma cells. *Cells,* **2023**, *12*(9), 1219.
[http://dx.doi.org/10.3390/cells12091219] [PMID: 37174618]

[148]   Almahayni, K.; Spiekermann, M.; Fiore, A.; Yu, G.; Pedram, K.; Möckl, L. Small molecule inhibitors of mammalian glycosylation. *Matrix Biology Plus,* **2022**, *16*, 100108.
[http://dx.doi.org/10.1016/j.mbplus.2022.100108] [PMID: 36467541]

[149]   Granchi, C.; Minutolo, F. Anticancer agents that counteract tumor glycolysis. *ChemMedChem,* **2012**, *7*(8), 1318-1350.
[http://dx.doi.org/10.1002/cmdc.201200176] [PMID: 22684868]

CHAPTER 7

2-Deoxy-D-Glucose as a Potential Antiviral and Anti-COVID-19 Drug

Pandeeswaran Santhoshkumar[1], Arunagiri Sivanesan Aruna Poorani[1], Mohamed Ibrahim Mohamed Ismail[1] and Palaniswamy Suresh[1,*]

[1] *Supramolecular and Catalysis Lab, Dept. of Natural Products Chemistry, School of Chemistry, Madurai Kamaraj University, Madurai-625021, Tamilnadu, India*

Abstract: The search for effective therapeutics has been unyielding in the relentless battle against the COVID-19 pandemic. A potential drug candidate is 2-deoxy-D-glucose (2-DG), which has been evaluated as a polypharmacological agent for antiviral therapy due to its influence on the glycolytic pathway. This chapter delves into the promising role of 2-deoxy-D-glucose (2-DG) as a potential anti-viral drug. With a focus on the biochemical and pharmacological aspects, this chapter explores how 2-DG may disrupt the viral life cycle and modulate host immune responses. An in-depth analysis of the current scientific evidence, including preclinical studies and clinical trials, will be highlighted to shed light on the drug's efficacy, safety, and potential as a treatment option. Furthermore, the challenges and prospects of 2-DG in the context of COVID-19 management will be elaborated. The COVID-19 pandemic has posed unprecedented challenges to global healthcare systems, demanding swift and innovative approaches to combat the virus. Amid this backdrop, the utilization of 2-deoxy-D-glucose (2-DG) as an anti-COVID-19 drug has emerged as a promising avenue for research and therapeutic development. This chapter offers an exhaustive exploration of the potential of 2-DG in the context of COVID-19 treatment. Additionally, action mechanisms and safety concerns associated with administering 2-DG in treating COVID-19 will be reviewed. This chapter aims to equip readers with a comprehensive understanding of 2-DG's role in the fight against COVID-19 and its place in the evolving the landscape of antiviral therapeutics.

Keywords: Antiviral therapy, Glycolytic, Polypharmacological agent, SARS-CoV-2, 2-DG.

1. INTRODUCTION

Energy is a basic need for all living things to continue to exist in the universe. Glucose serves as the primary energy source for all living things (including

---

* **Corresponding author Palaniswamy Suresh:** Supramolecular and Catalysis Lab, Dept. of Natural Products Chemistry, School of Chemistry, Madurai Kamaraj University, Madurai-625021, Tamilnadu, India; Tel: +919790296673; E-mail: suresh.chem@mkuniversity.ac.in

Raman Singh, Antresh Kumar & Kuldeep Singh (Eds.)
All rights reserved-© 2024 Bentham Science Publishers

plants), from primordial forms to multicellular, structured creatures. Cancer, viral infections, and COVID-19 are diseases that have been shown to rewire cell metabolism. As a result, the cell uses glycolysis primarily to meet the high energy requirement necessary for the rapid growth of diseased cells or viruses. While glycolysis does produce ATP, which is a form of energy, the primary reason cells, especially cancer cells or cells infected by viruses, rely heavily on glycolysis might be more related to their need for carbon. 2-Deoxy-D-glucose, commonly called, is a synthetic substitute for glucose. 2-Deoxy-D-glucose (2-DG) was discovered as a competitive inhibitor of glycolysis that is non-metabolizable and contains a hydrogen atom instead of the hydroxyl group found in C-2 carbon of glucose (Fig. **1**). Competitive inhibition is a specific kinetic term that refers to competition for the substrate binding site. It is not really applicable to a metabolic pathway with many enzymes.

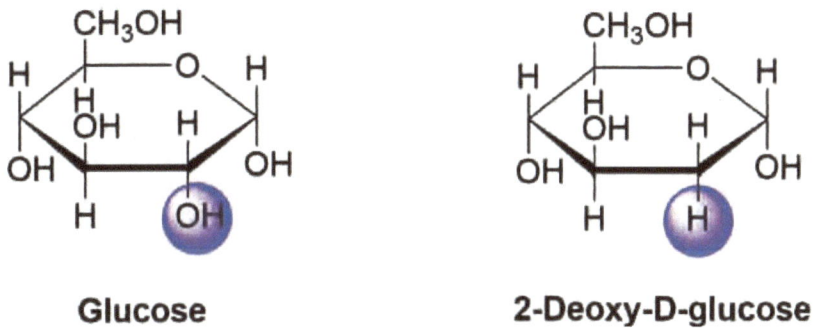

Fig. (1). Structure of Glucose and 2-Deoxy-D-glucose (2-DG) [1].

In the glycolysis process, glucose gets converted into pyruvate, which depends on enzymes such as hexokinase and phosphohexose isomerase, the structural difference in 2-DG inhibits both. Hexokinase readily phosphorylates 2DG to give 2DG-6P. This 2DG-6P can inhibit hexokinase at high concentrations. Consequently, 2-DG's suppression of glycolysis and subsequent adenosine triphosphate (ATP) depletion confirm 2-DG's status as an antimetabolite of glucose. Apart from its ability to inhibit glycolysis, 2-DG also exhibits its anticancer, anti-inflammatory, antiviral, and calorie restriction mimetic properties by modulating the adenosine monophosphate-activated protein kinase (AMPK), and tumour suppressor gene (p53), and protein N-glycosylation in the endoplasmic reticulum (ER) [1].

Despite the extensive use of 2-Deoxy-D-glucose (2-DG) under various situations and physiological applications, the role of this synthetic analogue of glucose has simply been speculated based on a poor metabolic rate and impaired protein glycosylation. In order to understand its role in biological systems, various studies, such as interference with glycolysis, nutritional deprivation conditions, and energy depletion like feeding cells with low or no glucose, and simulation *via in-vitro* culture or in animals by adding 2-deoxy-D-glucose to the medium, have been carried out [2].

2. BIOLOGICAL EFFECTS OF 2-DG

The 2-Deoxy-D-Glucose has a diverse biological effect on metabolic processes. For example, oxidative stress is caused by various metabolic processes of 2-DG, such as the inhibition of 2-DG on glycolysis and ATP generation, disruption of protein N-glycosylation, reduction in energy metabolism and NADPH levels, and interference with cellular thiol metabolism. By impression of this metabolic disruption, 2-DG is identified as an effective cytotoxic agent and has little influence on the viability of healthy cells. The molecule possesses multiple functions, encompassing antiviral, anti-inflammatory, anticancer, and antiepileptic properties, among others. Additionally, it serves as a tracer and a hypoglycemic agent, functioning as both a D-glucose and D-mannose mimic [3]. Its adverse effects stem from its capability to inhibit glycosylation while leaving glycolysis unaffected. Reported experimental results revealed that 2-DG is relatively harmless at lower doses but can lower the blood pressure and slow breathing under higher doses [4].

2-DG can consult neuroprotection to the central nervous system (CNS) of the neurons but sources increased cell death in the existence of hypoxia [4]. In the CNS, microglia cells serve as the macrophages. In *in-vitro* models, 2-DG inhibits the microglia's glycolysis, resulting in ATP depletion and causing cell death. The reason behind the selective impact of 2-DG on microglia is their heightened reliance on glycolysis during activation. In contrast, neurons primarily rely on mitochondria to fulfil their ATP needs. Therefore, in animal models of disorders such as Parkinson's disease, Alzheimer's disease, stroke, meningitis, trauma, and epilepsy that are associated with microglial activation-related neuronal loss, neurons are mostly unaffected by the actions of the treatment. Neuroprotection is not absolute, and pathological conditions linked to hypoxia, such as trauma, vascular dementia, and stroke, have been linked to increased neuronal death. Most studies indicate that a clinically tolerable dose of 2-DG is up to 63 mg/kg/day [3, 5 - 7].

3. 2-DG IN VIRAL REPLICATION

Since the late 1950s, experimentation with 2-DG in viral replication was reported [8]. Kilbourne's initial publication in 1959 noted a considerable decrease in influenza virus load in the chorioallantoic membrane of embryonated chicken eggs [8]. Following that, 2-DG was investigated as an antiviral agent against a variety of viruses, including Herpesviridae [9, 10], Flaviviridae [11], and Orthomyxoviridae [12, 13], Rhabdoviridae [14], Retroviridae, Paramyxoviridae [14] Togaviridae [12], and Picornaviridae. Table **1** summarizes the action of 2-DG on several viruses [15]. The mechanism of 2-DG's antiviral activity includes (i) the erroneous incorporation of 2-DG into the viral capsid structure, compromising the virus's infectious nature, and (ii) interference in the folding process of glycoproteins in the endoplasmic reticulum.

Table 1. Effects of 2-DG on virus replication of various viruses [15].

S. No.	Virus Family	Virus Studied	Species Affected	Model Understudied	Effect of 2-DG on the Viral Impact of Replication	Highlights of the Study Involved	References
1.	Adenoassociated virus	Adeno-associated virus along with Herpes Simplex virus coinfection.	Humans	Hep-2 cells	+/-	• Inhibited early viral protein synthesis. • **Inhibited assembly of the virus into capsid configuration.**	[18]
2.	Caliciviridae	Murine Noroviruses (MNV)	Humans	RAW 264.7 cells	-	• No significant inhibition.	[19]
3.	Flaviviridae	Japanese B encephalitis virus	Humans	BHK-21 cells	+	• **Inhibited assembly of virus and further maturation into infectious form.**	[11]
4.	Flaviviridae	Zika Virus (ZIK V)	Humans	HReEC cells	+	• Absence of the viral protein ZIKV NS3, after treatment. • **Significantly inhibited the viral replication.**	[20 - 22]
5.	Hepadnaviridae	Hepatitis B Virus (HBV)	Humans	HepG2.2.15 cells	+	• **Significantly inhibited the viral replication.**	[23 - 26]

(Table 1) cont.....

S. No.	Virus Family	Virus Studied	Species Affected	Model Understudied	Effect of 2-DG on the Viral Impact of Replication	Highlights of the Study Involved	References
6.	Herpesviridae	Cytomegalovirus	Humans	Diploid human embryonic lung cells	+	• Interfered with mRNA synthesis essential for viral replication. • **Depleted UTP pool**	[13]
7.	Herpesviridae	Herpes Simplex virus	Humans	Vero cells	+	• **Attachment and penetration of virus to host cell are decreased, resulting in reduced infectivity.**	[27 - 29]
8.	Herpesviridae	Herpes Simplex virus	Humans	BSC1 cells	+	• **Yield of infectious viral particles reduced.**	[9]
9.	Herpesviridae	Herpes Simplex virus	Humans	Rabbits	+	• **Reduction in the ocular herpetic keratitis lesions was observed.**	[30]
10.	Herpesviridae	Herpes Simplex virus – 1	Humans	Mice and Guinea pigs	-	• No effect was observed on skin lesions. • **Did not clear the infection.**	[13]
11.	Herpesviridae	Herpes Simplex virus – 1	Humans	Women	+	• **Infection was cleared in more than 85% of the women infected with Herpes virus.**	[31]

(Table 1) cont.....

S. No.	Virus Family	Virus Studied	Species Affected	Model Understudied	Effect of 2-DG on the Viral Impact of Replication	Highlights of the Study Involved	References
12.	Herpesviridae	Infectious bovine rhinotracheitis viral infection	Bovine	Calves	+/-	• Injection of 2DG on a daily basis – No protection. **• Ocular instillation – Reduced viral-**	[32]
13.	Herpesviridae	Pseudorabies	Porcine	Primary rabbit kidney cells	+	• Production of non-infectious viral particles. **• Fusion of virus into host cell is inhibited.**	[33, 34]
14.	Human Herpesviridae	Herpes Simplex Virus 1 (HSV 1)	Humans	HEL cells	+	**• Significantly inhibited the viral replication.**	[35 - 39]
15.	Orthomyxoviridae	Fowl plague virus	Avian	Primary chicken fibroblast cells	+	**• Significantly inhibited the production of viral particles.**	[12]
16.	Orthomyxoviridae	Influenza virus	Humans	The chorio-allantoic membrane of chicken embryo	+	**• Viral concentration was 8 to 32-fold lesser upon comparison with control at 8 hours post inoculation.**	[8]
17.	Papillomaviridae	Human Pathogenic Papillomavirus type 18 (HPV 18)	Humans	HeLa cells	+	**• Significantly inhibited the production of viral particles.**	[40]

(Table 1) cont.....

S. No.	Virus Family	Virus Studied	Species Affected	Model Understudied	Effect of 2-DG on the Viral Impact of Replication	Highlights of the Study Involved	References
18.	Paramyxoviridae	Bovine respiratory syncytial virus	Bovine	Bovine turbinate cell cultures	+	• Replication and cytopathic effects – reversibly inhibited • **Mature virions lacked characteristic surface projections.**	[14]
19.	Paramyxoviridae	Newcastle disease virus	Avian	Primary chicken fibroblast cells	+	• Significantly inhibited the production of viral particles.	[14]
20.	Picornaviridae	Rhinoviruses (RV)	Humans	HeLa cells	+	• **Inhibited early viral protein synthesis.**	[41]
21.	Retroviridae	Human Immunodeficiency Virus	Humans	HUT H9 / CEM / -78 / MT-4	+	• Blocked the formation of syncytia Inhibits viral fusion, attachment and penetration.	[14]
22.	Rhabodoviridae	Vesicular stomatitis virus	Bovine and porcine	BHK or HeLa cells	+	• Significantly inhibited the production of viral particles.	[14]
23.	Togaviridae	Semliki Forest virus	Humans	BHK or HeLa cells	+	• Significantly inhibited the production of viral particles.	[42, 14]
24.	Togaviridae	Sindbis virus	Humans	BHK or HeLa cells	+	• Significantly inhibited the production of viral particles.	[43, 14]

*(+) - Inhibits the viral replication (-) - No significant inhibition.

This interference causes stress in the endoplasmic reticulum, activating the unfolded protein response, resulting in the shutdown of protein synthesis and the blocking of viral replication; (iii) inhibition of glycolysis, resulting in the deprivation of building blocks required for viral replication [16]. The mechanism of inhibition of SARS-related coronavirus-2 (SARS-CoV-2) involves the deprivation of building blocks. In this instance, both glycolysis, which provides energy, and glycosylation, which supplies glycoproteins for spike protein production, are suppressed. 2-DG is an effective cytotoxic drug that has been tried in diverse models of viral infections due to its ability to interface with multiple cellular processes. 2-DG has been investigated as a solo antiviral drug or clinically used with other antiviral medicines [17].

4. COVID-19

The world has been profoundly affected by the coronavirus disease-19 (COVID-19) pandemic, which was brought on by the severe acute respiratory syndrome coronavirus 2 (SARS CoV-2) [44]. The World Health Organization (WHO) designated the outbreak, which began as an epidemic in Wuhan province, China, in February 2020, to be a global pandemic on March 11, 2020 [45]. SARS CoV-2 is a respiratory tract virus, just like SARS and MERS coronaviruses. It was first discovered in 1965 using human tracheal cell culture [46]. Human-to-human droplets are the primary way the virus spreads, yet new research also points to aerosol production as a possible route [47]. Owing to the infection's high contagiousness and current ease of travel, it spreads quickly worldwide. One major obstacle is that many infected people have either minimal or no symptoms at all, but they can still spread the infection. The illness presents with symptoms that include fever, cough, sore throat, headache, and exhaustion, similar to viral pneumonia or a regular cold [48]. The infection is difficult to detect because the clinical indications are mild. In addition to evaluating antibodies for prior infections, real-time polymerase chain reaction (RT PCR) or rapid antigen testing is required for identification [49, 50]. Treatment for COVID-19 individuals differs according to the severity of the illness (Fig. 4). The All-India Institute of Medical Sciences (AIIMS) protocol of the 17th of May 2021 states that in India, oxygen support and intravenous steroids are provided for moderate to severe cases, with selective recommendations for medications such as remdesivir and tocilizumab. Many medications have been tested all throughout the world, with varying degrees of success [51]. The effect of 2-DG on Covid-19 was initiated, as it has been already proven on the many other human viruses. Aligning with this, 2-deoxy-D-glucose (2DG) received approval from the Indian Council of Medical Research (ICMR) on May 1, 2021. During the first wave, India had successfully contained the spread and kept the death toll remarkably low [52].

The primary mechanism of action of 2-DG, a synthetic glucose analogue, is the inhibition of glycolysis. SARS-CoV-2 is a new coronavirus that increases glycolytic and other related processes to get essential substrates for its replication, structure, and function. This substance has shown promise in the treatment of viral infections, seizures, and cancer [20, 53]. The medication has the ability to cure COVID-19 by completely stopping SARS-CoV-2 multiplication in infected monocytes, therefore enhancing the effects of already prescribed medications [54].

4.1. Structure of COVID-19

Positive single-stranded RNA genomes, including SARS-CoV, MERS-CoV, and SARS-CoV-2, are found in the coronavirus envelopes. The SARS-CoV-2 virus particles (Fig. **2**) have a size range of 65 to 125 nm and are spherical to pleomorphic. The nucleocapsid (N) protein coats and tightly coils the 29,811 nucleotides of viral RNA inside the particle. The lipid outer membrane has three glycoproteins embedded in it: spike (S), membrane (M), and envelope (E) [58]. The distinctive "corona" is formed by homotrimers made of spike proteins that emerge from the lipid sheath. Spike proteins facilitate the entry of viruses into host cells by attaching to the angiotensin-converting enzyme 2 (ACE2) that is expressed in respiratory tract cells [55]. A loss of functionality may occur, resulting in viral inactivation, when these constituents alter their spatial and structural configurations. In actuality, there are two ways of viral disinfection: chemically, by treating the virus with organic solvents (alcohols), chlorine (sodium hypochlorite), surfactants, transition/noble metal ions, metal/metal oxide nanoparticles, *etc.*, or physically, by heating the virus to a temperature above 65 °C, by UV-C irradiation, by adjusting the relative humidity, *etc* [56].

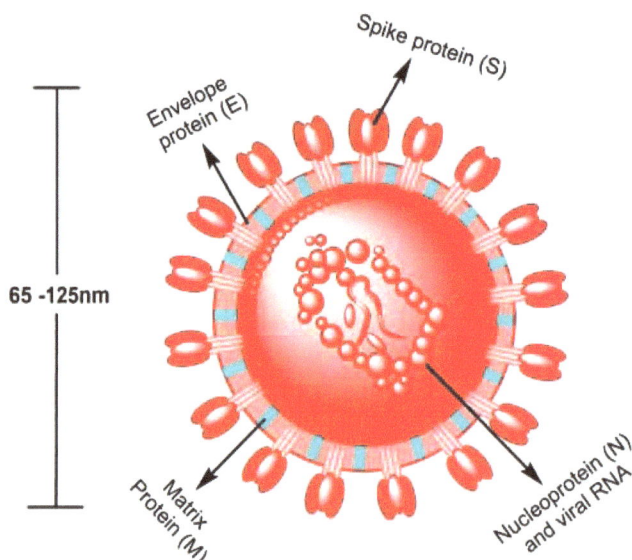

Fig. (2). Schematic representation of SARS-CoV-2 [58].

4.2. Metabolically, SARS-CoV-2 Affected Cells are Similar to Cancer Cells

The Warburg effect, known as aerobic glycolysis, manifests in tumour cells metabolizing glucose to lactate for ATP generation even in the existence of sufficient oxygen. This adaptation results from a hypoxic, poorly vascularized tumour environment and a compromised electron transport chain in the mitochondria. By providing ATP, lowering apoptotic death, and promoting tumour dissemination through lactate-induced extracellular matrix breakdown, it gives malignancies a survival advantage [57].

Monocyte-macrophages show a metabolic resemblance to cancer cells in regions of inflammation. Due to the higher metabolic demands of their pro-inflammatory phenotype, they have compromised mitochondrial function, and have shifted to glycolysis (M1) [59]. On the other hand, oxidative phosphorylation plays a significant role in the production of ATP and the repair of inflammatory damage in the monocyte-macrophage lineage's anti-inflammatory phenotype (M2). However, AMPK downregulation, p53 inactivation, and mitochondrial dysfunction caused by inflammatory mediators generated in COVID-19 impede this phenotype [60].

Pneumocytes of the alveolar-capillary barrier and endothelial cells infected with viruses exhibit increased aerobic glycolysis. Furthermore, especially in the early stages of the infection, alveolar epithelial cells are more vulnerable to SARS-CoV-2 infection than endothelial cells or monocytes [61].

In COVID-19, elevated glycolytic activity has been identified as a key mechanism promoting viral replication and the inflammatory response [54, 62]. Evidence suggests that higher glycolytic activity in SARS-CoV-2-infected monocytes is linked to the genetic overexpression of enzymes in the way (Fig. **3**) [63]. An important part of the viral entrance, replication, and inflammatory response is played by this increased glycolytic flux. The overexpression of the gene encoding the angiotensin-converting enzyme 2 (ACE2) promotes the entry of viruses into cells, provides a carbon source for the absorption of virions, and increases the expression of inflammatory mediators and damage to organs, such as IL-6T, NF-α, IFN, IL-1β, and α, β, and λ. Crucially, these modifications are independent of mitochondria, as demonstrated by the upregulation of ACE2 and inflammatory mediators following oligomycin-mediated ATP synthase proton channel blockage, which in turn impacts the citric acid cycle and electron transport chain [60].

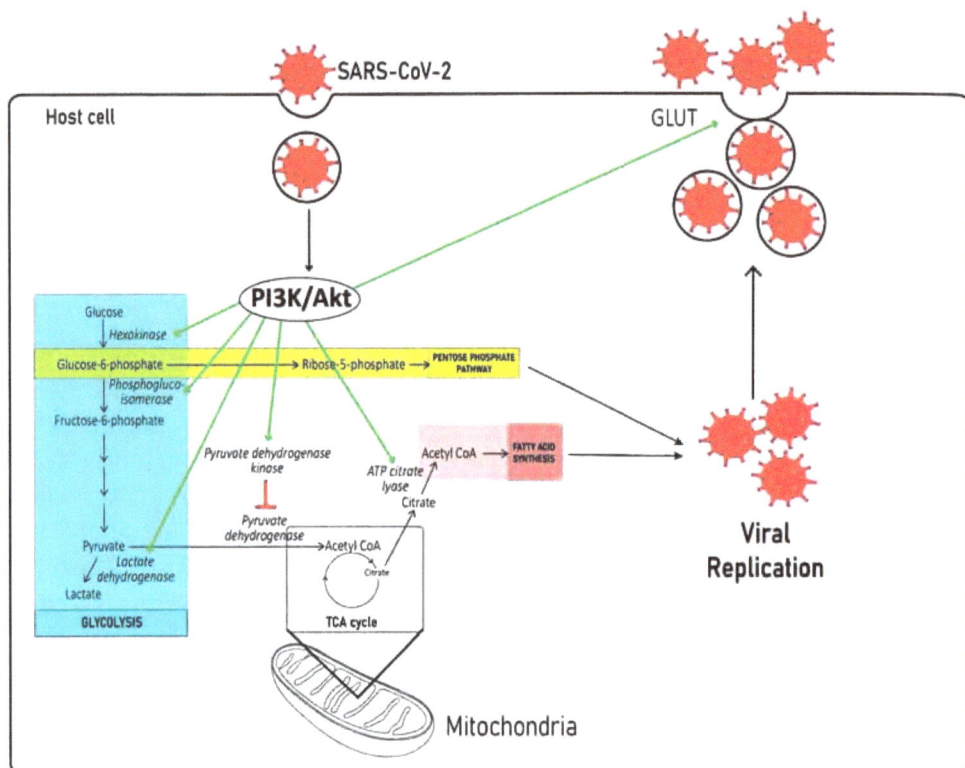

Fig. (3). Diverse Downstream Consequences of the SARS-CoV-2-Triggered PI3K/Akt Pathway [63].

Following a recent study, the monocytes from patient's peripheral blood who had COVID-19 pneumonia were mainly redistributed in favour of more intermediate or pro-inflammatory cells. Glycolysis and oxidative phosphorylation were reduced in these cells. Whether SARS-CoV-2 was present in these blood cells is still unknown. COVID-19 is linked to reduced blood virus detection rates, which suggests that the mediators released at the sites of inflammation may have distant impacts on metabolism [64 - 66].

4.3. Association between Blood Glucose and Viral Infection

Diabetes and COVID-19 are correlated in both directions. In individuals who are obese and have type II diabetes and insulin resistance, COVID-19 is more prevalent and severe. Additionally, it is linked to the development of new cases of diabetes as well as the aggravation of pre-existing diabetic metabolic problems, such as hyperosmolarity and diabetic ketoacidosis [67]. Several factors contribute to the multifactorial hyperglycemia linked to SARS-CoV-2 infection, including the stress response to a severe illness, insulin resistance, pancreatic beta-cell malfunction, and the use of steroids in treatment. Among these, the leading cause of hyperglycemia in COVID-19 is likely insulin resistance brought on by malfunctioning adipose tissue [68].

A *trans*-membrane protein of the Golgi apparatus is called Golgi protein 73 (GP73). Increased production of the protein is linked to hepatocyte injury and may be used as a prognostic and diagnostic indicator of liver impairment in patients with long-term HBV infection [69]. The serum concentration of the protein is correlated with the severity of COVID-19, and its levels are around two times higher in individuals with SARSCoV-2 infection compared to the reference group (p<0.0001). With little impact on glycogenolysis, its main mechanism of action is to increase hepatic and renal gluconeogenesis. The recent spike in blood glucose levels linked to SARS-CoV-2 infection may be caused by the increased expression of GP73. But as elevated liver enzymes are only seen in 14-53% of COVID-19 patients [70], GP73 GP73-mediated gluconeogenesis is unable to account for the elevated blood glucose levels linked to SARS-COV-2 infection in the absence of hepatocyte damage. Due to enhanced cellular uptake of glucose, elevated blood sugar levels in diabetes lead to malfunction and ultimately cell death. In people with diabetes, hexokinase-2 (HK2) mediated glycolytic flux can compromise cellular processes without changing transcription. The dicarbonyl stress, protein kinase C, and hexosamine pathways can all be triggered by an increase in glycolytic flux [71].

The PI3K/Akt/mTOR and ERK/MAPK signaling pathways influence MERS-CoV replication. Research indicates that SARS-CoV-2 infection is linked to elevated blood glucose levels and the activation of these ways, which impact host cell metabolism and supply the substrates for viral replication (Fig. **3**). Therefore, in SARS-CoV-2-infected cells, disruption of the glycolytic pathway can result in the total halt of viral replication [54, 72, 73].

4.4. 2-DG in COVID-19

4.4.1. Metabolic Insights and Therapeutic in COVID-19: 2-DG Clinical Trials

Numerous studies have reported metabolic changes associated with COVID-19 infection, indicating increased glucose reserve and glycolytic activity in immune cells, such as SARS-CoV-2-infected monocytes. This is not the case with respiratory syncytial virus (RSV). As a result, glycolysis is an essential source of ATP and carbon for sustaining these cells' metabolic processes. Furthermore, glucose is essential for replicating SARS CoV-2 in human-infected cells, involving the two most prevalent glucose metabolic pathways, glycolysis and glycosylation. According to reports, 2-DG-mediated suppression of glucose metabolism can prevent the glucose-dependent expression of inflammatory genes [54, 72, 74].

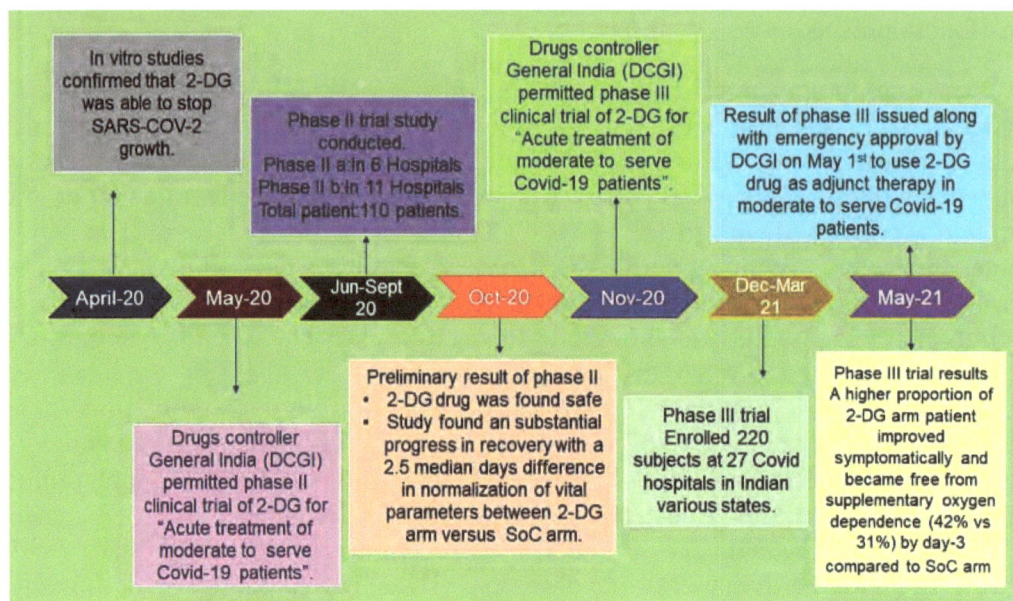

Fig. (4). A Timeline Analysis of the 2-DG Clinical Trial [51].

Based on these findings, the Defense Research and Development Organization (DRDO) research laboratory, the Institute of Nuclear Medicine and Allied Sciences, collaborated with Dr Reddy's Laboratories (DRLs) in Hyderabad to conduct a clinical trial on 2-DG to assess its efficacy against COVID-19 infection. Approved in May 2020 (CTRI/2020/06/025664), the Phase II trial was carried out from May to October 2020 with 110 COVID patients. Two hundred and twenty patients participated in the Phase III experiment from December 2020 to March 2021 at 27 COVID-19 facilities spread over several Indian cities. The findings revealed that a considerably greater percentage of patients—42% in the 2-DG group compared to 31% in the standard of care arm were improving symptomatically and weaning off oxygen assistance. Patients 65 years of age and older showed similar tendencies. Furthermore, the 2-DG arm exhibited a greater RT-PCR conversion rate. Ultimately, on May 8th, 2021, the Drug Controller General of India (DCGI) authorized 2-DG as a COVID therapy, with a focus on emergency use in COVID patients needing more oxygen support [75].

4.4.2. Clinical Trial of 2-DG in COVID-19

The 2-DG is a potential COVID-19 treatment studied in various clinical trials, including Phase I, II, and III. The drug has shown promising results in these trials, with faster recovery and improved outcomes in COVID-19 patients. Here is a summary of clinical trials:

Phase I: Based on permissibility data from prior clinical studies in patients with solid cancers, the first day-to-day dose of 2-DG was 63 mg kg^{-1} [77]. If no safety issues were noted at the beginning dose, the doses would be increased further, from 63 mg kg^{-1}to 90 mg kg^{-1}/day (almost 1.5 fold) and 126 mg kg^{-1}/day (about 2 fold) planned [76, 77].

Phase II: A multicenter, open-label, randomized, parallel-group clinical trial was conducted to assess the safety, tolerability, and effectiveness of 2-DG in addition to standard of care (SOC1 and SOC2) *vs* SOC alone in patients with moderate to severe COVID-19 [77]. The Drugs Controller General of India (DCGI) oversaw the trial, which the relevant ethics committees authorized. Given the novelty of the medicine and the dearth of published information about safety and effectiveness in patients who are not cancer patients, the sponsors and DCGI worked together to set the sample size for this evidence of concept study (110 patients, twenty-two individuals in each arm) [76, 77].

Between June 2019 and September 2020, 110 patients were randomly assigned to five therapeutic groups (Part A: 2-DG 63 mg and SOC1; Part B: 2-DG 90 mg, 2-DG 126 mg, and SOC2 groups) comprising 22 persons each [77]. Due to an adverse event, one patient in the 2-DG 126 mg group was discontinued before receiving any dose; the other 99 patients received doses (Fig. **5**) [77].

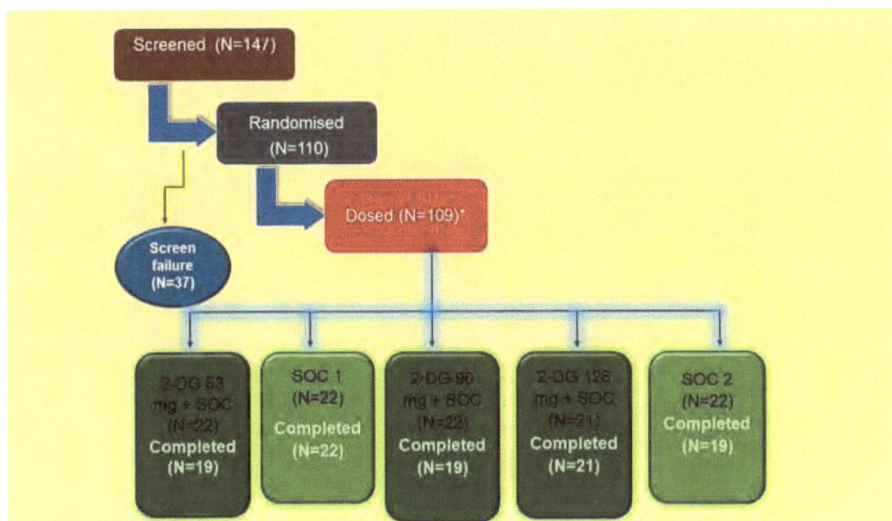

Fig. (5). Flowchart illustrates patient distribution across treatment groups: 2-DG, SOC, SOC1 (Part A), and SOC2 (Part B) of the study [77]..

The baseline and demographic parameters of the treatment groups were similar (Table **2**). For all randomized patients, the mean age (standard deviation) was 44.9 (10.90) years, and the mean weight (SD) was 68.6 (11.39) kg. Eighty-seven percent of the eighty-eight patients had an MSN. Certain baseline characteristics of the diseases varied across the patients participating in Parts A and B of the study. In section A, the mean (SD) number of days from the onset of early COVID-19 symptoms was 7.2 (2.58) days for persons in the SOC1 group and 6.6 (2.26) days for those in the 2-DG group of 63 mg. For Part B, it was 4.5 (1.41) days for the 2-DG 90 mg group, 4.3 (1.46) days for the 126 mg of 2-DG group, and 4.4 (1.40) days for the SOC2 group (Table **2**). With the exception of three patients whose severity information was missing, all enrolled patients were determined to have moderate COVID-19, as specified by the guideline [77].

Table 2. **Patient demographic and baseline characteristics [77].**

-		63mg of 2-DG +SOC N=22 n (%)	SOC1 N=22 n (%)	90 mg of 2-DG +SOC N=22 n (%)	126 mg of 2-DG +SOC N=21 n (%)	SOC2 N=22 n (%)	References
Age (years)	Mean	44.2 (12.71)	44.4 (9.59)	46.3 (11.00)	42.7 (9.33)	46.6 (11.96)	[77]
Gender (n %)	Woman	7 (31.8)	6 (27.3)	1 (4.5)	5 (23.8)	2 (9.1)	
	Man	15 (68.2)	16 (72.7)	21 (95.5)	16 (76.2)	20 (90.9)	
Days since the first COVID-19 symptom appeared	Mean (SD)	6.6 (2.26)	7.2 (2.58)	4.5 (1.41)	4.3 (1.46)	4.4 (1.40)	
Clinical severity status as defined by MoH&FW [n (%)]	Group 1 (Mild)	0	0	0	0	0	
	Group 2 (Moderate)	21 (95.5%)[a]	21 (95.5%)[a]	22 (100.0%)	21 (100.0%)	21 (95.5%)[a]	
	Group 3 (Severe)	0	0	0	0	0	

(Table 2) cont.....

-		63mg of 2-DG +SOC N=22 n (%)	SOC1 N=22 n (%)	90 mg of 2-DG +SOC N=22 n (%)	126 mg of 2-DG +SOC N=21 n (%)	SOC2 N=22 n (%)	References
Oxygen saturation (SpO$_2$%)	N	22	21	22	21	21	
	Mean (SD)	93.1 (2.39)	93.0 (1.82)	92.7 (1.55)	92.5 (1.47)	93.0(2.07)	
	Median	92.0	93.0	93.0	93.0	93.0	
Heart rate (per minute)	N	22	21	22	21	21	
	Mean (SD)	85.0 (11.32)	86.3 (15.17)	81.3 (10.39)	84.9 (11.57)	89.6 (8.48)	
	Median	80.0	84.0	80.0	88.0	89.0	[77]
Respiratory rate (per minute)	N	22	21	22	21	21	
	Mean (SD)	22.1 (3.04)	21.4 (3.20)	23.9 (2.41)	24.4 (2.09)	24.7±2.61	
	Median	24.0	22.0	25.0	25.0	25.0	
WHO clinical progression scale	N	22	22	22	21	22	
	Mean (SD)	5.1 (0.35)	5.0 (0.21)	4.3 (0.48)	4.3 (0.46)	4.3 (0.48)	
	Median	5.0	5.0	4.0	4.0	4.0	

SOC1=studied part A in SOC, SOC2= studied part B in SOC
N: The whole patient population within the designated treatment group
n: number of patients
MoH and FW: Ministry of Health and Family Welfare
[a] In all three groups, there was one patient for whom the severity assessment was absent.

Efficacy: The 2-DG 90 mg/day group had the shortest median time (2.5 days) to achieve and maintain SpO$_2 \geq 94\%$ on room air at sea level, closely followed by the 2-DG 126 mg/day group (3.0 days). For the other three groups - 63 mg/day, SOC1, and SOC2- the median duration to reach SpO$_2 \geq 94\%$ was 5.0 days (Table 3). When compared to the SOC2 group (Table 3) and the pooled SOC group, the 2-DG 90 mg/day group's Hazard ratio (95% CI) was 2.3 (1.14, 4.64) (p=0.0201) and 2.6 (1.49, 4.70) (p=0.0009), respectively. There was no statistically significant difference between 2-DG 63 mg/day and SOC1 or 2-DG 126 mg/day and SOC2 [77].

Table 3. Exploring Efficacy Endpoints: A Contrast between Active (2-DG) and SOC are Groups [77].

-		SOC + 2-DG 63 mg	SOC1	SOC + 2-DG 90 mg	SOC + 2-DG 126 mg	SOC2	Pooled SOC (SOC1+SOC2)	References
Time to achieve SpO$_2\geq$94% (days) (on two consecutive valuations on room air, at sea level)	N	22	22	22	21	22	44	
	Median	5	5	2.5	3	5	5	
	-	1.277 (2.477, 0.658)	-	2.3 (4.642, 1.14)	0.975 (1.925, 0.494)	-	-	
Time to discharge (days)	P-value	0.4698	-	0.0201	0.9415	-	-	
	Median	12	11	18	11	10	10	
	95% CI[a] (HR)	0.791 (1.504, 0.416)	-	2.238 (4.703 1.065)	0.679 (1.38, 0.334,)	-	-	[77]
Time to clinical recovery[b] (days)	P-value [a]	0.4746	-	0.0336	0.2847	-	-	
	Median	4.5	5	3	4	6	5	
	95% CI[a] (HR)	0.985 (1.846, 0.526)	-	3.837 (7.944, 1.853,)	1.881 (, 3.838, 0.922)	-	-	
Time to vital signs normalization[c] (days)	P-value [a]	0.9629	-	0.0003	0.0824	-	-	
	Median	7	7	5	10	8	7	
	95% CI[a] (HR)	0.889 (1.674, 0.472)	-	4.341 (11.294, 1.669)	1.024 (2.511, 0.418,)	-	-	
Days needed to enhance the WHO clinical progression by two points	P-value [a]	0.7162	-	0.0026	0.958	-	-	
	Median	11	10.5	5	5	6	8	[77]
	95% CI[a] (HR)	0.624 (1.224, 0.318,)	-	1.763 (3.363, 0.924,)	1.183 (2.221, 0.63,)	-	-	

[a] Every 2-DG+SOC group in the study's Parts A and B was associated with a matching SOC group. SOC2 was compared with the 90 mg/day and 126 mg/day groups, whereas SOC1 was compared with the 63 mg/day group.

[b] The composite endpoint known as "time to clinical recovery" measures the number of days required to attain and sustain a room air blood oxygen saturation of 94% as well as the time it takes to reach a 5-point Likert-type symptom severity score of $\leq$1 for all COVID-19-related symptoms after study treatment has begun.

[c] The time to vital signs normalization was the earliest date after the research therapy started on which all of the following vital sign criteria were met: body temperature < 98.9 °F, respiratory rate < 20 breaths per minute, blood oxygen saturation (SpO$_2$) > 95% on room air, and heart rate < 90 bpm.

Time to Clinical Recovery is a composite endpoint that counts the days it takes to reach and maintain a SpO_2 of $\geq 94\%$ on room air as well as the number of days it takes to reach a patient-assessed symptom severity score of ≤ 1 on a 5-point Likert-type scale for all COVID-19-related symptoms. In the 2-DG 63 mg/day, 2-DG 90 mg/day, and 2-DG 126 mg/day groups, the median time to clinical recovery was four and a half days, three days, and four days, respectively; in the SOC1 and SOC2 groups, it was five and six days, as shown in Table **3**. When comparing the 2-DG 90 mg/day group to the SOC2 group and the pooled SOC group, the HZ (95% CI) was 3.8 (1.85, 7.94) (p=0.0003) (Table **3**) [77].

Similarly, the time to normalize vital signs was significantly better in the 2-DG 90 mg/day group than in the SOC2 group. The median time to vital signs normalization was five days in the 2-DG 90 mg/day group compared to eight days in the contemporary SOC2 group, Hazard ratio (95% CI) from the CPH model=4.3 (1.67, 11.29) (p=0.0026) (Table **3**) [77].

In just five days, the 2-DG 90 mg/day and 2-DG 126 mg/day groups both demonstrated a median improvement in clinical status score of two points over baseline. On the other hand, the 2-DG 90 mg/day group (4 days) and the 2-DG 126 mg/day group (3 days) had the quickest median improvement. There was no statistically significant distinction between the SOC2 group and these two groups (Table **3**). The CPH model was used to calculate the time it took to achieve a 2-point improvement over standard in the clinical status. For the 2-DG 90 mg/day *vs.* SOC2 group, the resultant Hazard Ratio (95% Confidence Interval) was 1.8 (0.92, 3.36) (p=0.0852), and for the 2-DG 126 mg/day *vs.* SOC2 group, it was 1.18 (0.63, 2.22) (p=0.6021) (Table **3**). The only finding that was significant was the comparison of the median time to two points of improvement (HR=2.364; 95% CI: 1.33, 4.18; p=0.0032) between the 2-DG 90 mg/day group and the combined SOC group [77].

The median time until the initial conversion to a negative RT-PCR test for COVID-19 RNA was 5.0 days for the 2-DG 90 mg/day group (4.0 days from descriptive statistics) and 7.0 days for the 2-DG 63 mg/day group (6.0 days from expressive statistics) according to the CPH model. At 3.5 days, the SOC1 group had the quickest median time to this test. The median duration for the 2-DG 126 mg/day and SOC2 groups was 7.0 days. When compared to the corresponding SOC groups, none of the 2-DG groups displayed statistically important differences. With HR=2.0 (0.94, 4.25; p=0.0702), the 2-DG 90 mg/day group, however, showed a statistically superior tendency.

Finally, Phase II trial showed that 2-DG, at a dose of 90 mg/kg/day, demonstrated clinical benefit over standard of care (SOC) alone in treating moderate to severe

COVID-19. For COVID-19 medication development, reaching and maintaining a $SpO_2 \geq 94\%$ deemed a clinically significant endpoint. The findings of this investigation demonstrated the viability of 2-DG and supported the need for a critical Phase III trial to assess it [77].

The 2-DG 90 mg/day group had the shortest median time to discharge from the isolation ward (8.0 days), out of all the groups (Table **3**). When compared to the SOC2 group (Table **2**) and the pooled SOC, the 2-DG 90 mg/day group's Hazard ratio (95% CI) was 2.2 (1.07, 4.70) (p=0.0336) and 2.2 (1.21, 4.04) (p=0.01). Compared to their respective SOC groups, the other two dosage groups (2-DG 63 mg/day and 2-DG 126 mg/day groups) did not show statistical significance (Table **3**) [77].

Phase III: In November 2020, the Drug Controller General of India (DCGI) approved Phase III clinical studies after Phase II trial. Two hundred twenty patients participated in Phase-III trial from December 2020 to March 2021 at 27 COVID hospitals across several states. Compared to the Standard of Care (SOC), a considerably more significant proportion of patients in the 2-DG arm experienced symptomatic improvement and became independent of supplemental oxygen by Day 3 (42% *vs.* 31%), suggesting early release from oxygen therapy/dependency. Patients older than 65 showed signs of this encouraging trend as well. As a result, on May 1, 2021, the DCGI approved this medication's emergency use as an adjuvant treatment in moderate-to-severe COVID-19 instances. The medication may be easily manufactured and made broadly accessible nationwide because of its generic nature and structural similarity to glucose. When taken orally in the form of powder, the medication builds up in cells infected with viruses, impeding their ability to synthesize new DNA and produce energy. It differs due to its specific accumulation in infected cells. The medication is expected to save lives by reducing hospital stays for COVID-19 patients due to its particular mode of action in infected cells, as a spike in COVID-19 cases during the second wave resulted in high oxygen dependency and hospitalizations [78].

4.4.3. Mechanistic Insight into the Inhibition of Viral Replication by 2DG

The following crucial actions are involved in the mechanism by which 2-deoxy-D-glucose (2-DG) inhibits viral replication in hosts infected with SARS-CoV-2 (Fig. **6**).

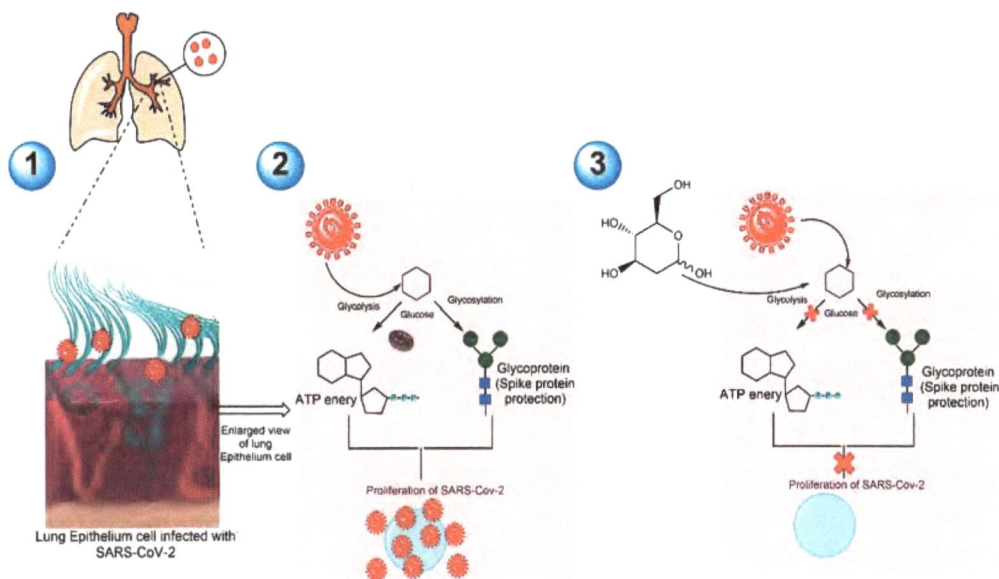

Fig. (6). Mechanism of viral replication inhibition by 2-deoxy-D-glucose (2-DG) in SARS-CoV-2 infected host [79].

Step I: Inflammatory Action in the Lower Respiratory Tract: When the lower respiratory tract becomes infected with SARS-CoV-2, lung epithelial cells, in particular, experience an inflammatory reaction.

Step II: Glucose Involvement in Viral Replication: Because glucose catalyzes the production of adenosine triphosphate (ATP), which gives energy to viral host cells, glucose is essential. Additionally, it promotes the synthesis of glycans, which helps glycoproteins during glycosylation. The reproduction of viruses depends on these glycoproteins.

Step III: 2-DG Inhibition: 2-DG interferes with regular cellular functioning by acting as an antimetabolite of glucose. It interferes with the virus's energy supply and prevents glycoprotein synthesis by inhibiting both glycolysis and glycosylation. Viral proliferation is inhibited as a result of this disturbance [79].

In summary, 2-DG disrupts the energy supply and essential processes necessary for viral replication, potentially hindering the proliferation of SARS-CoV-2 in infected host cells.

CONCLUSION

This chapter discusses the structural features and influence of 2-DG (2-Deoxy-D-Glucose) on the glycolytic pathway. All the reports summarise and narrate that

2-DG acts as a polypharmacological agent for antiviral therapy. It is clearly understood that 2-DG is a potential antiviral drug while administered under lower doses, but in higher doses, it leads to many disorders, which are discussed elaborately. The suggested dose level is up to 63 mg/kg/day from the reported values. Furthermore, primarily, how 2-DG shows its efficacy against the pandemic disease COVID-19 was presented, and how the corresponding clinical trial revealed the metabolic insight and opened the possible therapeutic options for the treatment of COVID-19 has been discussed briefly. In addition to that, the mechanism of action and safety concerns associated with administering 2-DG in treating COVID-19 were reviewed. These particulars divulge that 2-DG behaves as a potential antiviral as well as an anti-COVID-19 drug.

LIST OF ABBREVIATIONS

2-DG	- 2-Deoxy-D-Glucose
ACE2	- Angiotensin-converting enzyme 2
AIIMS	- All India Institute of Medical Sciences
AMP	- Adenosine monophosphate
AMPK	-Adenosine monophosphate-activated protein kinase
ATP	-Adenosine triphosphate
COVID-19	- Coronavirus disease-19
DCGI	- Drug Controller General of India
DNA	- Deoxyribonucleic acid
DRDO	- Defence Research and Development Organization
ER	- Endoplasmic reticulum
GLUT-1	- Glucose transporter 1
GP73	- Golgi protein 73
HBV	- Hepatitis B virus
HeLa	- Henrietta Lacks (Cervical Cancer Cell line)
HK2	- Hexokinase 2
HR	- Hazard ratio
HSV	- Herpes Simplex Virus
HPV	- Human papillomavirus
HPV18	- Human pathogenic papillomavirus type 18
IFN	- Interferon receptor
IL-1β	- Interleukin-1 beta
IL-6	- Interleukin-6
ICMR	- Indian Council of Medical Research

LHBS	- Large viral surface antigens	
mRNA	- Messenger ribonucleic acid	
MCT4	- Monocarboxylate transporter 4	
MERS	- Middle East respiratory syndrome	
MERS-CoV	- Middle East respiratory syndrome coronavirus	
MNV	- Murine norovirus	
NADPH	- Nicotinamide adenine dinucleotide phosphate hydrogen	
NoV	- Noroviruses	
OHPHOS	- Oxidative phosphorylation	
PI3K	- Phosphatidylinositol 3-kinase	
Akt	- Protein kinase B	
PPP	- Pentose phosphate pathway	
RV	- Rhinoviruses	
RNA	- Ribonucleic acid	
RT-PCR	- Real-time polymerase chain reaction	
SARS	- Severe acute respiratory syndrome	
SARS-CoV	- Severe acute respiratory syndrome coronavirus	
SD	- Standard deviation	
SOC	- Standard of care	
SpO$_2$	- Saturation of Peripheral Oxygen	
TCA	- Tricarboxylic acid cycle	
TNF-α	- Tumour Necrosis Factor alpha	
TPI	- Triosephosphate isomerase	
UV-C	- Ultra violet C	
WHO	- World Health Organization	
ZIKV	- Zika virus	

ACKNOWLEDGEMENTS

We gratefully acknowledge the financial support from MKU-RUSA 2.0, TANSCHE, and TNSCST, Tamil Nadu. Also, we thank DST-FIST-II, New Delhi.

FUNDING INFORMATION

This work was funded by Madurai Kamaraj University- Rashtriya Uchchatar Shiksha Abhiyan (MKU-RUSA) Ref No. 007-R2/MKU/SOC/2020-2021, Tamil Nadu State Council for Higher Education (TANCSHE) Ref No. 131/2019A dated 23-06-22, Tamil Nadu State Council for Science and Technology Ref No.

TNSCST/STP/Covid-19/2020-21-3682 and Department of Science and Technology Ref No. SR/FST/CS-II/2017/35(C).

REFERENCES

[1] Sols, A.; Crane, R.K. Substrate specificity of brain hexokinase. *J. Biol. Chem.,* **1954**, *210*(2), 581-595.
[http://dx.doi.org/10.1016/S0021-9258(18)65384-0] [PMID: 13211595]

[2] Xi, H.; Kurtoglu, M.; Liu, H.; Wangpaichitr, M.; You, M.; Liu, X.; Savaraj, N.; Lampidis, T.J. 2-Deoxy-d-glucose activates autophagy *via* endoplasmic reticulum stress rather than ATP depletion. *Cancer Chemother. Pharmacol.,* **2011**, *67*(4), 899-910.
[http://dx.doi.org/10.1007/s00280-010-1391-0] [PMID: 20593179]

[3] Singh, R.; Gupta, V.; Kumar, A.; Singh, K. 2-Deoxy-D-Glucose: A novel pharmacological agent for killing hypoxic tumor cells, oxygen dependence-lowering in covid-19, and other pharmacological activities. *Adv. Pharmacol. Pharm. Sci.,* **2023**, *2023*, 1-15.
[http://dx.doi.org/10.1155/2023/9993386] [PMID: 36911357]

[4] Pajak, B.; Siwiak, E.; Sołtyka, M.; Priebe, A.; Zieliński, R.; Fokt, I.; Ziemniak, M.; Jaśkiewicz, A.; Borowski, R.; Domoradzki, T.; Priebe, W. 2-Deoxy-d-glucose and its analogs: from diagnostic to therapeutic agents. *Int. J. Mol. Sci.,* **2019**, *21*(1), 234.
[http://dx.doi.org/10.3390/ijms21010234] [PMID: 31905745]

[5] Raez, L. E.; Papadopoulos, K.; Ricart, A. D.; Chiorean, E. G.; DiPaola, R. S.; Stein, M. N.; Rocha Lima, C. M.; Schlesselman, J. J.; Tolba, K.; Langmuir, V. K.; Kroll, S.; Jung, D. T.; Kurtoglu, M.; Rosenblatt, J.; Lampidis, T. J. A phase i dose-escalation trial of 2-deoxy-d-glucose alone or combined with docetaxel in patients with advanced solid tumors. *Cancer Chemother. Pharmacol.,* **2013**, *71*(2), 523530.
[http://dx.doi.org/10.1007/s00280-012-2045-1/]

[6] Bhatt, A. N.; Shenoy, S.; Munjal, S.; Chinnadurai, V.; Agarwal, A.; Kumar, A. V.; Shanavas, A.; Kanwar, R.; Chandna, S. 2-Deoxy-d-glucose as an adjunct to standard of care in the medical management of covid-19: a proof-of-concept & dose-ranging randomised clinical trial. *BioRxiv,* **2021**
[http://dx.doi.org/10.1101/2021.10.08.21258621]

[7] Fessel, J. Cure of Alzheimer's dementia requires addressing all of the affected brain cell types. *J. Clin. Med.,* **2023**, *12*(5), 2049.
[http://dx.doi.org/10.3390/jcm12052049]

[8] Kilbourne, E.D. Inhibition of influenza virus multiplication with a glucose antimetabolite (2-deoxy-D-glucose). *Nature,* **1959**, *183*(4656), 271-272.
[http://dx.doi.org/10.1038/183271b0] [PMID: 13622777]

[9] Courtney, R.J.; Steiner, S.M.; Benyesh-Melnick, M. Effects of 2-deoxy-d-glucose on herpes simplex virus replication. *Virology,* **1973**, *52*(2), 447-455.
[http://dx.doi.org/10.1016/0042-6822(73)90340-1] [PMID: 4350224]

[10] Radsak, K.D.; Weder, D. Effect of 2-deoxy-D-glucose on cytomegalovirus-induced DNA synthesis in human fibroblasts. *J. Gen. Virol.,* **1981**, *57*(1), 33-42.
[http://dx.doi.org/10.1099/0022-1317-57-1-33] [PMID: 6275020]

[11] Woodman, D.R.; Williams, J.C. Effects of 2-deoxy-D-glucose and 3 deazauridine individually and in combination on the replication of Japanese B encephalitis virus. *Antimicrob. Agents Chemother.,* **1977**, *11*(3), 475-481.
[http://dx.doi.org/10.1128/AAC.11.3.475] [PMID: 856001]

[12] Kaluza, G.; Scholtissek, C.; Rott, R. Inhibition of the multiplication of enveloped RNA-viruses by glucosamine and 2-deoxy-D-glucose. *J. Gen. Virol.,* **1972**, *14*(3), 251-259.
[http://dx.doi.org/10.1099/0022-1317-14-3-251] [PMID: 4336520]

[13] Kern, E.R.; Glasgow, L.A.; Klein, R.J.; Friedman-Kien, A.E. Failure of 2-deoxy-D-glucose in the

treatment of experimental cutaneous and genital infections due to herpes simplex virus. *J. Infect. Dis.,* **1982**, *146*(2), 159-166.
[http://dx.doi.org/10.1093/infdis/146.2.159] [PMID: 6286785]

[14]   Tripathy, R.N.; Mohanty, S.B. Effect of 2-deoxy-D-glucose and glucosamine on bovine respiratory syncytial virus. *Am. J. Vet. Res.,* **1979**, *40*(9), 1288-1293.
[PMID: 525934]

[15]   Padmanath, K.; Rajasekaran, R.; Jagatheesan, P.N.R. Use of 2-deoxy-D-glucose in virology research: A mini review. *International Journal of Veterinary Sciences and Animal Husbandry,* **2023**, *8*(2), 43-46.
[http://dx.doi.org/10.22271/veterinary.2023.v8.i2a.490]

[16]   Mesri, E.A.; Lampidis, T.J. 2-Deoxy- D -glucose exploits increased glucose metabolism in cancer and viral-infected cells: Relevance to its use in INDIA against SARS-COV -2. *IUBMB Life,* **2021**, *73*(10), 1198-1204.
[http://dx.doi.org/10.1002/iub.2546] [PMID: 34418270]

[17]   Pająk, B.; Zieliński, R.; Manning, J.T.; Matejin, S.; Paessler, S.; Fokt, I.; Emmett, M.R.; Priebe, W. The antiviral effects of 2-deoxy-d-glucose (2-dg), a dual d-glucose and d-mannose mimetic, against sars-cov-2 and other highly pathogenic viruses. *Molecules,* **2022**, *27*(18), 5928.
[http://dx.doi.org/10.3390/molecules27185928] [PMID: 36144664]

[18]   Xi, H.; Kurtoglu, M.; Lampidis, T.J. The wonders of 2-deoxy- D -glucose. *IUBMB Life,* **2014**, *66*(2), 110-121.
[http://dx.doi.org/10.1002/iub.1251] [PMID: 24578297]

[19]   Passalacqua, K. D.; Lu, J.; Goodfellow, I.; Kolawole, A. O.; Arche, J. R.; Maddox, R. J.; Carnahan, K. E.; O'Riordan, M. X. D.; Wobus, C. E. Glycolysis is an intrinsic factor for optimal replication of a norovirus. *mBio,* **2019**, *10*(2), 10.
[http://dx.doi.org/10.1128/mBio.02175-18]

[20]   Lin, S.C.; Chen, M.C.; Liu, S.; Callahan, V.M.; Bracci, N.R.; Lehman, C.W.; Dahal, B.; de la Fuente, C.L.; Lin, C.C.; Wang, T.T.; Kehn-Hall, K. Phloretin inhibits Zika virus infection by interfering with cellular glucose utilisation. *Int. J. Antimicrob. Agents,* **2019**, *54*(1), 80-84.
[http://dx.doi.org/10.1016/j.ijantimicag.2019.03.017] [PMID: 30930299]

[21]   Spivack, J.G.; Prusoff, W.H.; Tritton, T.R. A study of the antiviral mechanism of action of 2-deoxy-d-glucose: Normally glycosylated proteins are not strictly required for herpes simplex virus attachment but increase viral penetration and infectivity. *Virology,* **1982**, *123*(1), 123-138.
[http://dx.doi.org/10.1016/0042-6822(82)90300-2] [PMID: 6293188]

[22]   Pang, H.; Jiang, Y.; Li, J.; Wang, Y.; Nie, M.; Xiao, N.; Wang, S.; Song, Z.; Ji, F.; Chang, Y.; Zheng, Y.; Yao, K.; Yao, L.; Li, S.; Li, P.; Song, L.; Lan, X.; Xu, Z.; Hu, Z. Aberrant NAD$^+$ metabolism underlies Zika virus–induced microcephaly. *Nat. Metab.,* **2021**, *3*(8), 1109-1124.
[http://dx.doi.org/10.1038/s42255-021-00437-0] [PMID: 34385701]

[23]   Shawa, I.T. Hepatitis B and C viruses. In: *Hepatitis B and C*; IntechOpen, **2019**.
[http://dx.doi.org/10.5772/intechopen.82772]

[24]   Masson, J.J.R.; Billings, H.W.W.; Palmer, C.S. Metabolic reprogramming during hepatitis B disease progression offers novel diagnostic and therapeutic opportunities. *Antivir. Chem. Chemother.,* **2017**, *25*(2), 53-57.
[http://dx.doi.org/10.1177/2040206617701372] [PMID: 28768434]

[25]   Wu, Y.H.; Yang, Y.; Chen, C.H.; Hsiao, C.J.; Li, T.N.; Liao, K.J.; Watashi, K.; Chen, B.S.; Wang, L.H.C. Aerobic glycolysis supports hepatitis B virus protein synthesis through interaction between viral surface antigen and pyruvate kinase isoform M2. *PLoS Pathog.,* **2021**, *17*(3), e1008866.
[http://dx.doi.org/10.1371/journal.ppat.1008866] [PMID: 33720996]

[26]   Liang, T.J.; Hepatitis, B. Hepatitis B: The virus and disease. *Hepatology,* **2009**, *49*(S5) Suppl., S13-S21.

[http://dx.doi.org/10.1002/hep.22881] [PMID: 19399811]

[27] Tayyar, R.; Ho, D. Herpes simplex virus and varicella zoster virus infections in cancer patients. *Viruses,* **2023**, *15*(2), 439.
[http://dx.doi.org/10.3390/v15020439]

[28] Zhu, S.; Viejo-Borbolla, A. Pathogenesis and virulence of herpes simplex virus. *Virulence,* **2021**, *12*(1), 2670-2702.
[http://dx.doi.org/10.1080/21505594.2021.1982373] [PMID: 34676800]

[29] Tsurumi, T.; Lehman, I.R. Release of RNA polymerase from vero cell mitochondria after herpes simplex virus type 1 infection. *J. Virol.,* **1990**, *64*(1), 450-452.
[http://dx.doi.org/10.1128/jvi.64.1.450-452.1990] [PMID: 2152832]

[30] Ray, E.; Halpern, B.L.; Levitan, D.B.; Blough, H. A new approach to viral chemotherapy. Inhibitors of glycoprotein synthesis. *Lancet,* **1974**, *304*(7882), 680-683.
[http://dx.doi.org/10.1016/S0140-6736(74)93261-9] [PMID: 4142959]

[31] Blough, H.A.; Giuntoli, R.L. Successful treatment of human genital herpes infections with 2-deoxy-D-glucose. *JAMA,* **1979**, *241*(26), 2798-2801.
[http://dx.doi.org/10.1001/jama.1979.03290520022018] [PMID: 221691]

[32] Mohanty, S.B.; Rockemann, D.D.; Tripathy, R.N. Chemotherapeutic value of 2-deoxy-D-glucose in infectious bovine rhinotracheitis viral infection in calves. *Am. J. Vet. Res.,* **1980**, *41*(7), 1049-1051.
[PMID: 6254407]

[33] Zheng, H.H.; Fu, P.F.; Chen, H.Y.; Wang, Z.Y. Pseudorabies virus: from pathogenesis to prevention strategies. *Viruses,* **2022**, *14*(8), 1638.
[http://dx.doi.org/10.3390/v14081638] [PMID: 36016260]

[34] Ludwig, H.; Rott, R. Effect of 2-deoxy-D-glucose on herpesvirus-induced inhibition of cellular DNA synthesis. *J. Virol.,* **1975**, *16*(2), 217-221.
[http://dx.doi.org/10.1128/jvi.16.2.217-221.1975] [PMID: 168399]

[35] Subak-Sharpe, J.H.; Dargan, D.J. HSV molecular biology: general aspects of herpes simplex virus molecular biology. *Virus Genes,* **1998**, *16*(3), 239-251.
[http://dx.doi.org/10.1023/A:1008068902673] [PMID: 9654678]

[36] https://www.who.int/news-room/fact-sheets/detail/herpes-simplex-virus

[37] Varanasi, S.K.; Donohoe, D.; Jaggi, U.; Rouse, B.T. Manipulating glucose metabolism during different stages of viral pathogenesis can have either detrimental or beneficial effects. *J. Immunol.,* **2017**, *199*(5), 1748-1761.
[http://dx.doi.org/10.4049/jimmunol.1700472] [PMID: 28768727]

[38] Shannon, W.M.; Arnett, G.; Drennen, D.J. Lack of efficacy of 2-deoxy-D-glucose in the treatment of experimental herpes genitalis in guinea pigs. *Antimicrob. Agents Chemother.,* **1982**, *21*(3), 513-515.
[http://dx.doi.org/10.1128/AAC.21.3.513] [PMID: 7201777]

[39] Knowles, R.W.; Person, S. Effects of 2-deoxyglucose, glucosamine, and mannose on cell fusion and the glycoproteins of herpes simplex virus. *J. Virol.,* **1976**, *18*(2), 644-651.
[http://dx.doi.org/10.1128/jvi.18.2.644-651.1976] [PMID: 178901]

[40] Kang, H.T.; Ju, J.W.; Cho, J.W.; Hwang, E.S. Down-regulation of Sp1 activity through modulation of O-glycosylation by treatment with a low glucose mimetic, 2-deoxyglucose. *J. Biol. Chem.,* **2003**, *278*(51), 51223-51231.
[http://dx.doi.org/10.1074/jbc.M307332200] [PMID: 14532290]

[41] Gualdoni, G.A.; Mayer, K.A.; Kapsch, A.M.; Kreuzberg, K.; Puck, A.; Kienzl, P.; Oberndorfer, F.; Frühwirth, K.; Winkler, S.; Blaas, D.; Zlabinger, G.J.; Stöckl, J. Rhinovirus induces an anabolic reprogramming in host cell metabolism essential for viral replication. *Proc. Natl. Acad. Sci. USA,* **2018**, *115*(30), E7158-E7165.
[http://dx.doi.org/10.1073/pnas.1800525115] [PMID: 29987044]

[42]   Garoff, H.; Wilschut, J.; Liljeström, P.; Wahlberg, J.M.; Bron, R.; Suomalainen, M.; Smyth, J.; Salminen, A.; Barth, B.U.; Zhao, H.; Forsell, K.; Ekström, M. Assembly and entry mechamisms of semliki forest virus. In: *Positive-Strand RNA Viruses*; Springer Vienna: Vienna, **1994**; pp. 329-338.
         [http://dx.doi.org/10.1007/978-3-7091-9326-6_33]

[43]   Gylfe, Å.; Ribers, Å.; Forsman, O.; Bucht, G.; Alenius, G.M.; Wållberg-Jonsson, S.; Ahlm, C.; Evander, M. Mosquitoborne sindbis virus infection and long-term illness. *Emerg. Infect. Dis.,* **2018**, *24*(6), 1141-1142.
         [http://dx.doi.org/10.3201/eid2406.170892] [PMID: 29781426]

[44]   Lebow, J.L. Family in the Age of COVID-19. *Fam. Process,* **2020**, *59*(2), 309-312.
         [http://dx.doi.org/10.1111/famp.12543] [PMID: 32412686]

[45]   dos Santos, W.G. Natural history of COVID-19 and current knowledge on treatment therapeutic options. *Biomed. Pharmacother.,* **2020**, *129*, 110493.
         [http://dx.doi.org/10.1016/j.biopha.2020.110493] [PMID: 32768971]

[46]   Kahn, J.S.; McIntosh, K. History and recent advances in coronavirus discovery. *Pediatr. Infect. Dis. J.,* **2005**, *24*(11) Suppl., S223-S227.
         [http://dx.doi.org/10.1097/01.inf.0000188166.17324.60] [PMID: 16378050]

[47]   Zhang, R.; Li, Y.; Zhang, A.L.; Wang, Y.; Molina, M.J. Identifying airborne transmission as the dominant route for the spread of COVID-19. *Proc. Natl. Acad. Sci. USA,* **2020**, *117*(26), 14857-14863.
         [http://dx.doi.org/10.1073/pnas.2009637117] [PMID: 32527856]

[48]   https://www.thelancet.com/journals/lancet/article/PIIS0140-6736(20)30211-7/fulltext

[49]   Goudouris, E.S. Laboratory diagnosis of COVID-19. *J. Pediatr. (Rio J.),* **2021**, *97*(1), 7-12.
         [http://dx.doi.org/10.1016/j.jped.2020.08.001] [PMID: 32882235]

[50]   Banerjee, P.; Sarma, I.D.; Sekhar, D.H.; Brahma, D.K.; Surong, M. 2-Deoxy-D-Glucose: A ray of hope in COVID pandemic. *J. Pharmacol. Pharmacother.,* **2021**, *12*(3), 107-109.
         [http://dx.doi.org/10.4103/jpp.jpp_69_21]

[51]   Sahu, K.; Kumar, R. Role of 2-Deoxy-D-Glucose (2-DG) in COVID-19 disease: A potential game-changer. *J. Family Med. Prim. Care,* **2021**, *10*(10), 3548-3552.
         [http://dx.doi.org/10.4103/jfmpc.jfmpc_1338_21] [PMID: 34934645]

[52]   Sahu, K.K.; Pal, R.K.; Naik, G.; Rathore, V.; Kumar, R. Comparison between two different successful approaches to COVID-19 pandemic in India (Dharavi *versus* Kerala). *J. Family Med. Prim. Care,* **2020**, *9*(12), 5827-5832.
         [http://dx.doi.org/10.4103/jfmpc.jfmpc_1860_20] [PMID: 33681002]

[53]   Kossoff, E.H.; Zupec-Kania, B.A.; Auvin, S.; Ballaban-Gil, K.R.; Christina Bergqvist, A.G.; Blackford, R.; Buchhalter, J.R.; Caraballo, R.H.; Cross, J.H.; Dahlin, M.G.; Donner, E.J.; Guzel, O.; Jehle, R.S.; Klepper, J.; Kang, H-C.; Lambrechts, D.A.; Liu, Y.M.C.; Nathan, J.K.; Nordli, D.R., Jr; Pfeifer, H.H.; Rho, J.M.; Scheffer, I.E.; Sharma, S.; Stafstrom, C.E.; Thiele, E.A.; Turner, Z.; Vaccarezza, M.M.; van der Louw, E.J.T.M.; Veggiotti, P.; Wheless, J.W.; Wirrell, E.C. Optimal clinical management of children receiving dietary therapies for epilepsy: Updated recommendations of the International Ketogenic Diet Study Group. *Epilepsia Open,* **2018**, *3*(2), 175-192.
         [http://dx.doi.org/10.1002/epi4.12225]

[54]   Codo, A.C.; Davanzo, G.G.; Monteiro, L.B.; de Souza, G.F.; Muraro, S.P.; Virgilio-da-Silva, J.V.; Prodonoff, J.S.; Carregari, V.C.; de Biagi Junior, C.A.O.; Crunfli, F.; Jimenez Restrepo, J.L.; Vendramini, P.H.; Reis-de-Oliveira, G.; Bispo dos Santos, K.; Toledo-Teixeira, D.A.; Parise, P.L.; Martini, M.C.; Marques, R.E.; Carmo, H.R.; Borin, A.; Coimbra, L.D.; Boldrini, V.O.; Brunetti, N.S.; Vieira, A.S.; Mansour, E.; Ulaf, R.G.; Bernardes, A.F.; Nunes, T.A.; Ribeiro, L.C.; Palma, A.C.; Agrela, M.V.; Moretti, M.L.; Sposito, A.C.; Pereira, F.B.; Velloso, L.A.; Vinolo, M.A.R.; Damasio, A.; Proença-Módena, J.L.; Carvalho, R.F.; Mori, M.A.; Martins-de-Souza, D.; Nakaya, H.I.; Farias, A.S.; Moraes-Vieira, P.M. Elevated glucose levels favor sars-cov-2 infection and monocyte response through a HIF-1α/Glycolysis-dependent axis. *Cell Metab.,* **2020**, *32*(3), 437-446.e5.

[http://dx.doi.org/10.1016/j.cmet.2020.07.007] [PMID: 32697943]

[55]   Huang, H.; Fan, C.; Li, M.; Nie, H.L.; Wang, F.B.; Wang, H.; Wang, R.; Xia, J.; Zheng, X.; Zuo, X.; Huang, J. COVID-19: A call for physical scientists and engineers. *ACS Nano,* **2020**, *14*(4), 3747-3754.
[http://dx.doi.org/10.1021/acsnano.0c02618] [PMID: 32267678]

[56]   Wigginton, K.R.; Pecson, B.M.; Sigstam, T.; Bosshard, F.; Kohn, T. Virus inactivation mechanisms: impact of disinfectants on virus function and structural integrity. *Environ. Sci. Technol.,* **2012**, *46*(21), 12069-12078.
[http://dx.doi.org/10.1021/es3029473] [PMID: 23098102]

[57]   Sanchez, W.Y.; McGee, S.L.; Connor, T.; Mottram, B.; Wilkinson, A.; Whitehead, J.P.; Vuckovic, S.; Catley, L. Dichloroacetate inhibits aerobic glycolysis in multiple myeloma cells and increases sensitivity to bortezomib. *Br. J. Cancer,* **2013**, *108*(8), 1624-1633.
[http://dx.doi.org/10.1038/bjc.2013.120] [PMID: 23531700]

[58]   Ruiz-Hitzky, E.; Darder, M.; Wicklein, B.; Ruiz-Garcia, C.; Martín-Sampedro, R.; del Real, G.; Aranda, P. Nanotechnology responses to COVID-19. *Adv. Healthc. Mater.,* **2020**, *9*(19), 2000979.
[http://dx.doi.org/10.1002/adhm.202000979] [PMID: 32885616]

[59]   Kramer, P.A.; Ravi, S.; Chacko, B.; Johnson, M.S.; Darley-Usmar, V.M. A review of the mitochondrial and glycolytic metabolism in human platelets and leukocytes: Implications for their use as bioenergetic biomarkers. *Redox Biol.,* **2014**, *2*, 206-210.
[http://dx.doi.org/10.1016/j.redox.2013.12.026] [PMID: 24494194]

[60]   Icard, P.; Lincet, H.; Wu, Z.; Coquerel, A.; Forgez, P.; Alifano, M.; Fournel, L. The key role of Warburg effect in SARS-CoV-2 replication and associated inflammatory response. *Biochimie,* **2021**, *180*, 169-177.
[http://dx.doi.org/10.1016/j.biochi.2020.11.010] [PMID: 33189832]

[61]   Mangge, H.; Herrmann, M.; Meinitzer, A.; Pailer, S.; Curcic, P.; Sloup, Z.; Holter, M.; Prüller, F. Increased kynurenine indicates a fatal course of COVID-19. *Antioxidants,* **2021**, *10*(12), 1960.
[http://dx.doi.org/10.3390/antiox10121960] [PMID: 34943063]

[62]   Ajaz, S.; McPhail, M.J.; Singh, K.K.; Mujib, S.; Trovato, F.M.; Napoli, S.; Agarwal, K. Mitochondrial metabolic manipulation by SARS-CoV-2 in peripheral blood mononuclear cells of patients with COVID-19. *Am. J. Physiol. Cell Physiol.,* **2021**, *320*(1), C57-C65.
[http://dx.doi.org/10.1152/ajpcell.00426.2020] [PMID: 33151090]

[63]   Malgotra, V.; Sharma, V. *2-Deoxy-d-Glucose inhibits replication of novel coronavirus (SARS-CoV-2) with adverse effects on host cell metabolism*; preprint; medicine & pharmacology **2021**.
[http://dx.doi.org/10.20944/preprints202106.0333.v1]

[64]   Huang, Y.; Chen, S.; Yang, Z.; Guan, W.; Liu, D.; Lin, Z.; Zhang, Y.; Xu, Z.; Liu, X.; Li, Y. SARS-CoV-2 viral load in clinical samples from critically ill patients. *Am. J. Respir. Crit. Care Med.,* **2020**, *201*(11), 1435-1438.
[http://dx.doi.org/10.1164/rccm.202003-0572LE] [PMID: 32293905]

[65]   Ling, Y.; Xu, S.B.; Lin, Y.X.; Tian, D.; Zhu, Z.Q.; Dai, F.H.; Wu, F.; Song, Z.G.; Huang, W.; Chen, J.; Hu, B.J.; Wang, S.; Mao, E.Q.; Zhu, L.; Zhang, W.H.; Lu, H.Z. Persistence and clearance of viral RNA in 2019 novel coronavirus disease rehabilitation patients. *Chin. Med. J. (Engl.),* **2020**, *133*(9), 1039-1043.
[http://dx.doi.org/10.1097/CM9.0000000000000774] [PMID: 32118639]

[66]   Wölfel, R.; Corman, V.M.; Guggemos, W.; Seilmaier, M.; Zange, S.; Müller, M.A.; Niemeyer, D.; Jones, T.C.; Vollmar, P.; Rothe, C.; Hoelscher, M.; Bleicker, T.; Brünink, S.; Schneider, J.; Ehmann, R.; Zwirglmaier, K.; Drosten, C.; Wendtner, C. Virological assessment of hospitalized patients with COVID-2019. *Nature,* **2020**, *581*(7809), 465-469.
[http://dx.doi.org/10.1038/s41586-020-2196-x] [PMID: 32235945]

[67]   Rubino, F.; Amiel, S.A.; Zimmet, P.; Alberti, G.; Bornstein, S.; Eckel, R.H.; Mingrone, G.; Boehm, B.; Cooper, M.E.; Chai, Z.; Del Prato, S.; Ji, L.; Hopkins, D.; Herman, W.H.; Khunti, K.; Mbanya,

J.C.; Renard, E. New-onset diabetes in Covid-19. *N. Engl. J. Med.,* **2020**, *383*(8), 789-790.
[http://dx.doi.org/10.1056/NEJMc2018688] [PMID: 32530585]

[68]   Reiterer, M.; Rajan, M.; Gómez-Banoy, N.; Lau, J.D.; Gomez-Escobar, L.G.; Gilani, A.; Alvarez-
       Mulett, S.; Sholle, E.T.; Chandar, V.; Bram, Y.; Hoffman, K.; Rubio-Navarro, A.; Uhl, S.; Shukla,
       A.P.; Goyal, P.; tenOever, B.R.; Alonso, L.C.; Schwartz, R.E.; Schenck, E.J.; Safford, M.M.; Lo, J.C.
       Hyperglycemia in acute COVID-19 is characterized by adipose tissue dysfunction and insulin
       resistance. *bioRxiv,* **2021**, 2021.03.21.21254072.

[69]   Xu, Z.; Liu, L.; Pan, X.; Wei, K.; Wei, M.; Liu, L.; Yang, H.; Liu, Q. Serum golgi protein 73 (GP73)
       is a diagnostic and prognostic marker of chronic HBV liver disease. *Medicine (Baltimore),* **2015**,
       94(12), e659.
       [http://dx.doi.org/10.1097/MD.0000000000000659] [PMID: 25816035]

[70]   Zhang, C.; Shi, L.; Wang, F.S. Liver injury in COVID-19: management and challenges. *Lancet
       Gastroenterol. Hepatol.,* **2020**, *5*(5), 428-430.
       [http://dx.doi.org/10.1016/S2468-1253(20)30057-1] [PMID: 32145190]

[71]   Rabbani, N.; Thornalley, P.J. Hexokinase-2 glycolytic overload in diabetes and ischemia–reperfusion
       injury. *Trends Endocrinol. Metab.,* **2019**, *30*(7), 419-431.
       [http://dx.doi.org/10.1016/j.tem.2019.04.011] [PMID: 31221272]

[72]   Bojkova, D.; Klann, K.; Koch, B.; Widera, M.; Krause, D.; Ciesek, S.; Cinatl, J.; Münch, C.
       Proteomics of SARS-CoV-2-infected host cells reveals therapy targets. *Nature,* **2020**, *583*(7816), 469-
       472.
       [http://dx.doi.org/10.1038/s41586-020-2332-7] [PMID: 32408336]

[73]   Karam, B.S.; Morris, R.S.; Bramante, C.T.; Puskarich, M.; Zolfaghari, E.J.; Lotfi-Emran, S.;
       Ingraham, N.E.; Charles, A.; Odde, D.J.; Tignanelli, C.J. mTOR inhibition in COVID-19: A
       commentary and review of efficacy in RNA viruses. *J. Med. Virol.,* **2021**, *93*(4), 1843-1846.
       [http://dx.doi.org/10.1002/jmv.26728] [PMID: 33314219]

[74]   Ghosh, B.; Roy, S.; Singh, J.K. The mode of therapeutic action of 2-deoxy d-glucose: anti- viral or
       glycolysis blocker? *ChemRxiv,* **2021**.
       [http://dx.doi.org/10.26434/chemrxiv-2021-2z6ln]

[75]   https://pib.gov.in/PressReleasePage.aspx?PRID=1717007

[76]   https://www.mohfw.gov.in/pdf/UpdatedDetailedClinicalManagementProtocolforCOVID19adultsdated
       24052021.pdf

[77]   Bhatt, A.N.; Shenoy, S.; Munjal, S.; Chinnadurai, V.; Agarwal, A.; Vinoth Kumar, A.; Shanavas, A.;
       Kanwar, R.; Chandna, S. 2-deoxy-d-glucose as an adjunct to standard of care in the medical
       management of COVID-19: a proof-of-concept and dose-ranging randomised phase II clinical trial.
       BMC Infect. Dis., **2022**, *22*(1), 669.
       [http://dx.doi.org/10.1186/s12879-022-07642-6] [PMID: 35927676]

[78]   https://pib.gov.in/pib.gov.in/Pressreleaseshare.aspx?PRID=1717007

[79]   Huang, Z.; Chavda, V.P.; Vora, L.K.; Gajjar, N.; Apostolopoulos, V.; Shah, N.; Chen, Z.S. 2-Deox-
       -D-Glucose and its derivatives for the COVID-19 treatment: an update. *Front. Pharmacol.,* **2022**, *13*,
       899633.
       [http://dx.doi.org/10.3389/fphar.2022.899633] [PMID: 35496298]

CHAPTER 8

Prospects for Cancer Diagnosis, Treatment, and Surveillance: [18F]FDG PET/CT and Innovative Molecular Imaging to Direct Immunotherapy in Cancer

Juhi Rais[1], **Manish Ora**[1] and **Manish Dixit**[1,*]

[1] *Department of Nuclear Medicine, Sanjay Gandhi Postgraduate Institute of Medical Sciences, Lucknow-226014, Uttar Pradesh, India*

Abstract: Positron Emission Tomography (PET), a noninvasive technique, is most suitable for quantitative evaluation of *in vivo* tumor biology. Based on its metabolic activity, the accumulation of F-18 fluorodeoxyglucose ([18F]FDG), a positron emitter radionuclide, is most explored indicative of tumor features. Quantitative evaluation of FDG uptake is frequently used for treatment monitoring following chemotherapy or chemoradiotherapy. Several investigations showed that FDG PET, which measures metabolic change, was a more sensitive marker than CT or MRI, which measures morphological change. [18F]FDG is now frequently used to assess tumor metabolism as well as to track the effectiveness of immunotherapy, which is a useful treatment for several malignancies. With the use of *in vivo* whole-body CD^{8+} T cell and PD-L1 expression imaging, for instance, radiopharmaceuticals that are novel in nature offer the rare chance to characterize the immunological tumor microenvironment (TME) and more accurately forecast which patients may react to therapy. Longitudinal molecular imaging may also aid in clarifying potent changes, especially in instances of resistance that occurred during immunotherapy, and aid in guiding a more individualized therapeutic strategy. To categorize, forecast, and track treatment response and molecular dynamics in areas of therapeutic need, this review focuses on new and existing uses of [18F]FDG for imaging.

Keywords: Checkpoint inhibitors, Immunotherapy, Positron emission tomography (PET), Tumor metabolism, [18F]FDG.

1. INTRODUCTION

An essential tool for detecting and treating cancer, the glucose analog PET radiotracer [18F]FDG detects glucose consumption [1, 2]. Modern clinical and

* **Corresponding author Manish Dixit:** Department of Nuclear Medicine, Sanjay Gandhi Postgraduate Institute of Medical Sciences, Lucknow-226014, Uttar Pradesh, India; E-mail: dixitm@sgpgi.ac.in

research applications encompass all major disciplines of human health, including neurology, cancer, cardiology, and infection/inflammatory diseases as hybrid PET/computed tomography (PET/CT) is commercially available. For instance, [^{18}F]FDG PET imaging is helpful in the early staging of lung, colorectal, and esophageal malignancies and in detecting recurrences [1]. Furthermore, preclinical and clinical research indicates that modifications in the amount of [^{18}F]FDG accumulated in tumors following specific treatments may be highly predictive and serve as an early biomarker of treatment effectiveness [3, 4]. The therapeutic efficacy of [^{18}F]FDG PET in the treatment of cancer has been established, and the metabolic process by which [^{18}F]FDG detects glucose consumption is well characterized. Nevertheless, there is still a dearth of comprehensive knowledge on the signaling pathways that govern glucose consumption and [^{18}F]FDG accumulation in cancer. By comprehending these signaling pathways, it may be possible to link the amount of [^{18}F]FDG accumulation to specific and potentially targetable changes in a given cancer type. This could also help identify additional therapies for which [^{18}F]FDG PET could be used as an early predictor of therapeutic efficacy.

The present scenario of [^{18}F]FDG PET/CT in systemic and tumoral immune response monitoring is the primary focus of this chapter. This review recognizes the limitations of morphological imaging in the systemic monitoring of immunotherapy response, with an elaboration of investigation of the incremental benefit of [^{18}F]FDG PET/CT as a molecular biomarker.

2. CURRENT STATUS OF [^{18}F]FDG AND ITS MECHANISM OF ACTION IN VARIOUS DISEASES

Positron emission tomography (PET) is used in conjunction with 2-deoxy-2-[^{18}F]fluoro-D-glucose ([^{18}F]FDG), a positron-emitting radiotracer, to diagnose and track a variety of disorders. Standard imaging technologies like CT, MRI, and X-rays enable very detailed observation of both healthy and unhealthy tissue. Functional imaging methods such as PET scans can be used in addition to structural modalities to address some of these shortcomings. [^{18}F]FDG is therefore a well-recognized biomarker with further advantages for a range of biological research.

2.1. Neurology

The FDA has authorized the use of FDG in neurology to locate aberrant glucose metabolism foci connected to epileptic seizure foci. Additionally, FDG can aid in the visualization of different brain regions for variations in glucose metabolism, which aids in the diagnosis of a variety of neurological disorders such as brain damage and other neurological disorders like dementia, Parkinson's disease, Alzheimer's disease, *etc* [5 - 7] (Fig. **1**).

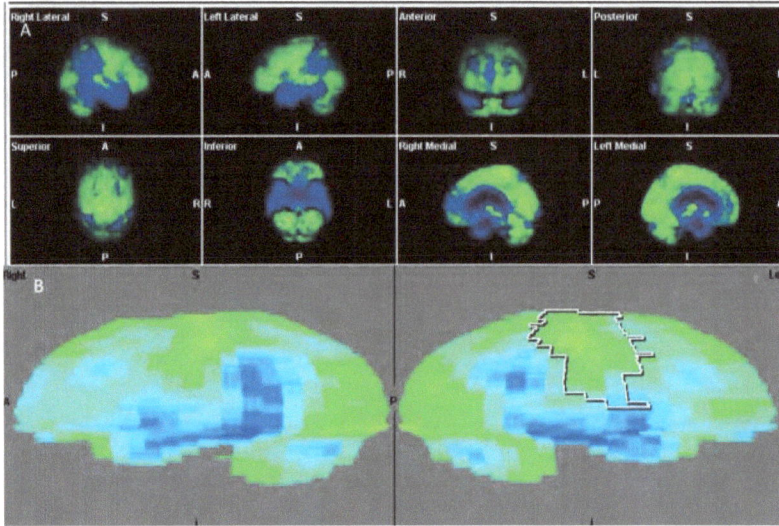

Fig. (1). 56 year male presented with progressive forgetfulness for 1 year. (**A**) Brain FDG PET/CT 3-D volumetric images revealed hypometabolism in the temporoparietal region. (**B**) SPM images revealed significant symmetrical hypometabolism in the temporoparietal region. The findings were consistent with Alzheimer's Disease.

The main fuel for the brain is glucose, which can help diagnose some pathologic disorders by showing differences in glucose usage from the normal metabolic rhythm and FDG can help in identifying the locations of seizure foci. FDG-PET can not only pinpoint the locations of seizure foci but also reveal details regarding the overall functional state of the brain [8].

2.2. Cardiology

When coupled with myocardial perfusion imaging, FDG shows which left ventricular myocardium has residual glucose metabolism and how much left ventricular dysfunction is present. The buildup of macrophages and myocardial ischemia that causes atherosclerosis can also be seen using FDG [9]. A heart that is in good health uses free fatty acids as its primary energy source, but anaerobic glucose metabolism replaces fatty acid metabolism in ischemia myocardial tissue. The myocardium that is hibernating among patients with coronary artery disease and left ventricular dysfunction is identified by FDG-PET in nuclear medicine when the patients are scheduled for coronary revascularization. The principle behind its use is that while myocytes that have suffered reversible injuries can utilize glucose, those that have suffered irreversible injuries cannot. Systolic function in the area with reduced perfusion can be reversed if blood flow is restored, as indicated by the accumulation of FDG in such places. A perfusion-metabolism mismatch is a term used to describe the observed pattern of reduced blood flow and higher glucose metabolism. Consequently, areas with scarring or irreversible loss of systolic function exhibit matching patterns of reduced FDG accumulation and decreased perfusion. In such patterns, the likelihood of functional return after revascularization is limited. With FDG uptake, myocardial perfusion is somewhat reduced by a non-transmural match pattern. It is a non-transmural scar that is unlikely to heal unless it is associated with reversibility caused by stress. Revascularization should not, however, be decided only on the basis of FDG-PET since effective coronary revascularization is necessary to restore systolic function [10]. The atherosclerotic arteries absorb FDG, and large vessels such as the aorta and other major arteries have a considerable presence within their intima. The uptake of FDG is caused by the macrophages in the atherosclerotic plaque having increased metabolic activity. PET allows visualization of smooth muscles in artery walls, which absorb FDG [11]. Fig. (2). shows hibernating myocardium in the LAD territory.

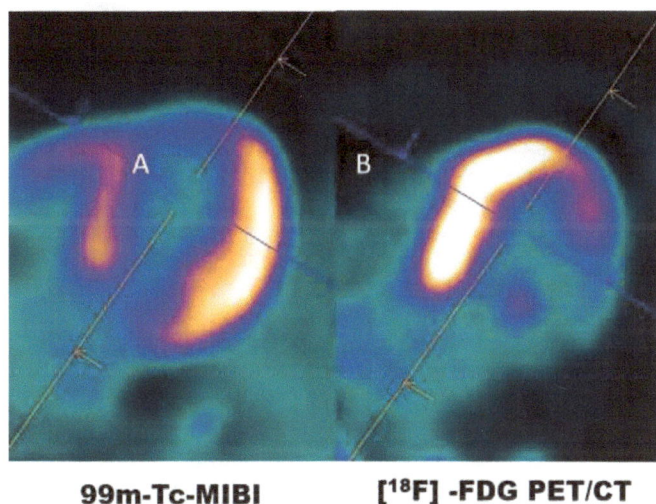

99m-Tc-MIBI   [18F] -FDG PET/CT

Fig. (2). A 48-year male presented with a sudden onset of chest pain and shortness of breath. The ECG was suggestive of Acute MI. ECHO revealed significant hypokinesia in the LAD territory. Angiography revealed a significant (~90%) lesion in the Left anterior descending artery (not shown). Rest perfusion study (**A**) revealed a large area of hypoperfusion in the LAD territory. Corresponding FDG image (**B**) shows preserved metabolism. The scan findings are suggestive of hibernating myocardium in the LAD territory.

2.3. Inflammatory Disorders

Orthopedic infections, autoimmune arteritis, rheumatologic disorders, osteomyelitis, ileitis, and vasculitis are among the inflammatory diseases for which FDG is clinically applied (Figs. **3 - 5**) [9, 12]. Because inflammatory cells have high rates of glycolysis thus FDG accumulates in these cells. FDG-PET is utilized to identify areas of inflammation and infection, especially orthopedic infections associated with implanted prostheses and osteomyelitis. In such complex and challenging clinical situations, FDG-PET is a valuable biomarker and is repeatedly used for study. Other inflammatory conditions such as sarcoidosis, vasculitis, rheumatologic disorders, and localized ileitis can also be detected using FDG-PET [12].

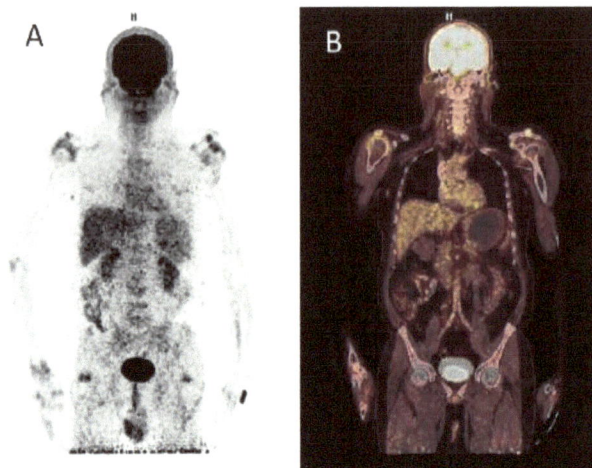

Fig. (3). A 49-year male presented with pyrexia of unknown origin since 10 weeks. **A-** MIP image of FDG PET/CT revealed symmetrical focal areas of increased uptake in the shoulder, wrist, hands, and hip joint region. Coronal Fused PET/CT images revealed increased uptake in the corresponding joints. Scan features were suggestive of inflammatory polyarthritis.

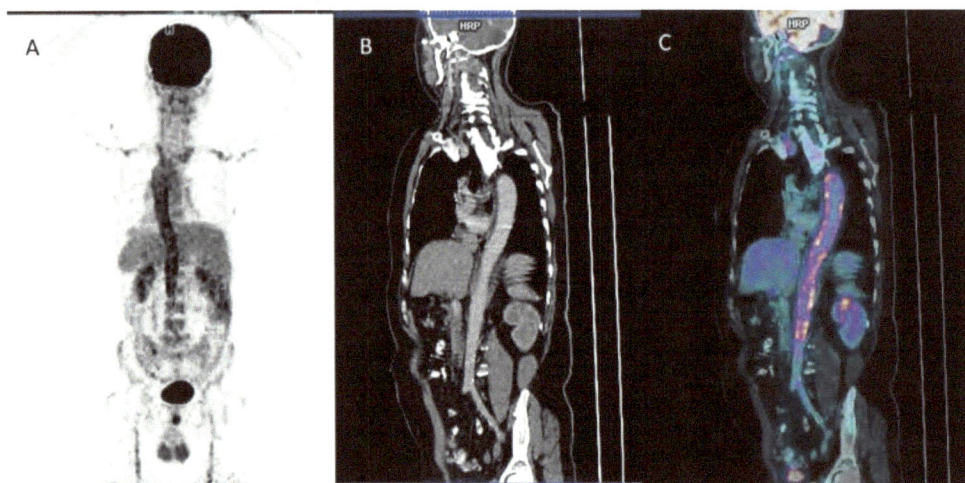

Fig. (4). A 29-year-old male presented with vague chest pain and weakness in both upper limbs. His ESR and CRP were raised. FDG PET/CT MIP (**A**) images show increased uptake along the arch of the aorta, thoracic aorta, and abdominal aorta. Increased uptake is also seen along both subclavian arteries. Sagittal curved reformatted CT and fused PET/CT images (**B** and **C**) reveal increased uptake in the walls of the vessels. Scan findings are suggestive of aortoarteritis.

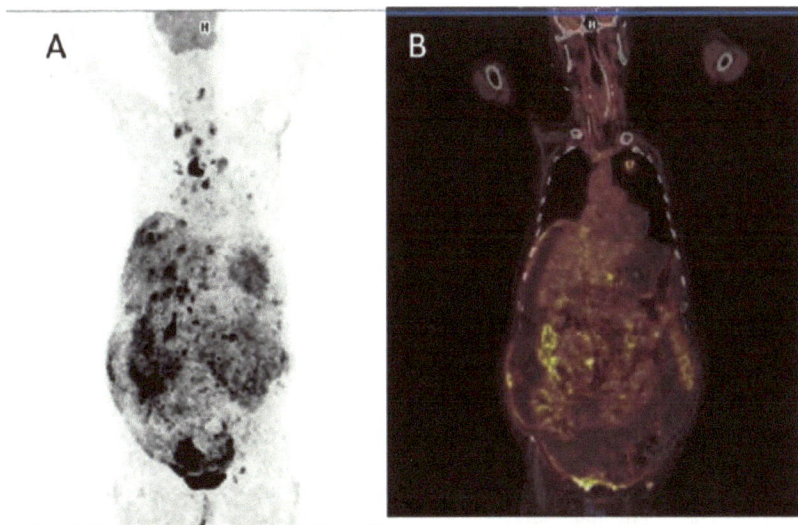

Fig. (5). A 69-year-old male presented with progressive abdominal distention and fever. Multiple Fluid cytology was negative for malignancy. An MIP image of FDG PET/CT revealed Diffuse increased uptake in the abdominal cavity and mediastinum. B Fused coronal PET/CT shows diffuse increased uptake in the peritoneum. FDG avid lesion is noted in the left lung. Biopsy from the mediastinal revealed tuberculosis.

2.4. Oncology

For the assessment, staging, and follow-up of cancer treatments for a variety of cancers, including lymphomas and colorectal cancer, as well as cancers of the breast, thyroid, esophagus, colon, malignant melanoma, and non-small cell lung cancer, FDG has FDA approval [13, 14]. FDG/PET is a useful diagnostic and therapeutic response monitoring tool in oncology because metabolic changes in neoplastic cells usually happen before an increase in tumor growth [15]. To produce phospholipids, triglycerides, cholesterol esters, and acylated proteins for rapid cell division, cancer cells require a high concentration of NADPH (Fig. **6**). The Warburg effect dictates that aerobic glycolysis must be activated in response to the elevated need for NADPH. The process of making lactate when oxygen is present and mitochondria are active is known as aerobic glycolysis.

Higher expression of hexokinases, decreased expression of glucose-6-phosphatase, and higher activity of glucose transporters all contribute to this process [16]. Malignant cells absorb FDG more readily, and the PET scan can identify this FDG buildup. Additionally, in patients who have received prior cerebral radiation therapy, FDG-PET can assist in the differentiation of radiation necrosis, edema, and tumor recurrence. Greater amounts of FDG are absorbed by tumors than by healthy tissue; it is absent in necrosis and reduced in edematous areas [17].

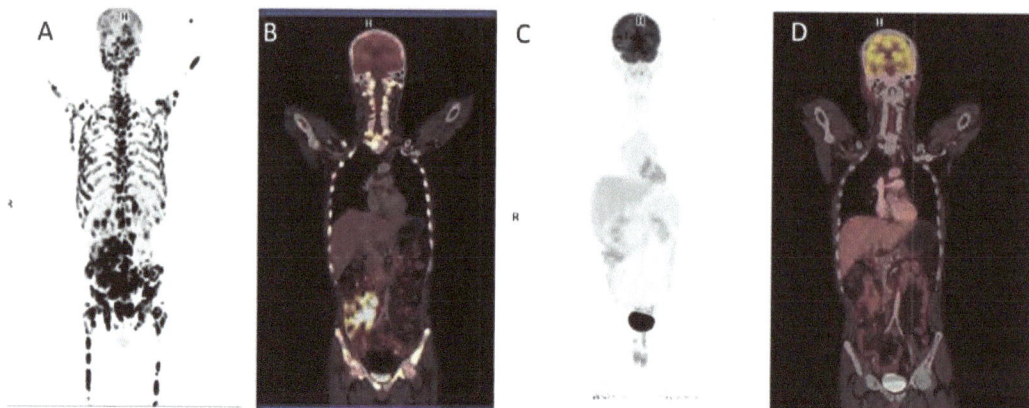

Fig. (6). A 28-year-old male presented with pancytopenia. Abdominal ultrasound revealed mesenteric lymphadenopathy. Bone marrow biopsy was suggestive of Burkitt's Lymphoma. (**A-B**) Baseline MIP and Coronal fused whole–body FDG PET-CT revealed extensive uptake in the visualized bone marrow. The patient received 3 cycles of chemotherapy. Interim PET/CT shows (**C-D**) complete resolution of the lesion-Complete metabolic response.

2.5. Planning and Treatment Strategy

A number of oncology therapy domains can benefit from the application of quantitative PET imaging [18]. First, the treatment plan is determined by the FDG PET scans, which represent the tumor's genetic and/or histological condition [19]. Secondly, because quantitative pictures frequently offer excellent tumor-to-background contrast, they are employed for more precise delineation of specific volumes in radiation planning [20]. Thirdly, response monitoring and therapy stratification can be achieved by using quantitative imaging to determine the optimal treatment mode and dosage [21, 22]. Fourthly, dose painting—a technique in which the radiation dosage is spatially distributed throughout the target volume—could be carried out using quantitative imaging based on the quantitative parameter maps [23]. It is possible to use quantitative assessment of aspects such as partial response, complete response, stable illness, and tumour progression to properly determine the impact of treatment [24]. For the following stage of therapy planning, appropriate treatment monitoring is essential (Fig. 7).

With long-lasting effects in conditions that were previously linked to a dismal prognosis, immunotherapy has drastically altered the landscape of cancer treatment. The number of clinical trials and the ensuing approval of anticancer immunotherapies have increased significantly [25]. Patient selection is one of the most difficult issues since there is a pressing unmet clinical demand for biomarkers that support tailored treatment approaches and inform medication development. Molecular imaging can provide non-invasive therapy by providing real-time information on an evolving immune microenvironment. Predictive biomarkers are a critical unmet therapeutic need, and patient selection is still tricky. [^{18}F]FDG PET/CT may help evaluate the response, classify patients for therapy, and identify and track immune-related toxicities due to the heterogeneity of immune response within lesions, which poses an additional hurdle.

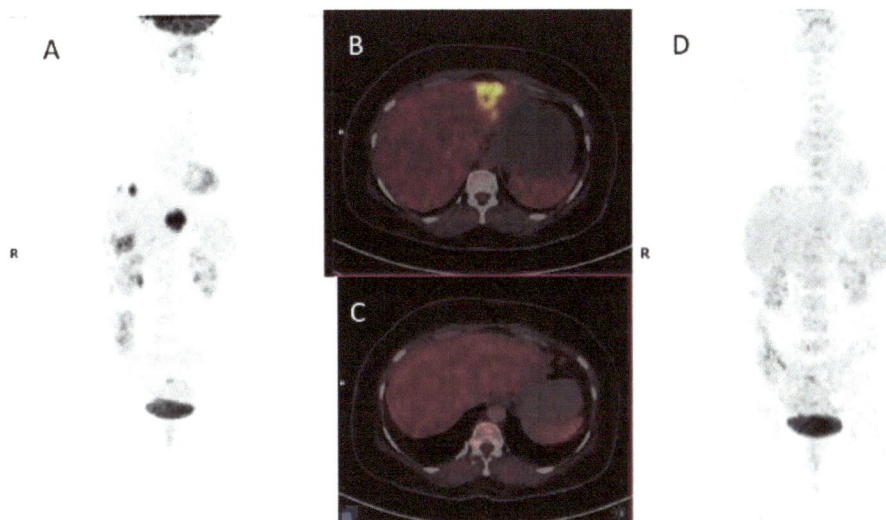

Fig. (7). A 52-year-old patient had a history of Carcinoma Left breast T2N1M0 in 2015. She underwent breast conservative surgery followed by chemotherapy, radiotherapy and trastuzumab. She presented with multiple liver lesions on FDG PET/CT (**A-B**). She was started on Lapatinib, which is a Dual tyrosine kinase inhibitor that interrupts HER2/neu and epidermal growth factor receptors. She had a complete metabolic response in the follow-up scan (**C-D**).

Although a small percentage of patients experience complete and lasting responses to conventional immunotherapy regimens, the majority of patients do not respond; hence, novel predictors of response and resistance mechanisms need to be developed. The limitations of standard response evaluation faced by unexpected reactions have been highlighted by numerous reclassifications of response criteria based on CT or MRI, as a result of strong data presented by large-scale clinical trials using morphologic imaging [26]. The total response of the immune system to therapy may be monitored noninvasively with molecular imaging. On the other hand, employing tracers targeted at cell-specific lineage targets or activation indicators may enhance our comprehension of the immune system. Although there are obstacles, the utility of [^{18}F]FDG PET/CT, which is generally available globally, is being further defined and improved.

3. BIOCHEMISTRY OF ACCUMULATION OF [^{18}F]FDG

Facilitated glucose transporters (GLUTs) carry [^{18}F] FDG across the cell membrane, at which point hexokinase enzymes phosphorylate it to form [^{18}F] FDG-6-phosphate [27]. Glucose transporters and related substances are the 14 isoforms that comprise the broad family of transporters known as GLUTs [28]. GLUT1 and GLUT3, which are extensively expressed in a range of malignancies, are the primary transporters of [^{18}F] FDG in most cancer cell types. [29]. Although it is unclear how exactly these transporters contribute to glucose flow in cancer as for sodium-dependent glucose transporters, [^{18}F] FDG is not a substrate [30]. Four distinct hexokinases are expressed by cells [31]. The majority of cancer cells express hexokinase 1 (HK1) and hexokinase 2 (HK2), either singly or in combination, and are thought to be the primary enzymes responsible for phosphorylating [^{18}F]FDG to [^{18}F]FDG-6-phosphate in cancer cells [31]. GLUTs can carry [^{18}F]FDG-6-phosphate outside of the cell after dephosphorylation by glucose-6-phosphatase [32].

It is likely context-dependent whether these metabolic processes are the primary cause of [^{18}F]FDG accumulation, and tumors that accumulate high levels of [^{18}F]FDG frequently have increased levels of GLUTs, glucose-6-phosphatase, or hexokinase enzymes. For instance, in non-small cell lung cancer, the levels of GLUT1 and GLUT3 exhibit a stronger correlation with [^{18}F] FDG accumulation than do the levels of HK1 and HK2 [33]. HK2 levels correlate with [^{18}F]FDG accumulation in pheochromocytomas and paragangliomas more strongly than GLUT1 or GLUT3 levels [34]. Both gastric and breast tumors have varied [^{18}F] FDG accumulation, and GLUT1 levels are correlated with [^{18}F]FDG accumulation in both cases [35, 36]. In low-grade hepatocellular carcinoma tumors, low [^{18}F] FDG accumulation is linked to high glucose-6-phosphatase activity and low hexokinase activity [37] (Fig. **8**).

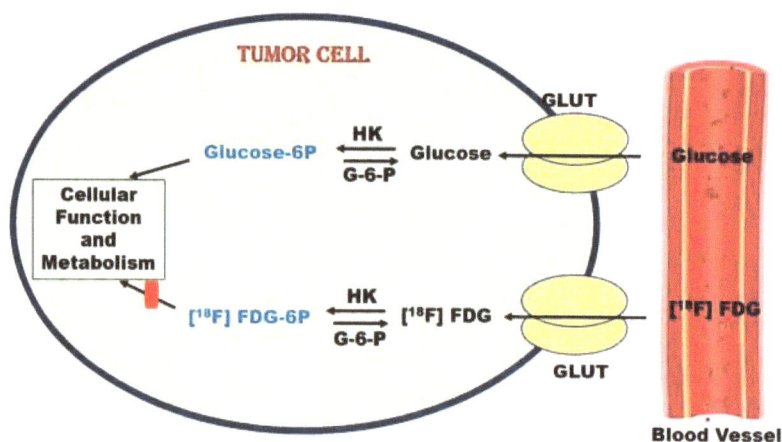

Fig. (8). Glucose and [^{18}F]FDG Metabolism and Cellular Uptake. Both enter the cells through the glucose transporter membrane proteins. After entering the cell, both are phosphorylated by hexokinase (HK), which can be reversed if glucose-6-phosphatase (G-6-P) is present. The cell can continue to metabolize phosphorylated glucose (Glucose-6 P), but phosphorylated [^{18}F]FDG ([^{18}F]FDG -6 P) is "trapped" because it cannot be further metabolized.

4. THE SIGNALING PATHWAYS AND [¹⁸F]FDG ACCUMULATION IN CANCER CELLS

There are numerous established techniques for calculating the amount of glucose consumed, such as monitoring the levels of 2-DG-6-phosphate in cells treated with 2-DG, the radioactivity accumulated in cells treated with a radiolabeled glucose analog, or the variations in glucose concentrations in cell culture media [38]. Most studies have discovered signaling mechanisms that control the transcriptional and posttranslational levels of GLUT proteins and hexokinase enzymes, hence regulating glucose consumption and [¹⁸F]FDG accumulation.

Novel transcriptional regulators of GLUT1 and GLUT3 are diverse and complex to classify. The transcription factors p63 and SOX2 stimulate glucose intake in squamous cell carcinoma cell lines by attaching to an enhancer region of the GLUT1 gene and promoting the production of GLUT1 messenger RNA (mRNA) and protein [39]. In melanoma cells, lysine methyl transferase KMT2D loss-of-function mutants upregulate the expression of GLUT1 and HK1 mRNA while downregulating the expression of IGFBP5, a negative regulator of insulin signaling [40]. Pax5 and IKZF1 act as tumor suppressors in pre-B-cell acute lymphoblastic leukemia by downregulating the amounts of GLUT1 and HK2 mRNA. [41]. When breast and colorectal cancer cells divide, the protein kinase SGK1 enhances the synthesis of GLUT1 mRNA, increasing the amount of GLUT1 protein and glucose uptake [42]. The transmembrane mucin glycoprotein MUC13 activates nuclear factor-kB in pancreatic cancer, which raises glucose intake and GLUT1 mRNA expression [43]. Over the past five years, research has focused on the transcription factor c-Myc's function in controlling the amounts of HK2 mRNA, which highlights its continued significance in controlling glucose consumption. On the other hand, serotonin stimulates the uptake of glucose by pancreatic cancer cells through binding to its receptor HTR2B, raising HIF1a and c-Myc protein levels, and elevating HK2 mRNA expression [44]. In lymphoma cell lines, inhibition of mTOR and c-Myc reduces glucose consumption, lowers GLUT1 mRNA levels, and raises glucose-6-phosphatase mRNA levels [45]. Gremlin-1 increases the amount of HK2 mRNA in breast cancer cells by triggering the reactive oxygen species–PKB (Akt)–STAT3 pathway [46]. miR-34c-3p inhibits guanylate kinase MAGI3 to increase glucose consumption in hepatocellular carcinoma cell lines, MAGI3 suppresses the transcriptional activity of b-catenin, and a reduction in MAGI3 levels raises the levels of HK2 mRNA and glucose consumption [47].

Studies that have identified extra regulators of TXNIP levels have confirmed the importance of TXNIP in controlling glucose consumption *i.e.*, higher glucose intake and higher GLUT1 at the plasma membrane are caused by lower TXNIP levels [48]. In non-small cell lung cancer cell lines, PI3K/Akt signaling promotes glucose intake and lowers TXNIP expression. Growth factors cause PI3K/Akt signaling to be activated in a hepatocellular carcinoma cell line, which phosphorylates TXNIP and reduces its association with GLUT1 to cause fast glucose uptake [49, 50]. In a range of cancer cell lines, lowering hyaluronan levels triggers receptor tyrosine kinase signaling, which causes the zinc finger protein ZNF36 to be induced and breaks down TXNIP mRNA [51]. Furthermore, ZNF36 binds to and aids in the degradation of HK2 mRNA [52], indicating that ZNF36 may control glucose consumption *via* various pathways. By decreasing the amounts of 6-phosphogluconate, the substrate of phosphogluconate dehydrogenase, the metabolic enzyme increases glucose consumption in metastatic pancreatic cancer cells.

5. IMMUNE CYCLE OF CANCER IN BRIEF

The process by which immune stimulatory substances result in immune activation, cancer cell detection, and eradication is referred to as the "cancer immunity cycle" [53]. Co-inhibitory signals enable self-tolerance by reducing the immunological response.

Neoantigens created by cancer cells or discharged into the Tumor Microenvironment (TME) upon cancer cell death serve as immunogenic signatures. T cell activation is moderated by co-inhibitory molecule expression on the surface of dendritic cells, such as CD80, CD86, programmed death-ligand 1 (PD-L1), and/or programmed death-ligand-2. After becoming activated, CD^{8+} T cells upregulate chemokine receptors, which leads to their migration into the TME, where they infiltrate and initiate a cytotoxic response [54]. Even though the cytotoxic immune response can be very successful, the immunological TME may become dysfunctional due to increased activation of regulatory T cells and upregulation of co-inhibitory molecules, such as PD-L1, CD80, and/or CD86, and cytokines [55]. Similar to dendritic cells, tumor cells can interact with T cells by producing co-inhibitory signals that cause the function of cytotoxic effector T cells to be downregulated or "switched off." Cancer, therefore, takes advantage of the delicate balance between immune costimulatory and co-inhibitory processes that preserve self-tolerance as a crucial strategy for immune resistance, subversion, and cancer cell survival [56, 57].

In nuclear medicine imaging, the primary PET radiotracer is [^{18}F]FDG, which investigates glucose metabolism. Nevertheless, [^{18}F]FDG targets immune cells as well as malignant cells. Immunotherapy induces an inflammatory response, which makes it challenging to distinguish between [^{18}F]FDG uptakes caused by inflammation and those associated with tumor cells. To go beyond this restriction, it can be helpful to comprehend the workings of immune checkpoint inhibitors (ICI) to find possible novel targets for nuclear medicine imaging [58].

6.   [^{18}F]FDGPET/CT   AND   ITS   STANDARD   THERAPEUTIC ASSESSMENT SCALES

[^{18}F]FDG PET/CT is a commonly used modality for evaluating malignancies for treatment. However, because this radiotracer exhibits an uptake in both the case of active cancer and inflammation, ICIs, which treat cancer by producing inflammation, raise doubts about its interpretation and the timing of execution [58]. Analogous difficulties are noted for anatomical pictures. The morphological imaging method for assessing the therapeutic effectiveness of cytotoxic chemotherapy is based on the finding that lesions that worsen with time or that develop new lesions after treatment are signs of a failed treatment [59]. Many criteria are available for evaluating a therapy for morphological imaging, including Response Evaluation Criteria in Solid Tumors (RECIST) 1.1, which employs single-diameter measurements that are unidimensional [60]. Comparing functional imaging to morphological imaging, such as CT, allows for an earlier assessment of response, as demonstrated by [^{18}F]FDG PET/CT. Functional imaging utilizing [^{18}F]FDG PET may offer a treatment assessment significantly earlier than morphological imaging in the case of gastrointestinal stromal tumors (GISTs) treated with imatinib. Anatomical responses can be predicted by [^{18}F]FDG PET in a matter of days to a week, but morphological imaging (CT) often requires several months to measure [61].

7. [^{18}F]FDG PET/CT FOR IMMUNOTHERAPY AGAINST CANCER

The multifunctional PET/CT radiotracer [^{18}F]FDG is used to study glucose metabolism, including tumor metabolism and inflammation. It is a well-respected nuclear medicine test used to investigate cancer, particularly for the extension assessment [62]. Apart from evaluating the extension, another important statistic to take into account may be the baseline [^{18}F]FDG total metabolic tumor volume (TMTV), which is acquired by segmenting every tumor on PET imaging. This is because of its semi-automated determination and strong prognostic value for a range of malignancies and treatments, including immunotherapy (Fig. 9). As a result, patients with high TMTV (10.8 months, 95% CI 5.9–15.8 months) had a significantly lower median overall survival (OS) than patients with low TMTV (26.0 months, 95% CI 3.0–49.2 months) in a trial by Ito *et al.* of 142 melanoma patients taking ipilimumab [60]. Comparable outcomes have been noted for ICI-treated non-small cell lung cancer (NSCLC) [63]. In addition to its utility in the preliminary extension evaluation, [^{18}F]FDG PET may also help assess the PD-1/PD-L1 status, which is a factor in the immunotherapy response. In tumor cells,

PD-L1 effectively stimulates glycolytic metabolism, and tumor glucose consumption metabolically limits T lymphocytes, primarily by decreasing their glycolytic potential [64].

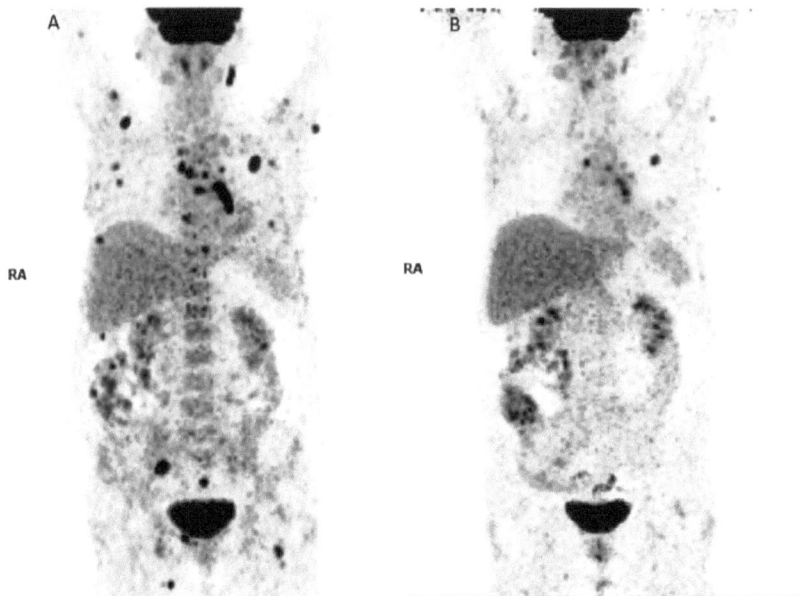

Fig. (9). A 63-year-old female presented with recurrent carcinoma breast after 4 years of initial management. Her FDG PET/CT MIP image reveals extensive skeletal metastases. She was started on Palbocilib, which is an inhibitor of CDK4 and CDK6. She had a partial metabolic response to the therapy (B).

Strong correlations were observed between the expression of PD-L1 protein and glucose transporter 1 (GLUT1), the latter of which is in charge of transporting [^{18}F]FDG in lung adenocarcinomas [65, 66] and squamous-cell carcinomas [67]. In a meta-analysis of three studies (718 patients), the maximum standardized uptake value (SUVmax) of [^{18}F]FDG PET reflecting tumor activity and PD-L1 expression revealed a weak correlation related to lung cancer; however, this low value precludes the SUVmax from being used as a stand-in for the PDL1 status in lung cancer [68]. Furthermore, a study including 63 patients discovered that the SUVmax values of bladder cancer patients who were tested positive for PD-1/PD-L1 were significantly greater. Furthermore, the study found that a cut-off value of 22.7 could be used to predict the presence of PD-1 and PD-L1 with accuracies of 71.4% and 77.8%, respectively [69]. It should be noted that, when immune-checkpoint inhibitors are taken into account, [^{18}F]FDG SUV has a substantial correlation not only with PD-1/PD-L1 status but also with other biomarkers of relevance, such as CD8$^+$tumor infiltration by lymphocytes (TILs) [70]. Moreover, [^{18}F]FDG PET/CT may be utilized to identify indirect predictors of immunotherapy treatment response. This suggests that the gut microbiota, whose analysis could help forecast the effect of immunotherapy treatment, may be reflected in this study, as the gut microbiota seems linked to the therapeutic response [71].

A retrospective pilot study involving 14 patients with metastatic melanoma treated with ipilimumab in the first line revealed that colonic, pre-therapeutic [^{18}F]FDG PET SUVmax appears lower for responding patients as a result. The mean SUVmax for those with complete response, partial response, and progressive disease was 1.33 ± 0.04, 2.2 ± 0.46, and 3.33 ± 2.67, respectively [72]. This may be explained by the discovery that, in low-bacterial environments, colonic metabolism switches from producing short-chain fatty acids through bacterial production to metabolizing glycolysis, which raises physiologic colonic [^{18}F]FDG uptake [73].

8. FUNCTION OF [^{18}F]FDG PET/CT AS AN INDICATOR OF PROGNOSIS

T-cell activation and function are significantly influenced by glycolytic metabolism, and there is a strong correlation between the expression of PD-L1 and glucose transporter 1 on the cell surface [74] (Fig. **10**). As a result, [^{18}F]FDG PET/CT may contribute to the TME's definition in addition to merely making tumor metabolism assessment easier. As an illustration, research on 55 patients with early non-small-cell lung cancer revealed a significant correlation between [^{18}F]FDG uptake (maximum standardized uptake value [SUVmax] and mean standardized uptake value) and cytotoxic CD^{8+}tumor-infiltrating lymphocytes (r = 0.31, P =.027 for both parameters) with disease-free survival (P =.002 and P =.004, respectively) [75]. Furthermore, the relationship between PD-L1 immunohistochemistry and SUVmax and other metabolic markers is also demonstrated [76]. On the other hand, no relationship was observed between the [^{18}F]FDG PET/CT metabolic characteristics and the PD-L1 tumor percentage score in research involving 100 patients with early-stage NSCLC [77]. Numerous investigations have examined the association between prognosis and immunotherapy response concerning semiquantitative and volume-based [^{18}F]FDG PET/CT metabolic characteristics; this research has been conducted primarily in malignant melanoma and non-small cell lung cancer.

According to an analysis of 27 patients with advanced NSCLC receiving CPIs (Check-point Inhibitors), the correlation was weak with low specificity (38.9% and 33.3%, respectively) [78]. On the other hand, in the setting of CPIs, several studies spanning different tumor types found no independent relationship between prognosis and baseline SUVmax [79]. SUVmax and maximal SUL were not observed to be associated with prognosis in a meta-analysis of [^{18}F]FDG PET/CT metabolic parameters in malignant melanoma [80]. Alternatively, a number of researchers have looked into the connection between CPI results and tumor load. Tumor burden markers such as high MTV (mean standardized uptake value), whole lesion glycolysis, their whole-body derivatives, and whole-body SUVmax have been consistently linked to suboptimal response to CPIs. Notwithstanding variations in research methodologies, a meta-analysis that combined the hazard ratios for MTV and TLG to forecast melanoma patients' response to immunotherapy produced a noteworthy predictive value (P>0.01, P>.001) [81]. It has also been proven that the metabolic response during CPI therapy, as assessed by MTV and TLG, correlates with circulating tumor cells [82]. Combining whole-body MTV with biochemical markers, such as lactate dehydrogenase, has further demonstrated potential in risk-stratifying patients. The hematopoietic compartment's [^{18}F]FDG uptake indicates a pro-inflammatory state. It may be useful in identifying patients who do not respond to CPIs or determining the appropriateness of innovative combination methods targeting myeloid-derived suppressor cells [83]. Ratios of the spleen to the liver and bone marrow to the liver were measured at baseline. Surrogate markers of hematopoiesis, [^{18}F]FDG PET/CT, have been demonstrated in multiple studies to have prognostic significance in patients undergoing CPI for metastatic melanoma and NSCLC. Though thought-provoking, there are still several obstacles to overcome, such as the absence of defined methods for measurement, the need for segmentation automation to streamline the transfer to clinical settings, and the distinction between low and high tumor burden.

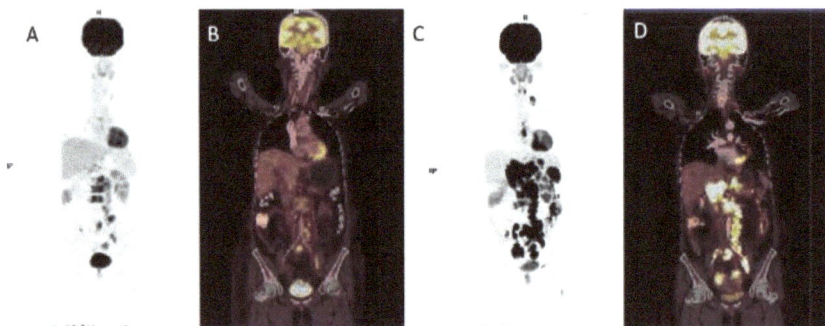

Fig. (10). A 71-year-old presented with recurrent renal cell carcinoma. She had a history of right nephrectomy 3 years back. Her FDG PET/CT scan revealed multiple retroperitoneal and pelvis lymph nodes (**A-B**). She was started on Nivolumab. It is a human IgG4 monoclonal antibody that blocks PD-1. Her follow-up scan (**C-D**) revealed extensive left supraclavicular, mediastinal, and pelvic lymphadenopathy. Overall scan findings are suggestive of disease progression.

9. ROLE OF[^{18}F]FDG PET/CT IN EVALUATING TOXICITY

Immune-related adverse events (irAEs) are special side effects linked to CPIs. All tissues or organs can become inflamed by CPIs, and the side-effect profiles of different medications and drug combinations differ in which tissue or organ is most likely to be impacted, when, how often, and how severe the effects are [84]. irAEs can happen days or more than a year after therapy ends, with a typical start of 2-16 weeks [85]. The severity of adverse events (AEs) can vary from highly tolerable (grades 1-2 may require oral corticosteroids) to hospitalization, therapy withdrawal (grades 3-5), and even death. Along with clinical symptoms and biological markers, conventional CT and MRI are valuable tools for identifying and tracking irAEs. [^{18}F]FDG PET/CT might offer a unique perspective on the inflammatory process. Up to 22% of patients on CPIs experience colitis, one of the more frequent irAEs [86]. Preventing complications, such as perforation and death, requires early discovery and treatment. There have been reports of diffusion, segmentation, and isolated rectosigmoid patterns of ^{18}F FDG uptake. Research revealed a substantial correlation between higher [^{18}F]FDG uptake and clinically severe diarrhea in patients receiving ipilimumab therapy for melanoma [87]. Reports of [^{18}F]FDG uptake have also been linked to less frequent immune-related upper gastrointestinal damage, such as gastritis, duodenitis, and esophagitis [88, 89]. Most common are hepatic irAEs, which are typically linked to localized increases in transaminases rather than occult radiologic abnormalities. However, there have been reports of diffusely increased [^{18}F]FDG uptake in the liver parenchyma as well as hepatomegaly [90].

As an adjuvant, when durvalumab is used after chemoradiotherapy for stage III non-small cell lung cancer (NSCLC), patients are more likely to develop pneumonia, a relatively uncommon but potentially fatal adverse event (irAE) that is more common with anti-PD-1 and anti-PD-L1 therapies (34%). It is well known that sarcoid-like reactions are frequently asymptomatic and cause increased [^{18}F]FDG uptake in the form of bilateral mediastinal and hilar lymphadenopathy [91].

Skin reactions that resemble sarcoids are possible, although they seldom affect the extrathoracic nodes. Diffuse or multifocal absorption of [^{18}F]FDG in the liver or spleen, as well as organomegaly, should also be a cause for concern. Endocrinopathies are prevalent adverse events (irAEs). Thyroiditis, which is typically asymptomatic but can exhibit diffuse [^{18}F]FDG uptake and cause a hypothyroid condition necessitating hormone replacement, affects up to 22% of patients [92]. Although rare, hypophysitis has been documented in as many as 8% of individuals using anti-CTLA-4 [93]. Although increased focal [^{18}F]FDG uptake in the pituitary fossa has been reported; background brain uptake makes it simple to overlook without a close examination. With CPIs, myalgia and arthralgia are comparatively prevalent (4%–8%) [94]. Since irAEs can occur even after stopping CPI, a role for [^{18}F]FDG PET/CT in predicting them is intriguing and merits more research. This information could help inform surveillance tactics for high-risk patients. Potential irAEs must, nevertheless, be identified and reported during [^{18}F]FDG PET/CT surveillance of immunotherapy patients.

CONCLUSION

[^{18}F]FDG is becoming increasingly important for diagnosing many infectious and inflammatory disorders and for monitoring therapy. PET images can be analyzed using numerical indices, which include volumetric parameters within the tumors, in addition to qualitative assessment. Improved clinical guidance for immunotherapies and theranostic prospects could result from the multilevel integration of imaging and other biomarkers. The use of immunotherapy in cancer treatment has changed the field of medical oncology and posed new difficulties for diagnostic imaging. With the use of novel radiotracers, such as *in vivo* whole-body programmed death-ligand 1 and CD^{8+} T cell distribution, it is possible to evaluate tumor morbidity and the immunological tumor microenvironment to more accurately predict which patients may react to treatment. In cases of immunotherapy resistance, in particular, longitudinal imaging may assist in characterizing alterations in a more detailed manner and guide a customized therapeutic approach. The TME and all the dynamic mechanisms underlying tumor genesis and proliferation, including the interaction between tumor cells and invading immune cells in the TME, have become better understood in the last few decades due to the remarkable advancements in translational medicine.

By revealing aspects of the tumor and TME, molecular imaging with [^{18}F]FDG PET/CT may be used to supplement traditional morphologic imaging. Although the majority of these novel radiotracers are still in the preclinical stage, they will undoubtedly expand the theragnostic horizon by offering supplementary data to the clinically employed [^{18}F]FDG PET/CT for the prediction of immunotherapy response in the context of personalized medicine. Although [^{18}F]FDG PET/CT is currently a widely used technique for tumor staging and response assessment, it has known disadvantages, including increased inflammatory component activity and pseudo progression. There are disadvantages, though, and it's more likely that molecular imaging will enhance rather than replace existing markers. Furthermore, novel opportunities could be presented by radiomics, artificial intelligence in imaging, and liquid biopsies that contain circulating tumor DNA.

ABBREVIATIONS

[^{18}F]FDG   2-deoxy-2-[^{18}F]fluoro-D-glucose

CPIs   Checkpoint Inhibitors

CT   Computed tomography

GLUTs   Glucose transporters

G-6-P	Glucose-6-phosphatase
GISTs	Gastrointestinal stromal tumors
HK	Hexokinase
ICI	Immune check-point inhibitors
irAEs	Immune-related adverse events
PET	Positron emission tomography
PD-L1	Programmed death-ligand 1
RECIST	Response Evaluation Criteria in Solid Tumors
TME	Tumor microenvironment
TMTV	Total metabolic tumor volume

ACKNOWLEDGMENTS

The authors would like to convey their heartfelt gratitude to the Department of Nuclear Medicine, SGPGIMS, Lucknow, for providing the resources necessary to compose and submit the book chapter for publication.

REFERENCES

[1]   Kostakoglu, L.; Agress, H., Jr; Goldsmith, S.J. Clinical role of FDG PET in evaluation of cancer patients. *Radiographics,* **2003**, *23*(2), 315-340.
[http://dx.doi.org/10.1148/rg.232025705] [PMID: 12640150]

[2]   Phelps, M.E. Positron emission tomography provides molecular imaging of biological processes. *Proc. Natl. Acad. Sci. USA,* **2000**, *97*(16), 9226-9233.
[http://dx.doi.org/10.1073/pnas.97.16.9226] [PMID: 10922074]

[3]   de Geus-Oei, L.F.; Vriens, D.; van Laarhoven, H.W.M.; van der Graaf, W.T.A.; Oyen, W.J.G. Monitoring and predicting response to therapy with ^{18}F-FDG PET in colorectal cancer: a systematic review. *J. Nucl. Med.,* **2009**, *50* Suppl. 1, 43S-54S.
[http://dx.doi.org/10.2967/jnumed.108.057224] [PMID: 19403879]

[4]   Mai, W.X.; Gosa, L.; Daniels, V.W.; Ta, L.; Tsang, J.E.; Higgins, B.; Gilmore, W.B.; Bayley, N.A.; Harati, M.D.; Lee, J.T.; Yong, W.H.; Kornblum, H.I.; Bensinger, S.J.; Mischel, P.S.; Rao, P.N.; Clark, P.M.; Cloughesy, T.F.; Letai, A.; Nathanson, D.A. Cytoplasmic p53 couples oncogene-driven glucose metabolism to apoptosis and is a therapeutic target in glioblastoma. *Nat. Med.,* **2017**, *23*(11), 1342-1351.
[http://dx.doi.org/10.1038/nm.4418] [PMID: 29035366]

[5]   Tai, Y.F.; Piccini, P. Applications of positron emission tomography (PET) in neurology. *J. Neurol. Neurosurg. Psychiatry,* **2004**, *75*(5), 669-676.
[http://dx.doi.org/10.1136/jnnp.2003.028175] [PMID: 15090557]

[6]   Reivich, M.; Kuhl, D.; Wolf, A.; Greenberg, J.; Phelps, M.; Ido, T.; Casella, V.; Fowler, J.; Hoffman, E.; Alavi, A.; Som, P.; Sokoloff, L. The [^{18}F]fluorodeoxyglucose method for the measurement of local cerebral glucose utilization in man. *Circ. Res.,* **1979**, *44*(1), 127-137.
[http://dx.doi.org/10.1161/01.RES.44.1.127] [PMID: 363301]

[7]   Newberg, A.; Alavi, A.; Reivich, M. Determination of regional cerebral function with FDG-PET imaging in neuropsychiatric disorders. *Semin. Nucl. Med.,* **2002**, *32*(1), 13-34.
[http://dx.doi.org/10.1053/snuc.2002.29276] [PMID: 11839066]

[8]   Sarikaya, I. PET studies in epilepsy. *Am. J. Nucl. Med. Mol. Imaging,* **2015**, *5*(5), 416-430.
       [PMID: 26550535]

[9]   Anagnostopoulos, C.; Georgakopoulos, A.; Pianou, N.; Nekolla, S.G. Assessment of myocardial
       perfusion and viability by Positron Emission Tomography. *Int. J. Cardiol.,* **2013**, *167*(5), 1737-1749.
       [http://dx.doi.org/10.1016/j.ijcard.2012.12.009] [PMID: 23313467]

[10]   Khalaf, S.; Chamsi-Pasha, M.; Al-Mallah, M.H. Assessment of myocardial viability by PET. *Curr.*
       Opin. Cardiol., **2019**, *34*(5), 466-472.
       [http://dx.doi.org/10.1097/HCO.0000000000000652] [PMID: 31393420]

[11]   Rosenbaum, D.; Millon, A.; Fayad, Z.A. Molecular imaging in atherosclerosis: FDG PET. *Curr.*
       Atheroscler. Rep., **2012**, *14*(5), 429-437.
       [http://dx.doi.org/10.1007/s11883-012-0264-x] [PMID: 22872371]

[12]   Jamar, F.; Buscombe, J.; Chiti, A.; Christian, P.E.; Delbeke, D.; Donohoe, K.J.; Israel, O.; Martin-
       Comin, J.; Signore, A. EANM/SNMMI guideline for ^{18}F-FDG use in inflammation and infection. *J.*
       Nucl. Med., **2013**, *54*(4), 647-658.
       [http://dx.doi.org/10.2967/jnumed.112.112524] [PMID: 23359660]

[13]   Rohren, E.M.; Turkington, T.G.; Coleman, R.E. Clinical applications of PET in oncology. *Radiology,*
       2004, *231*(2), 305-332.
       [http://dx.doi.org/10.1148/radiol.2312021185] [PMID: 15044750]

[14]   Otsuka, H.; Graham, M.; Kubo, A.; Nishitani, H. Clinical utility of FDG PET. *J. Med. Invest.,* **2004**,
       51(1-2), 14-19.
       [http://dx.doi.org/10.2152/jmi.51.14] [PMID: 15000251]

[15]   Groheux, D. Role of fludeoxyglucose in breast cancer. *PET Clin.,* **2018**, *13*(3), 395-414.
       [http://dx.doi.org/10.1016/j.cpet.2018.02.003] [PMID: 30100078]

[16]   Liberti, M.V.; Locasale, J.W. The warburg effect: How does it benefit cancer cells? *Trends Biochem.*
       Sci., **2016**, *41*(3), 211-218.
       [http://dx.doi.org/10.1016/j.tibs.2015.12.001] [PMID: 26778478]

[17]   Doyle, W.K.; Budinger, T.F.; Valk, P.E.; Levin, V.A.; Gutin, P.H. Differentiation of cerebral radiation
       necrosis from tumor recurrence by [^{18}F]FDG and 82Rb positron emission tomography. *J. Comput.*
       Assist. Tomogr., **1987**, *11*(4), 563-570.
       [http://dx.doi.org/10.1097/00004728-198707000-00001] [PMID: 3496366]

[18]   Kessler, L.G.; Barnhart, H.X.; Buckler, A.J.; Choudhury, K.R.; Kondratovich, M.V.; Toledano, A.;
       Guimaraes, A.R.; Filice, R.; Zhang, Z.; Sullivan, D.C. The emerging science of quantitative imaging
       biomarkers terminology and definitions for scientific studies and regulatory submissions. *Stat.*
       Methods Med. Res., **2015**, *24*(1), 9-26.
       [http://dx.doi.org/10.1177/0962280214537333] [PMID: 24919826]

[19]   Mu, W.; Jiang, L.; Zhang, J.; Shi, Y.; Gray, J.E.; Tunali, I.; Gao, C.; Sun, Y.; Tian, J.; Zhao, X.; Sun,
       X.; Gillies, R.J.; Schabath, M.B. Non-invasive decision support for NSCLC treatment using PET/CT
       radiomics. *Nat. Commun.,* **2020**, *11*(1), 5228.
       [http://dx.doi.org/10.1038/s41467-020-19116-x] [PMID: 33067442]

[20]   Greco, C.; Rosenzweig, K.; Cascini, G.L.; Tamburrini, O. Current status of PET/CT for tumour
       volume definition in radiotherapy treatment planning for non-small cell lung cancer (NSCLC). *Lung*
       Cancer, **2007**, *57*(2), 125-134.
       [http://dx.doi.org/10.1016/j.lungcan.2007.03.020] [PMID: 17478008]

[21]   Panje, C.; Panje, T.; Putora, P.M.; Kim, S.; Haile, S.; Aebersold, D.M.; Plasswilm, L. Guidance of
       treatment decisions in risk-adapted primary radiotherapy for prostate cancer using multiparametric
       magnetic resonance imaging: a single center experience. *Radiat. Oncol.,* **2015**, *10*(1), 47.
       [http://dx.doi.org/10.1186/s13014-015-0338-3] [PMID: 25880635]

[22]   Jaffray, D.A. Image-guided radiotherapy: from current concept to future perspectives. *Nat. Rev. Clin.*

Oncol., **2012,** *9*(12), 688-699.
[http://dx.doi.org/10.1038/nrclinonc.2012.194] [PMID: 23165124]

[23] Michaelidou, A.; Adjogatse, D.; Suh, Y.; Pike, L.; Thomas, C.; Woodley, O.; Rackely, T.; Palaniappan, N.; Jayaprakasam, V.; Sanchez-Nieto, B.; Evans, M.; Barrington, S.; Lei, M.; Guerrero Urbano, T. ^{18}F-FDG-PET in guided dose-painting with intensity modulated radiotherapy in oropharyngeal tumours: A phase I study (FiGaRO). *Radiother. Oncol.,* **2021,** *155,* 261-268.
[http://dx.doi.org/10.1016/j.radonc.2020.10.039] [PMID: 33161013]

[24] Chen, D.L.; Ballout, S.; Chen, L.; Cheriyan, J.; Choudhury, G.; Denis-Bacelar, A.M.; Emond, E.; Erlandsson, K.; Fisk, M.; Fraioli, F.; Groves, A.M.; Gunn, R.N.; Hatazawa, J.; Holman, B.F.; Hutton, B.F.; Iida, H.; Lee, S.; MacNee, W.; Matsunaga, K.; Mohan, D.; Parr, D.; Rashidnasab, A.; Rizzo, G.; Subramanian, D.; Tal-Singer, R.; Thielemans, K.; Tregay, N.; van Beek, E.J.R.; Vass, L.; Vidal Melo, M.F.; Wellen, J.W.; Wilkinson, I.; Wilson, F.J.; Winkler, T. Consensus recommendations on the use of [18] F-FDG PET/CT in lung disease. *J. Nucl. Med.,* **2020,** *61*(12), 1701-1707.
[http://dx.doi.org/10.2967/jnumed.120.244780] [PMID: 32948678]

[25] Hughes, D.J.; Subesinghe, M.; Taylor, B.; Bille, A.; Spicer, J.; Papa, S.; Goh, V.; Cook, G.J.R. [18]F FDG PET/CT and novel molecular imaging for directing immunotherapy in cancer. *Radiology,* **2022,** *304*(2), 246-264.
[http://dx.doi.org/10.1148/radiol.212481] [PMID: 35762888]

[26] Seymour, L.; Bogaerts, J.; Perrone, A.; Ford, R.; Schwartz, L.H.; Mandrekar, S.; Lin, N.U.; Litière, S.; Dancey, J.; Chen, A.; Hodi, F.S.; Therasse, P.; Hoekstra, O.S.; Shankar, L.K.; Wolchok, J.D.; Ballinger, M.; Caramella, C.; de Vries, E.G.E. iRECIST: guidelines for response criteria for use in trials testing immunotherapeutics. *Lancet Oncol.,* **2017,** *18*(3), e143-e152.
[http://dx.doi.org/10.1016/S1470-2045(17)30074-8] [PMID: 28271869]

[27] Phelps, M.E. Positron emission tomography provides molecular imaging of biological processes. *Proc. Natl. Acad. Sci. USA,* **2000,** *97*(16), 9226-9233.
[http://dx.doi.org/10.1073/pnas.97.16.9226] [PMID: 10922074]

[28] Adekola, K.; Rosen, S.T.; Shanmugam, M. Glucose transporters in cancer metabolism. *Curr. Opin. Oncol.,* **2012,** *24*(6), 650-654.
[http://dx.doi.org/10.1097/CCO.0b013e328356da72] [PMID: 22913968]

[29] Jadvar, H.; Alavi, A.; Gambhir, S.S. ^{18}F-FDG uptake in lung, breast, and colon cancers: molecular biology correlates and disease characterization. *J. Nucl. Med.,* **2009,** *50*(11), 1820-1827.
[http://dx.doi.org/10.2967/jnumed.108.054098] [PMID: 19837767]

[30] Wright, E.M.; Loo, D.D.F.; Hirayama, B.A. Biology of human sodium glucose transporters. *Physiol. Rev.,* **2011,** *91*(2), 733-794.
[http://dx.doi.org/10.1152/physrev.00055.2009] [PMID: 21527736]

[31] Xu, S.; Herschman, H.R. A tumor agnostic therapeutic strategy for hexokinase 1–null/hexokinase 2–positive cancers. *Cancer Res.,* **2019,** *79*(23), 5907-5914.
[http://dx.doi.org/10.1158/0008-5472.CAN-19-1789] [PMID: 31434645]

[32] Phelps, M.E.; Huang, S.C.; Hoffman, E.J.; Selin, C.; Sokoloff, L.; Kuhl, D.E. Tomographic measurement of local cerebral glucose metabolic rate in humans with (F-18)2-fluoro-2-deoxy- D-glucose: Validation of method. *Ann. Neurol.,* **1979,** *6*(5), 371-388.
[http://dx.doi.org/10.1002/ana.410060502] [PMID: 117743]

[33] de Geus-Oei, L.F.; Krieken, J.H.J.M.; Aliredjo, R.P.; Krabbe, P.F.M.; Frielink, C.; Verhagen, A.F.T.; Boerman, O.C.; Oyen, W.J.G. Biological correlates of FDG uptake in non-small cell lung cancer. *Lung Cancer,* **2007,** *55*(1), 79-87.
[http://dx.doi.org/10.1016/j.lungcan.2006.08.018] [PMID: 17046099]

[34] Van Berkel, A.; Rao, J.U.; Kusters, B.; Demir, T.; Visser, E.; Mensenkamp, A.R.; van der Laak, J.A.W.M.; Oosterwijk, E.; Lenders, J.W.M.; Sweep, F.C.G.J.; Wevers, R.A.; Hermus, A.R.; Langenhuijsen, J.F.; Kunst, D.P.M.; Pacak, K.; Gotthardt, M.; Timmers, H.J.L.M. Correlation between

in vivo ^{18}F-FDG PET and immunohistochemical markers of glucose uptake and metabolism in pheochromocytoma and paraganglioma. *J. Nucl. Med.,* **2014**, *55*(8), 1253-1259.
[http://dx.doi.org/10.2967/jnumed.114.137034] [PMID: 24925884]

[35]   Alakus, H.; Batur, M.; Schmidt, M.; Drebber, U.; Baldus, S.E.; Vallböhmer, D.; Prenzel, K.L.; Metzger, R.; Bollschweiler, E.; Hölscher, A.H.; Mönig, S.P. Variable ^{18}F-fluorodeoxyglucose uptake in gastric cancer is associated with different levels of GLUT-1 expression. *Nucl. Med. Commun.,* **2010**, *31*(6), 532-538.
[http://dx.doi.org/10.1097/MNM.0b013e32833823ac] [PMID: 20220543]

[36]   Bos, R.; van der Hoeven, J.J.M.; van der Wall, E.; van der Groep, P.; van Diest, P.J.; Comans, E.F.I.; Joshi, U.; Semenza, G.L.; Hoekstra, O.S.; Lammertsma, A.A.; Molthoff, C.F.M. Biologic correlates of (18)fluorodeoxyglucose uptake in human breast cancer measured by positron emission tomography. *J. Clin. Oncol.,* **2002**, *20*(2), 379-387.
[http://dx.doi.org/10.1200/JCO.2002.20.2.379] [PMID: 11786564]

[37]   Mossberg, K.; Taegtmeyer, H. *In vivo* assessment of skeletal muscle glucose metabolism with positron emitting 18-F-2-deoxy-2-fluoro-D-glucose (FDG). *J. Mol. Cell. Cardiol.,* **1987**, *19*, S50-S50.
[http://dx.doi.org/10.1016/S0022-2828(87)80775-7]

[38]   TeSlaa, T.; Teitell, M.A. Techniques to monitor glycolysis. *Methods Enzymol.,* **2014**, *542*, 91-114.
[http://dx.doi.org/10.1016/B978-0-12-416618-9.00005-4] [PMID: 24862262]

[39]   Hsieh, M.H.; Choe, J.H.; Gadhvi, J.; Kim, Y.J.; Arguez, M.A.; Palmer, M.; Gerold, H.; Nowak, C.; Do, H.; Mazambani, S.; Knighton, J.K.; Cha, M.; Goodwin, J.; Kang, M.K.; Jeong, J.Y.; Lee, S.Y.; Faubert, B.; Xuan, Z.; Abel, E.D.; Scafoglio, C.; Shackelford, D.B.; Minna, J.D.; Singh, P.K.; Shulaev, V.; Bleris, L.; Hoyt, K.; Kim, J.; Inoue, M.; DeBerardinis, R.J.; Kim, T.H.; Kim, J. p63 and SOX2 dictate glucose reliance and metabolic vulnerabilities in squamous cell carcinomas. *Cell Rep.,* **2019**, *28*(7), 1860-1878.e9.
[http://dx.doi.org/10.1016/j.celrep.2019.07.027] [PMID: 31412252]

[40]   Maitituoheti, M.; Keung, E.Z.; Tang, M.; Yan, L.; Alam, H.; Han, G.; Singh, A.K.; Raman, A.T.; Terranova, C.; Sarkar, S.; Orouji, E.; Amin, S.B.; Sharma, S.; Williams, M.; Samant, N.S.; Dhamdhere, M.; Zheng, N.; Shah, T.; Shah, A.; Axelrad, J.B.; Anvar, N.E.; Lin, Y.H.; Jiang, S.; Chang, E.Q.; Ingram, D.R.; Wang, W.L.; Lazar, A.; Lee, M.G.; Muller, F.; Wang, L.; Ying, H.; Rai, K. Enhancer reprogramming confers dependence on glycolysis and IGF signaling in KMT2D mutant melanoma. *Cell Rep.,* **2020**, *33*(3), 108293.
[http://dx.doi.org/10.1016/j.celrep.2020.108293] [PMID: 33086062]

[41]   Chan, L.N.; Chen, Z.; Braas, D.; Lee, J.W.; Xiao, G.; Geng, H.; Cosgun, K.N.; Hurtz, C.; Shojaee, S.; Cazzaniga, V.; Schjerven, H.; Ernst, T.; Hochhaus, A.; Kornblau, S.M.; Konopleva, M.; Pufall, M.A.; Cazzaniga, G.; Liu, G.J.; Milne, T.A.; Koeffler, H.P.; Ross, T.S.; Sánchez-García, I.; Borkhardt, A.; Yamamoto, K.R.; Dickins, R.A.; Graeber, T.G.; Müschen, M. Metabolic gatekeeper function of B-lymphoid transcription factors. *Nature,* **2017**, *542*(7642), 479-483.
[http://dx.doi.org/10.1038/nature21076] [PMID: 28192788]

[42]   Mason, J.A.; Cockfield, J.A.; Pape, D.J.; Meissner, H.; Sokolowski, M.T.; White, T.C.; Valentín López, J.C.; Liu, J.; Liu, X.; Martínez-Reyes, I.; Chandel, N.S.; Locasale, J.W.; Schafer, Z.T. SGK1 signaling promotes glucose metabolism and survival in extracellular matrix detached cells. *Cell Rep.,* **2021**, *34*(11), 108821.
[http://dx.doi.org/10.1016/j.celrep.2021.108821] [PMID: 33730592]

[43]   Kumari, S.; Khan, S.; Gupta, S.C.; Kashyap, V.K.; Yallapu, M.M.; Chauhan, S.C.; Jaggi, M. MUC13 contributes to rewiring of glucose metabolism in pancreatic cancer. *Oncogenesis,* **2018**, *7*(2), 19.
[http://dx.doi.org/10.1038/s41389-018-0031-0] [PMID: 29467405]

[44]   Jiang, S.H.; Li, J.; Dong, F.Y.; Yang, J.Y.; Liu, D.J.; Yang, X.M.; Wang, Y.H.; Yang, M.W.; Fu, X.L.; Zhang, X.X.; Li, Q.; Pang, X.F.; Huo, Y.M.; Li, J.; Zhang, J.F.; Lee, H.Y.; Lee, S.J.; Qin, W.X.; Gu, J.R.; Sun, Y.W.; Zhang, Z.G. Increased serotonin signaling contributes to the warburg effect in pancreatic tumor cells under metabolic stress and promotes growth of pancreatic tumors in mice.

Gastroenterology, **2017**, *153*(1), 277-291.e19.
[http://dx.doi.org/10.1053/j.gastro.2017.03.008] [PMID: 28315323]

[45]   Broecker-Preuss, M.; Becher-Boveleth, N.; Bockisch, A.; Dührsen, U.; Müller, S. Regulation of glucose uptake in lymphoma cell lines by c-MYC- and PI3K-dependent signaling pathways and impact of glycolytic pathways on cell viability. *J. Transl. Med.*, **2017**, *15*(1), 158.
[http://dx.doi.org/10.1186/s12967-017-1258-9] [PMID: 28724379]

[46]   Kim, N.H.; Sung, N.J.; Youn, H.S.; Park, S.A. Gremlin-1 activates Akt/STAT3 signaling, which increases the glycolysis rate in breast cancer cells. *Biochem. Biophys. Res. Commun.*, **2020**, *533*(4), 1378-1384.
[http://dx.doi.org/10.1016/j.bbrc.2020.10.025] [PMID: 33097188]

[47]   Weng, Q.; Chen, M.; Yang, W.; Li, J.; Fan, K.; Xu, M.; Weng, W.; Lv, X.; Fang, S.; Zheng, L.; Song, J.; Zhao, Z.; Fan, X.; Ji, J. Integrated analyses identify miR-34c-3p/MAGI3 axis for the Warburg metabolism in hepatocellular carcinoma. *FASEB J.*, **2020**, *34*(4), 5420-5434.
[http://dx.doi.org/10.1096/fj.201902895R] [PMID: 32080912]

[48]   Sullivan, W.J.; Mullen, P.J.; Schmid, E.W.; Flores, A.; Momcilovic, M.; Sharpley, M.S.; Jelinek, D.; Whiteley, A.E.; Maxwell, M.B.; Wilde, B.R.; Banerjee, U.; Coller, H.A.; Shackelford, D.B.; Braas, D.; Ayer, D.E.; de Aguiar Vallim, T.Q.; Lowry, W.E.; Christofk, H.R. Extracellular matrix remodeling regulates glucose metabolism through TXNIP destabilization. *Cell*, **2018**, *175*(1), 117-132.e21.
[http://dx.doi.org/10.1016/j.cell.2018.08.017] [PMID: 30197082]

[49]   Hong, S.Y.; Yu, F.X.; Luo, Y.; Hagen, T. Oncogenic activation of the PI3K/Akt pathway promotes cellular glucose uptake by downregulating the expression of thioredoxin-interacting protein. *Cell. Signal.*, **2016**, *28*(5), 377-383.
[http://dx.doi.org/10.1016/j.cellsig.2016.01.011] [PMID: 26826652]

[50]   Waldhart, A.N.; Dykstra, H.; Peck, A.S.; Boguslawski, E.A.; Madaj, Z.B.; Wen, J.; Veldkamp, K.; Hollowell, M.; Zheng, B.; Cantley, L.C.; McGraw, T.E.; Wu, N. Phosphorylation of txnip by akt mediates acute influx of glucose in response to insulin. *Cell Rep.*, **2017**, *19*(10), 2005-2013.
[http://dx.doi.org/10.1016/j.celrep.2017.05.041] [PMID: 28591573]

[51]   Kim, D.J.; Vo, M.T.; Choi, S.H.; Lee, J.H.; Jeong, S.Y.; Hong, C.H.; Kim, J.S.; Lee, U.H.; Chung, H.M.; Lee, B.J.; Cho, W.J.; Park, J.W. Tristetraprolin-mediated hexokinase 2 expression regulation contributes to glycolysis in cancer cells. *Mol. Biol. Cell*, **2019**, *30*(5), 542-553.
[http://dx.doi.org/10.1091/mbc.E18-09-0606] [PMID: 30650008]

[52]   Chen, D.S.; Mellman, I. Oncology meets immunology: the cancer-immunity cycle. *Immunity*, **2013**, *39*(1), 1-10.
[http://dx.doi.org/10.1016/j.immuni.2013.07.012] [PMID: 23890059]

[53]   Reynders, N.; Abboud, D.; Baragli, A.; Noman, M.Z.; Rogister, B.; Niclou, S.P.; Heveker, N.; Janji, B.; Hanson, J.; Szpakowska, M.; Chevigné, A. The distinct roles of cxcr3 variants and their ligands in the tumor microenvironment. *Cells*, **2019**, *8*(6), 613.
[http://dx.doi.org/10.3390/cells8060613] [PMID: 31216755]

[54]   Trujillo, J.A.; Sweis, R.F.; Bao, R.; Luke, J.J. T cell–inflamed *versus* non-t cell–inflamed tumors: a conceptual framework for cancer immunotherapy drug development and combination therapy selection. *Cancer Immunol. Res.*, **2018**, *6*(9), 990-1000.
[http://dx.doi.org/10.1158/2326-6066.CIR-18-0277] [PMID: 30181337]

[55]   Zitvogel, L.; Tesniere, A.; Kroemer, G. Cancer despite immunosurveillance: immunoselection and immunosubversion. *Nat. Rev. Immunol.*, **2006**, *6*(10), 715-727.
[http://dx.doi.org/10.1038/nri1936] [PMID: 16977338]

[56]   Pardoll, D.M. The blockade of immune checkpoints in cancer immunotherapy. *Nat. Rev. Cancer*, **2012**, *12*(4), 252-264.
[http://dx.doi.org/10.1038/nrc3239] [PMID: 22437870]

[57]   Decazes, P.; Bohn, P. Immunotherapy by immune checkpoint inhibitors and nuclear medicine

imaging: current and future applications. *Cancers (Basel)*, **2020**, *12*(2), 371.
[http://dx.doi.org/10.3390/cancers12020371] [PMID: 32041105]

[58]   Somarouthu, B.; Lee, S.I.; Urban, T.; Sadow, C.A.; Harris, G.J.; Kambadakone, A. Immune-related
       tumour response assessment criteria: a comprehensive review. *Br. J. Radiol.*, **2018**, *91*(1084),
       20170457.
       [http://dx.doi.org/10.1016/j.cell.2015.08.016] [PMID: 26321679]

[59]   Chang, C.H.; Qiu, J.; O'Sullivan, D.; Buck, M.D.; Noguchi, T.; Curtis, J.D.; Chen, Q.; Gindin, M.;
       Gubin, M.M.; van der Windt, G.J.W.; Tonc, E.; Schreiber, R.D.; Pearce, E.J.; Pearce, E.L. Metabolic
       competition in the tumor microenvironment is a driver of cancer progression. *Cell*, **2015**, *162*(6),
       1229-1241.
       [http://dx.doi.org/10.1007/s00259-018-4211-0] [PMID: 30488098]

[60]   Frasca, D.; Diaz, A.; Romero, M.; Thaller, S.; Blomberg, B.B. Secretion of autoimmune antibodies in
       the human subcutaneous adipose tissue. *PLoS One*, **2018**, *13*(5), e0197472.
       [http://dx.doi.org/10.1371/journal.pone.0197472] [PMID: 29768501]

[61]   Eisenhauer, E.A.; Therasse, P.; Bogaerts, J.; Schwartz, L.H.; Sargent, D.; Ford, R.; Dancey, J.;
       Arbuck, S.; Gwyther, S.; Mooney, M.; Rubinstein, L.; Shankar, L.; Dodd, L.; Kaplan, R.; Lacombe,
       D.; Verweij, J. New response evaluation criteria in solid tumours: Revised RECIST guideline (version
       1.1). *Eur. J. Cancer*, **2009**, *45*(2), 228-247.
       [http://dx.doi.org/10.1016/j.ejca.2008.10.026] [PMID: 19097774]

[62]   Ito, K.; Schöder, H.; Teng, R.; Humm, J.L.; Ni, A.; Wolchok, J.D.; Weber, W.A. Prognostic value of
       baseline metabolic tumor volume measured on 18F-fluorodeoxyglucose positron emission
       tomography/computed tomography in melanoma patients treated with ipilimumab therapy. *Eur. J.
       Nucl. Med. Mol. Imaging*, **2019**, *46*(4), 930-939.
       [http://dx.doi.org/10.1007/s00259-018-4211-0] [PMID: 30488098]

[63]   Seban, R.D.; Mezquita, L.; Berenbaum, A.; Dercle, L.; Botticella, A.; Le Pechoux, C.; Caramella, C.;
       Deutsch, E.; Grimaldi, S.; Adam, J.; Ammari, S.; Planchard, D.; Leboulleux, S.; Besse, B. Baseline
       metabolic tumor burden on FDG PET/CT scans predicts outcome in advanced NSCLC patients treated
       with immune checkpoint inhibitors. *Eur. J. Nucl. Med. Mol. Imaging*, **2020**, *47*(5), 1147-1157.
       [http://dx.doi.org/10.1007/s00259-019-04615-x] [PMID: 31754795]

[64]   Koh, Y.W.; Lee, S.J.; Han, J.H.; Haam, S.; Jung, J.; Lee, H.W. PD-L1 protein expression in non
       small-cell lung cancer and its relationship with the hypoxia-related signaling pathways: A study based
       on immunohistochemistry and RNA sequencing data. *Lung Cancer*, **2019**, *129*, 41-47.
       [http://dx.doi.org/10.1016/j.lungcan.2019.01.004] [PMID: 30797490]

[65]   Kaira, K.; Shimizu, K.; Kitahara, S.; Yajima, T.; Atsumi, J.; Kosaka, T.; Ohtaki, Y.; Higuchi, T.;
       Oyama, T.; Asao, T.; Mogi, A. 2-Deoxy-2-[fluorine-18] fluoro-d-glucose uptake on positron emission
       tomography is associated with programmed death ligand-1 expression in patients with pulmonary
       adenocarcinoma. *Eur. J. Cancer*, **2018**, *101*, 181-190.
       [http://dx.doi.org/10.1016/j.ejca.2018.06.022] [PMID: 30077123]

[66]   Kasahara, N.; Kaira, K.; Bao, P.; Higuchi, T.; Arisaka, Y.; Erkhem-Ochir, B.; Sunaga, N.; Ohtaki, Y.;
       Yajima, T.; Kosaka, T.; Oyama, T.; Yokobori, T.; Asao, T.; Nishiyama, M.; Tsushima, Y.; Kuwano,
       H.; Shimizu, K.; Mogi, A. Correlation of tumor-related immunity with 18F-FDG-PET in pulmonary
       squamous-cell carcinoma. *Lung Cancer*, **2018**, *119*, 71-77.
       [http://dx.doi.org/10.1016/j.lungcan.2018.03.001] [PMID: 29656756]

[67]   Surov, A.; Meyer, H.J.; Wienke, A. Standardized uptake values derived from 18 F-FDG PET may
       predict lung cancer microvessel density and expression of KI 67, VEGF, and HIF-1 α but not
       expression of cyclin D1, PCNA, EGFR, PD L1, and p53. *Contrast Media Mol. Imaging*, **2018**, 1-10.
       [http://dx.doi.org/10.1155/2018/9257929] [PMID: 29983647]

[68]   Chen, R.; Zhou, X.; Liu, J.; Huang, G. Relationship between the expression of PD-1/PD-L1 and 18F
       FDG uptake in bladder cancer. *Eur. J. Nucl. Med. Mol. Imaging*, **2019**, *46*(4), 848-854.
       [http://dx.doi.org/10.1007/s00259-018-4208-8] [PMID: 30627815]

[69]   Lopci, E.; Toschi, L.; Grizzi, F.; Rahal, D.; Olivari, L.; Castino, G.F.; Marchetti, S.; Cortese, N.; Qehajaj, D.; Pistillo, D.; Alloisio, M.; Roncalli, M.; Allavena, P.; Santoro, A.; Marchesi, F.; Chiti, A. Correlation of metabolic information on FDG-PET with tissue expression of immune markers in patients with non-small cell lung cancer (NSCLC) who are candidates for upfront surgery. *Eur. J. Nucl. Med. Mol. Imaging*, **2016**, *43*(11), 1954-1961.
       [http://dx.doi.org/10.1007/s00259-016-3425-2] [PMID: 27251642]

[70]   Yi, M.; Jiao, D.; Xu, H.; Liu, Q.; Zhao, W.; Han, X.; Wu, K. Biomarkers for predicting efficacy of PD-1/PD-L1 inhibitors. *Mol. Cancer*, **2018**, *17*(1), 129.
       [http://dx.doi.org/10.1186/s12943-018-0864-3] [PMID: 30139382]

[71]   Boursi, B.; Werner, T.J.; Gholami, S.; Houshmand, S.; Mamtani, R.; Lewis, J.D.; Wu, G.D.; Alavi, A.; Yang, Y.X. Functional imaging of the interaction between gut microbiota and the human host: A proof-of-concept clinical study evaluating novel use for 18F-FDG PET-CT. *PLoS One*, **2018**, *13*(2), e0192747.
       [http://dx.doi.org/10.1371/journal.pone.0192747] [PMID: 29447210]

[72]   Popinat, G.; Cousse, S.; Goldfarb, L.; Becker, S.; Gardin, I.; Salaün, M.; Thureau, S.; Vera, P.; Guisier, F.; Decazes, P. Sub-cutaneous Fat Mass measured on multislice computed tomography of pretreatment PET/CT is a prognostic factor of stage IV non-small cell lung cancer treated by nivolumab. *OncoImmunology*, **2019**, *8*(5), e1580128.
       [http://dx.doi.org/10.1080/2162402X.2019.1580128] [PMID: 31069139]

[73]   Decazes, P.; Tonnelet, D.; Vera, P.; Gardin, I. Anthropometer3D: Automatic multi-slice segmentation software for the measurement of anthropometric parameters from CT of PET/CT. *J. Digit. Imaging*, **2019**, *32*(2), 241-250.
       [http://dx.doi.org/10.1007/s10278-019-00178-3] [PMID: 30756268]

[74]   Farag, S.; Geus-Oei, L.F.; van der Graaf, W.T.; van Coevorden, F.; Grunhagen, D.; Reyners, A.K.L.; Boonstra, P.A.; Desar, I.; Gelderblom, H.; Steeghs, N. Early Evaluation of response using 18 F-FDG PET influences management in gastrointestinal stromal tumor patients treated with neoadjuvant imatinib. *J. Nucl. Med.*, **2018**, *59*(2), 194-196.

[75]   Chang, Y.L.; Yang, C.Y.; Lin, M.W.; Wu, C.T.; Yang, P.C. High co-expression of PD-L1 and HIF-1α correlates with tumour necrosis in pulmonary pleomorphic carcinoma. *Eur. J. Cancer*, **2016**, *60*, 125-135
       [http://dx.doi.org/10.1016/j.ejca.2016.03.012] [PMID: 27107327]

[76]   Lopci, E.; Toschi, L.; Grizzi, F.; Rahal, D.; Olivari, L.; Castino, G.F.; Marchetti, S.; Cortese, N.; Qehajaj, D.; Pistillo, D.; Alloisio, M.; Roncalli, M.; Allavena, P.; Santoro, A.; Marchesi, F.; Chiti, A. Correlation of metabolic information on FDG-PET with tissue expression of immune markers in patients with non-small cell lung cancer (NSCLC) who are candidates for upfront surgery. *Eur. J. Nucl. Med. Mol. Imaging*, **2016**, *43*(11), 1954-1961.
       [http://dx.doi.org/10.1007/s00259-016-3425-2] [PMID: 27251642]

[77]   Takada, K.; Toyokawa, G.; Okamoto, T.; Baba, S.; Kozuma, Y.; Matsubara, T.; Haratake, N.; Akamine, T.; Takamori, S.; Katsura, M.; Shoji, F.; Honda, H.; Oda, Y.; Maehara, Y. Metabolic characteristics of programmed cell death-ligand 1-expressing lung cancer on [18] F-fluorodeoxyglucose positron emission tomography/computed tomography. *Cancer Med.*, **2017**, *6*(11), 2552-2561.
       [http://dx.doi.org/10.1002/cam4.1215] [PMID: 28980429]

[78]   Kaira, K.; Kuji, I.; Kagamu, H. Value of ^{18}F-FDG-PET to predict PD-L1 expression and outcomes of PD-1 inhibition therapy in human cancers. *Cancer Imaging*, **2021**, *21*(1), 11.
       [http://dx.doi.org/10.1186/s40644-021-00381-y] [PMID: 33441183]

[79]   Hughes, D.; Hunter, S.; Nonaka, D.; Goh, V.; Bille, A.; Karapanagiotou, E.; Cook, G. Correlation of ^{18}F-FDG-PET/CT metabolic parameters with PD-L1 tumour proportion score (TPS) in resected non-small cell lung cancer (NSCLC). *Lung Cancer*, **2021**, *156*, S3.
       [http://dx.doi.org/10.1016/S0169-5002(21)00205-1]

[80]   Ito, K.; Schöder, H.; Teng, R.; Humm, J.L.; Ni, A.; Wolchok, J.D.; Weber, W.A. Prognostic value of baseline metabolic tumor volume measured on ^{18}F-fluorodeoxyglucose positron emission tomography/computed tomography in melanoma patients treated with ipilimumab therapy. *Eur. J. Nucl. Med. Mol. Imaging,* **2019**, *46*(4), 930-939.
        [http://dx.doi.org/10.1007/s00259-018-4211-0] [PMID: 30488098]

[81]   Ayati, N.; Sadeghi, R.; Kiamanesh, Z.; Lee, S.T.; Zakavi, S.R.; Scott, A.M. The value of ^{18}F-FDG PET/CT for predicting or monitoring immunotherapy response in patients with metastatic melanoma: a systematic review and meta-analysis. *Eur. J. Nucl. Med. Mol. Imaging,* **2021**, *48*(2), 428-448.
        [http://dx.doi.org/10.1007/s00259-020-04967-9] [PMID: 32728798]

[82]   Castello, A.; Rossi, S.; Mazziotti, E.; Toschi, L.; Lopci, E. Hyperprogressive disease in patients with non–small cell lung cancer treated with checkpoint inhibitors: the role of [18] F-FDG PET/CT. *J. Nucl. Med.,* **2020**, *61*(6), 821-826.
        [http://dx.doi.org/10.2967/jnumed.119.237768] [PMID: 31862803]

[83]   De Cicco, P.; Ercolano, G.; Ianaro, A. The new era of cancer immunotherapy: targeting myeloid-derived suppressor cells to overcome immune evasion. *Front. Immunol.,* **2020**, *11*, 1680.
        [http://dx.doi.org/10.3389/fimmu.2020.01680] [PMID: 32849585]

[84]   Larkin, J.; Chiarion-Sileni, V.; Gonzalez, R.; Grob, J.J.; Rutkowski, P.; Lao, C.D.; Cowey, C.L.; Schadendorf, D.; Wagstaff, J.; Dummer, R.; Ferrucci, P.F.; Smylie, M.; Hogg, D.; Hill, A.; Márquez-Rodas, I.; Haanen, J.; Guidoboni, M.; Maio, M.; Schöffski, P.; Carlino, M.S.; Lebbé, C.; McArthur, G.; Ascierto, P.A.; Daniels, G.A.; Long, G.V.; Bastholt, L.; Rizzo, J.I.; Balogh, A.; Moshyk, A.; Hodi, F.S.; Wolchok, J.D. Five-year survival with combined nivolumab and ipilimumab in advanced melanoma. *N. Engl. J. Med.,* **2019**, *381*(16), 1535-1546.
        [http://dx.doi.org/10.1056/NEJMoa1910836] [PMID: 31562797]

[85]   Boutros, C.; Tarhini, A.; Routier, E.; Lambotte, O.; Ladurie, F.L.; Carbonnel, F.; Izzeddine, H.; Marabelle, A.; Champiat, S.; Berdelou, A.; Lanoy, E.; Texier, M.; Libenciuc, C.; Eggermont, A.M.M.; Soria, J.C.; Mateus, C.; Robert, C. Safety profiles of anti-CTLA-4 and anti-PD-1 antibodies alone and in combination. *Nat. Rev. Clin. Oncol.,* **2016**, *13*(8), 473-486.
        [http://dx.doi.org/10.1038/nrclinonc.2016.58] [PMID: 27141885]

[86]   Lang, D.; Wahl, G.; Poier, N.; Graf, S.; Kiesl, D.; Lamprecht, B.; Gabriel, M. Impact of PET/CT for assessing response to immunotherapy—a clinical perspective. *J. Clin. Med.,* **2020**, *9*(11), 3483.
        [http://dx.doi.org/10.3390/jcm9113483] [PMID: 33126715]

[87]   Johncilla, M.; Grover, S.; Zhang, X.; Jain, D.; Srivastava, A. Morphological spectrum of immune check-point inhibitor therapy-associated gastritis. *Histopathology,* **2020**, *76*(4), 531-539.
        [http://dx.doi.org/10.1111/his.14029] [PMID: 31692018]

[88]   Vindum, H.H.; Agnholt, J.S.; Nielsen, A.W.M.; Nielsen, M.B.; Schmidt, H. Severe steroid refractory gastritis induced by Nivolumab: A case report. *World J. Gastroenterol.,* **2020**, *26*(16), 1971-1978.
        [http://dx.doi.org/10.3748/wjg.v26.i16.1971] [PMID: 32390707]

[89]   Raad, R.A.; Pavlick, A.; Kannan, R.; Friedman, K.P. Ipilimumab-induced hepatitis on ^{18}F-FDG PET/CT in a patient with malignant melanoma. *Clin. Nucl. Med.,* **2015**, *40*(3), 258-259.
        [http://dx.doi.org/10.1097/RLU.0000000000000606] [PMID: 25290291]

[90]   Antonia, S.J.; Villegas, A.; Daniel, D.; Vicente, D.; Murakami, S.; Hui, R.; Yokoi, T.; Chiappori, A.; Lee, K.H.; de Wit, M.; Cho, B.C.; Bourhaba, M.; Quantin, X.; Tokito, T.; Mekhail, T.; Planchard, D.; Kim, Y.C.; Karapetis, C.S.; Hiret, S.; Ostoros, G.; Kubota, K.; Gray, J.E.; Paz-Ares, L.; de Castro Carpeño, J.; Wadsworth, C.; Melillo, G.; Jiang, H.; Huang, Y.; Dennis, P.A.; Özgüroğlu, M. Durvalumab after chemoradiotherapy in stage iii non–small-cell lung cancer. *N. Engl. J. Med.,* **2017**, *377*(20), 1919-1929.
        [http://dx.doi.org/10.1056/NEJMoa1709937] [PMID: 28885881]

[91]   Gkiozos, I.; Kopitopoulou, A.; Kalkanis, A.; Vamvakaris, I.N.; Judson, M.A.; Syrigos, K.N. Sarcoidosis-like reactions induced by checkpoint inhibitors. *J. Thorac. Oncol.,* **2018**, *13*(8), 1076-

1082.
[http://dx.doi.org/10.1016/j.jtho.2018.04.031] [PMID: 29763666]

[92]   Sachpekidis, C.; Kopp-Schneider, A.; Hakim-Meibodi, L.; Dimitrakopoulou-Strauss, A.; Hassel, J.C. ^{18}F-FDG PET/CT longitudinal studies in patients with advanced metastatic melanoma for response evaluation of combination treatment with vemurafenib and ipilimumab. *Melanoma Res.,* **2019**, *29*(2), 178-186.
[http://dx.doi.org/10.1097/CMR.0000000000000541] [PMID: 30653029]

[93]   Calabrese, L.H.; Calabrese, C.; Cappelli, L.C. Rheumatic immune-related adverse events from cancer immunotherapy. *Nat. Rev. Rheumatol.,* **2018**, *14*(10), 569-579.
[http://dx.doi.org/10.1038/s41584-018-0074-9] [PMID: 30171203]

[94]   Hashimoto, K.; Kaira, K.; Yamaguchi, O.; Mouri, A.; Shiono, A.; Miura, Y.; Murayama, Y.; Kobayashi, K.; Kagamu, H.; Kuji, I. Potential of FDG-PET as prognostic significance after anti-pd-1 antibody against patients with previously treated non-small cell lung cancer. *J. Clin. Med.,* **2020**, *9*(3), 725.
[http://dx.doi.org/10.3390/jcm9030725] [PMID: 32156047]

CHAPTER 9

2-Deoxy-D-Glucose as an Emerging Chemotherapeutic Agent in Cancer Management

Ashutosh Singh[1], Ravinsh Kumar[1] and Amrita Srivastava[1,*]

[1] *Department of Life Science, Central University of South Bihar, Gaya–824236, India*

Abstract: Cancer cells have a unique property of uncontrolled growth and thus they require a constant supply of energy. Warburg observed that tumor cells prefer glycolysis even under oxygenic conditions and the process is known as aerobic glycolysis. Hence, cancerous cells show an enhanced glucose-to-lactate conversion rate. As cancerous growth is accompanied by enhanced glucose uptake, this feature is best suited for the management of unwanted cell proliferation by blocking the glucose metabolism of cancer cells. 2-deoxy-D-glucose (2DG), a glucose antimetabolite is considered a competitive inhibitor of glucose transport and glucose phosphorylation. It inhibits the glycolytic pathway primarily due to the inhibition of phosphohexose isomerase by 2-deoxy-D-glucose-6-phosphate (2DG- 6P). Its chemical resemblance to 2-deoxymannose causes interruption in the initial steps of N-linked glycosylation leading to the misfolding of proteins resulting in endoplasmic reticulum stress. In addition to the two properties of 2DG namely, the prevention of glycolysis and selective storage in the tumor cells, there are several other attributes of 2DG apart from the ones mentioned above that make it an attractive target for use as an antitumor agent. Some properties include the capability of inducing autophagy in tumor cells, inhibiting genomic replication as well as mRNA expression of viral genes responsible for Omit the induction of oncogenesis, blocking pathological angiogenesis while being cautious towards established endothelial tubes and prominent anti-metastatic effect. In the present chapter, various aspects of the use of 2DG in cancer management have been discussed.

Keywords: Anticancer, Competitive inhibition, Chemotherapeutic drug, Glycolysis, Warburg effect, 2-deoxy-D-Glucose.

1. INTRODUCTION

Unicellular organisms have Omit the tendency to initiate their reproductive phase as soon as possible when nutrients are available. They possess a system that senses the nutrient supply and accordingly channelizes the metabolites to fulfill

* **Corresponding author Amrita Srivastava:** Department of Life Science, Central University of South Bihar, Gaya–824236, India; E-mail: amritasrivastava@cub.ac.in

Raman Singh, Antresh Kumar & Kuldeep Singh (Eds.)

their requirement of carbon, nitrogen, and free energy for preparing the building blocks required to produce a new cell. However, biomass production ceases when there is a scarcity of nutrients. Under such circumstances, organisms readjust their metabolism in such a way that maximum free energy is conserved in order to survive through the starvation period. Also, the cells prefer not to enter the proliferative stage without undergoing proper cell cycle checkpoints. For this, they possess a cellular mechanism to prevent the entry of excessive nutrients, if available, so that they may not cause unnecessary induction of cell proliferation. Mammalian cells utilize the nutrients present in the external environment only when stimulated by growth factors but the process of cell division in cancer cells becomes independent of growth factors due to some genetic mutations.

Dividing cells require replication/synthesis of all the chemical constituents that are essential to build macromolecules required for the synthesis of all cellular components such as DNA, RNA, proteins, glucose, and lipids. Precursors for cell division are provided in some form or the other through glucose. Therefore, glycolysis is upregulated to maintain the level of glycolytic intermediates needed to support biosynthesis in proliferating cells [1]. Owing to the profound role of glucose in cellular metabolism and proliferation, its analogs, such as 2-deoxy-D-glucose, which have a metabolic fate different from glucose can be employed to regulate widespread diseases such as cancer, epilepsy, aging-related issues, and viral infections.

2. GLUCOSE METABOLISM IN CANCER CELLS

In normal cells, glucose first gets metabolized in the glycolytic cycle to produce NADH and pyruvate. Both the end products of the glycolytic cycle, NADH and pyruvate are transported into the mitochondria where oxidation of pyruvate takes place through the TCA cycle while NADH is oxidized to NAD^+ in the electron transport chain [2]. The reducing equivalents produced in the TCA cycle are used to fuel oxidative phosphorylation to maximize the synthesis of adenosine triphosphate (ATP) [3].

When glucose is subjected to oxidation through the Krebs cycle and the transfer of electrons occurs through the electron transport chain, several-fold higher amounts of ATP are generated in terms of ATP generated per molecule of glucose oxidation as compared to aerobic glycolysis. Even then aerobic glycolysis is preferred over oxidative phosphorylation as it provides ATP at a faster rate. Analysis of data generated from a study on 31 cancer cell lines/tissues suggested that the average percentage of ATP contribution from glycolysis is 17% [4]. It is evident through a study on the reduced flux-balance model by Vazquez *et al.*

(2010) [5] that synthesizing ATP through aerobic glycolysis is of normal occurrence in a cell that tends to have more mitochondria than its threshold.

Since cancer cells have a peculiar feature of sustained proliferation, they overcome the feedback regulatory mechanisms to meet their anabolic demands. For the continuation of glycolysis, a constant supply of NAD^+ and ADP is required for the continuation of glycolysis. NAD^+ from NADH is generated during the conversion of pyruvate to lactate by lactate dehydrogenase. Enhanced rate of glycolysis that is encountered in cancer cells is fueled by this enzymatic activity [6]. Growth-regulating factors stimulate proliferation in normal cells of healthy tissues by binding to their respective transmembrane receptors. Nutrients and oxygen required for this purpose are made available through the blood supply [7]. In contrast to normal cells, which require mitogenic growth signals for their propagation, cancer cells depend on their growth factors so they have reduced requirement for extracellular growth factors. This implies that instead of the normally occurring paracrine mode of operation of growth factors, cancer cells mainly rely on the autocrine mode of growth factors utilization. Mutations in receptor-associated signaling molecules and insensitiveness towards anti-growth stimuli lead to independent cellular proliferation in tumor cells [8]. Unrestrained cellular proliferation of cancer cells places newly formed tumor cells away from the blood vessels in the area where the tumor is proliferating. Therefore, the availability of blood and glucose to the core of the tumor cells gets impaired. Partial oxygen pressure declines to extremely hypoxic values (≤ 0.5mm Hg) in avascular areas in a tumor [9]. Tumor cells experiencing hypoxia secrete a transcription factor known as Hypoxia-inducible factor-Iα (HIF-Iα), which, in turn, regulates tumor pH and angiogenesis.

The term angiogenesis is used for the formation of new blood vessels and is often found exacerbated in tumors. Vascular endothelial growth factor (VEGF) and Ang-2 are the two critical factors that are secreted in response to hypoxia and are involved in angiogenesis. HIF-Iα induces the expression of VEGF by binding to its promoter and thereby promotes tumor angiogenesis [10]. Transcriptional regulation of VEGF also takes place by Ras-ERK and PI(3)K–AKT pathways [11].

One of the enzymes of the glycolytic pathway-hexokinase (HK), which is involved on phosphorylation of glucose to produce glucose-6-phosphate by utilizing an ATP is also a target of HIF-Iα and hence it is responsible for high glycolytic rate in hypoxic solid tumors [12]. There are four types of HKs found in mammalian tissues that are encoded by different genes – *HK1, HK2, HK3,* and *HK4* [13]. Biochemical attributes of the above-mentioned hexokinases are comparable to each other but they show unique tissue localization and enzymatic behaviour. HK1 is ubiquitously expressed in most mammalian adult tissues while HK2 is abundantly expressed mostly in embryonic tissues. Increased expression of HK2 is evident only in adipose, skeletal, and cardiac muscles [14] and confers resistance to apoptosis [8]. HK1, HK2, and HK3 show a high affinity for glucose while HK4 (also known as glucokinase), with expression restricted to the liver and pancreas, has a lower affinity for glucose. Interestingly, glucose concentrations lying within the normal physiological range are known to inhibit HK3.

Hexokinases catalyse the first committed step of glycolysis to produce glucose 6-phosphate (G6P) and accordingly get inhibited when there is an excess of G6P. This step is the most crucial one because, at this stage, glucose gets trapped inside cells. If not phosphorylated, glucose gets exported outside the cell by transporters [15]. Binding of HK2 to voltage-dependent anion channel (VDAC) located within the outer mitochondrial membrane decreases its sensitivity towards G6P and thus renders it insensitive to product inhibition [16]. High HK2 expression in cancer cells and its decreased sensitivity when bound to VDAC causes rapid production of G6P. Latter, being a major source of carbon, is of great significance to tumor cells as it serves as a precursor for their growth and proliferation. Also, it contributes to generation of ATP through its conversion to lactate [17].

Abnormal glycolytic flux in cancer cells is not only activated in hypoxia. Normally, differentiated cells produce large amounts of lactate under anaerobic conditions but cancer cells have a unique property to produce large amounts of lactate even when sufficient oxygen is available. This mechanism is referred to as the "Warburg effect". According to the original idea of Otto Warburg, it was hypothesized that mitochondria become defective in cancer cells causing impaired aerobic respiration leading to more dependence on glycolytic mechanisms (Warburg, 1956) [18]. However, a further study rejected this hypothesis as mitochondria were found to remain functional in cancer cells.

Many oncogenes are held responsible for the Warburg effect. Products of these genes such as Ras, phosphoinositide 3-kinase (PI3K), protein kinase B (PKB/AKT), and Von Hippel-Lindau induce the expression of HIF-1α even in non-hypoxic conditions. HIF-Iα promotes glucose uptake *via* glucose transporter 1 (GLUT1) along with the upregulation of HK2. In tumor cells, high AKT and mTOR (mechanistic target of rapamycin) oncogenic activity promotes HIF-Iα expression that predominantly causes the synthesis of enzymes required for glycolysis and production of lactate. On one hand, HIF-Iα transcriptionally activates glycolytic enzymes but on the other hand, it inhibits the conversion of pyruvate to acetyl-CoA by activating pyruvate dehydrogenase kinase 1, which in turn inhibits the function of pyruvate dehydrogenase. In this way, the activity of

HIF-Iα pushes cancer cells to aerobic glycolysis [19]. Cancer cells do not switch to aerobic glycolysis due to mitochondrial dysfunction. Rather, they use glycolytic intermediates to support anabolic reactions in cells which provide advantages in cellular proliferation [20].

In addition to glycolysis, glycogenolysis acts as another source of energy to tumor cells facing nutrient stress as it produces G6P that enters the glycolytic pathway. Glucose is stored in the form of glycogen inside the cells. Although most tissues are capable of glycogen storage, the most abundant depot is present in the liver and skeletal muscles. Glycogen metabolism is found upregulated in several cancers such as renal, breast, bladder, uterine, ovarian, skin, and brain cancers. According to a recent study, RAB25 is considered a positive regulator of glycogen synthesis in cancer cells [21]. AGL is a glycogen-debranching enzyme that acts as a tumor suppressor in bladder cancer [22]. In hypoxic conditions, both glycogen synthesis and breakdown enzymes are induced [23]. Under hypoxic conditions, HIF-Iα induces several synthetic enzymes and regulatory proteins such as UTP: Glucose-1-Purydylyltransferase, glycogen synthase enzyme, glycogen branching enzyme, phosphoglucomutase, and PPP1R3C.

In renal carcinoma cell lines RCC4 and 786-O, defect in the tumor suppressor protein and HIF-negative regulator von Hippel–Lindau leads to constitutive expression of HIF-Iα and HIF- 2α, which in turn regulates the synthesis of glycogen [21]. Cancer cells experiencing prolonged hypoxia conditions lead to activation of enzymes responsible for glycogen breakdown [24]. The breakdown of glycogen contributes to the production of NADPH, an essential reducing agent for scavenging Reactive Oxygen Species (ROS) and nucleotide, amino acid, and lipid synthesis, as well as nucleotides needed for DNA repair and proliferation through the pentose phosphate pathway. It might be targeted to develop therapeutic drugs against cancer.

3. 2-DEOXY-D-GLUCOSE

3.1. Structure and Properties

The term 'glucose' was first coined by a French chemist Jean Baptiste Andre Dumas. A simple sugar consisting of 6 carbons is known as glucose. It has two functional groups, aldehyde and alcohol groups. A chemical reaction between the C-5 hydroxyl group and the aldehyde group present on the C-1 leads to cyclization resulting in the formation of α-D-glucopyranose and β-D-glucopyranose. Both these isomers differ only in the orientation of the –OH group. Polarimetric analysis of glucose by Kekule (in 1866) confirmed its dextrorotatory nature as it rotates the light in a clockwise direction. Thus, dextrorotatory glucose is represented as D-glucose [25]. When the –OH group present at the 2nd carbon is replaced by hydrogen, it becomes an analog of glucose known as 2-deoxy-D-glucose (2DG; Fig. **1**).

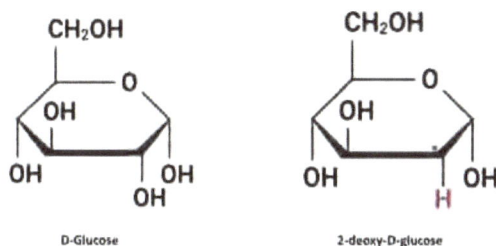

Fig. (1). Comparative structures of Glucose and 2-deoxy-D-glucose.

In this first step of glycolysis, glucose gets converted into glucose-6-phosphate (Fig. **2**). 2DG is a natural non-metabolizable glucose analog that gets phosphorylated by hexokinase and forms 2-deoxy-D-glucose-6-phosphate. As the latter does not act as a substrate for phosphohexose isomerase, further steps of glycolysis are inhibited leading to the intracellular accumulation of 2DG-6P (Fig. **3**).

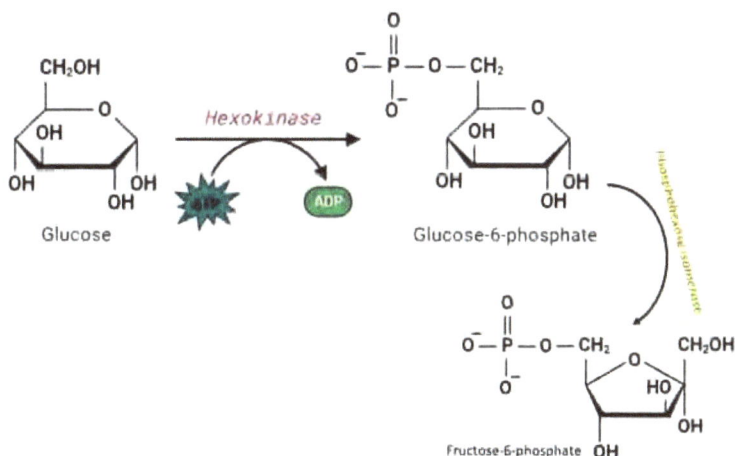

Fig. (2). First step in glycolytic conversion of glucose to form Glucose-6-phosphate.

Thus, in normal metabolism where glucose is converted to form pyruvate during glycolysis, further metabolism of 2DG beyond 2-deoxy-D-glucose-6-phosphate does not occur (Fig. **4**). In addition to glycolysis inhibition, 2DG activates adenosine-activated protein kinase (AMPK), induces autophagy, promotes apoptosis *via* activation of tumor suppressor gene p53, and interferes in N-glycosylation process leading to endoplasmic reticulum (ER) stress [26]. Alteration of the 2' carbon of glucose molecule decides its fate *i.e.* metabolic pathway and use within the cell. For example, in the naturally occurring glucose isomer mannose, the only difference is the orientation of the -OH group at 2' carbon that is opposite of glucose, and due to this, it acts as a substrate for N-glycosylation and not as an energy source.

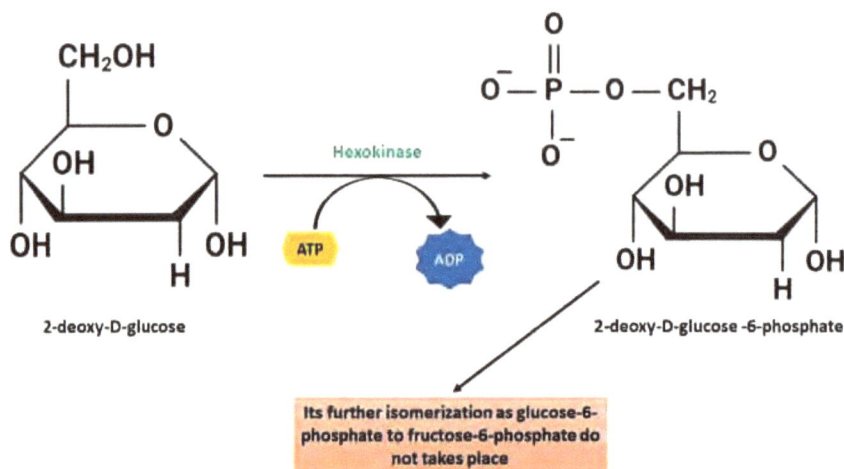

Fig. (3). First step in the glycolytic conversion of 2DG.

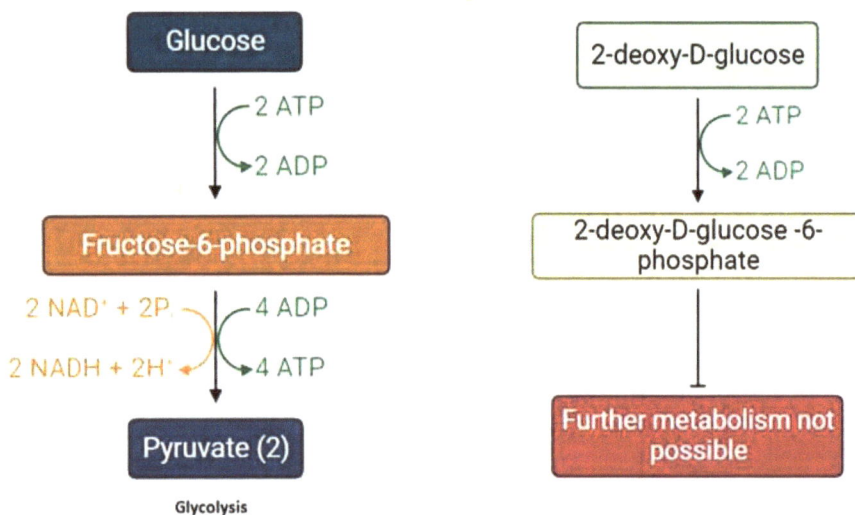

Fig. (4). Metabolic fate of glucose during glycolysis leading to the formation of pyruvate in contrast to glycolytic inhibition in case of 2DG.

3.2. A Brief Historical Perspective of 2DG

There were several studies reporting different methods for the synthesis of 2DG but most of them suffer from operational problems like low yield, low purity, and formation of a racemic mixture (see Chapter 2). 2-deoxy-2-fluoro-D-glucose (19FDG) is an analog of natural glucose that easily penetrates the cells and accumulates there. Initially, it was speculated that it would act as an anticancer agent but later it was found that its therapeutic Dosage was observed to affect both malignant as well as normal cells.

2DG in radiolabelled form plays a crucial role in PET imaging [27]. This aspect has been discussed in chapters 5 and 7. Cramer and Woodward in their study on the yeast model reported that 2DG has the ability to strongly inhibit the fermentation of glucose that occurs in the absence of oxygen [28]. Jha and Pohlit reported that 2DG inhibits the DNA double-strand break repair while it enhances radiation-induced cell killing [29]. 2-deoxy-D-glucose may differentially inhibit the repair of radiation damage in hypoxic tumour cells while the enhancement of repair processes could be expected in normal tissues. In the late 1980s, a combination of 2DG and rhodamine 123 (mitochondrial uncoupler) showed an effective result in both *in vitro* and *in vivo* models [30]. It was reported by Jain *et al.* (1985) that 2DG could be used to optimize the radiation effect by enhancing the radiation damage in cancer cells while reducing its damage in normal cells [31]. The application of 2DG as a prospective therapeutic against hypoxic cancer cells that had turned chemo-resistant began in the late 1990s [32]. Since very early 2DG has been consistently tested for its application as an anticancer agent. 2DG in combination with several other drugs has shown significant results in this regard [33]. So, it can be targeted as one of the strategies to combat cancer. Recently, it gained popularity in the pandemic. Codo *et al.* [34] confirmed that increased glucose levels and glycolysis promote SARS-CoV2 infection. Several patients affected by COVID had immense dependence on an external supply of oxygen which was shown to be considerably reduced upon administration of 2DG. It was therefore medically authorized by the Indian Drug Regulatory Authority in May 2020 during the COVID-19 pandemic (see chapter 7) [35].

4. THERAPEUTIC APPLICATIONS OF 2DG

Cancer cells employ diverse strategies for proliferation and invasion including non-requirement of growth signals, uncontrolled replicative behavior, averted angiogenesis, insensitivity to immune response, resistance to apoptotic cell death, non-responsive behavior towards growth inhibitors, genetic variability, chronic inflammation and changes in normal cell metabolism. Additionally, hypoxic conditions prevail in tumorigenic regions lying away from the core, which also face poor vascularization thereby promoting glycolysis as the primary ATP production pathway for cancer cells. Recognizing the immense need for glycolysis in cancerous cells provides a way of selectively eliminating cancer cells while sparing untransformed cells.

Tumor cells even in aerobic conditions exhibit the Warburg effect favoring glycolysis over oxidative phosphorylation for energy production [18]. The increased glucose demands for metabolic functions result in enhanced glucose transport into cancerous cells facilitated by the transcriptional activation of the Glut1 glucose transporter gene. Elevated Glut1 expression is prevalent in various human cancers notably in breast cancers where its high levels correlate with heightened proliferative activity and histological score. This association implies that escalated glucose uptake may act as a pivotal regulatory point impacting the growth of synthetic activity and suppression of apoptosis in malignant cells. Recently there has been a lot of emphasis on the importance of comprehending these metabolic pathways and introducing 2DG as a potential therapeutic agent targeting glucose metabolism in cancer treatment.

Aft *et al.* (2002) reported the potential role of the anti-metabolite 2DG in cancer treatment particularly emphasizing its impact on breast cancer cells [36]. The research indicates that 2DG disrupts glucose metabolism resulting in a dose-dependent inhibition of cell growth in human breast cancer cell lines. Treatment with 2DG leads to decreased cell viability and clonogenic survival pointing towards apoptosis. This is further supported by increased caspase3 activity and cleavage of poly (ADP-ribose) polymerase. Breast cancer cells exposed to 2DG exhibit elevated levels of Glut1 transporter protein and enhanced glucose uptake compared to untreated cells. Their study suggests that 2DG induces apoptosis in breast cancer cells by activating the apoptotic pathway. Additionally, they propose that treated breast cancer cells expedite their demise by upregulating glucose transporter proteins facilitating heightened 2DG uptake and subsequently triggering cell death. Their findings underscore the potential of targeting glucose metabolism specifically through agents like 2DG as a promising strategy for chemotherapeutic intervention in breast cancer.

Due to its structural similarity to glucose, it competitively binds to the receptor and enters inside the cell where it gets phosphorylated by hexokinase. As 2DG-6P is not a substrate for phosphohexose isomerase, it gets accumulated intracellularly to a concentration capable of inhibiting hexokinase. Inhibition of hexokinase suppresses glycolysis and ATP production leading to a depletion of cellular energy [37]. Consequently, the pathogen is unable to obtain the required energy because of energy depletion in the host itself. This deprived cellular microenvironment results in the deactivation of the pathogen. Moreover, the lowered concentration of ATP triggers AMP (adenosine monophosphate)-mediated protein kinase activation leading to the phosphorylation of mTOR kinase (the mechanistic target of rapamycin kinase) and tuberous sclerosis (TSC 1). Consequently, autophagy of infected cells and cell death occur due to the inhibition of the G1 phase in the cell cycle [38].

2DG could be of potential use in cancer diagnostics [39, 40]. The Warburg effect in cancer cells characterized by increased glucose consumption has driven the development of 2DG radioisotope analogs for detecting transformed cells. Positron emission tomography utilizing 18F-DG, a radiolabeled glucose analog is widely employed for cancer detection, staging, treatment response monitoring, and recurrence detection. 2DG's ability to penetrate the blood-brain barrier suggests its potential in brain tumor diagnostics. Initiated in 1969, Louis Sokoloff's research led to the synthesis of 18F-DG, a highly utilized radiotracer today. PET scanning with 18F-DG reflects glucose metabolism, offering visualization and diagnosis, particularly in organs with intensive glucose metabolism or excretion.

5. IMPLICATIONS OF 2DG IN CANCER

2DG has a profound effect on various biochemical and physiological modifications as observed in cancerous cells. Some 2DG-mediated modulations in oncogenic processes have been summarized below (Fig. **5**).

5.1. Effects on Angiogenesis

The tumor microenvironment plays a crucial role in tumorigenesis. The growth and metastasis of tumor depend on angiogenesis. Endothelial cells are mostly in a quiescent state and rarely divide but in a diseased condition, the activation of VEGF changes the state of endothelial cells from quiescent to highly proliferative. Angiogenesis acts as an important factor in cancer progression. This process takes place in four steps – In the first step, the basement membrane in the tissues gets injured leading to hypoxia followed by the activation of endothelial cells by angiogenic factors in the second step. Angiogenic factors activate the proliferation of endothelial cells in the third step and finally, the angiogenesis process continues under the influence of angiogenic factors. Angiogenic activators such as angiogenin, basic fibroblast growth factor, granulocyte colony-stimulating factor, epidermal growth factor, placental growth factor, interleukin-8, hepatocyte growth factor, platelet-derived endothelial growth factor, transforming growth factor-α, transforming growth factor-β, tumor necrosis factor (TNF)-α and VEGF are involved in angiogenesis [41]. Growing tumor cells increases the distance of the core of the tumor from the vessels resulting in hypoxia. This condition activates the HIF-Iα, which in turn activates the VEGF and promotes angiogenesis.

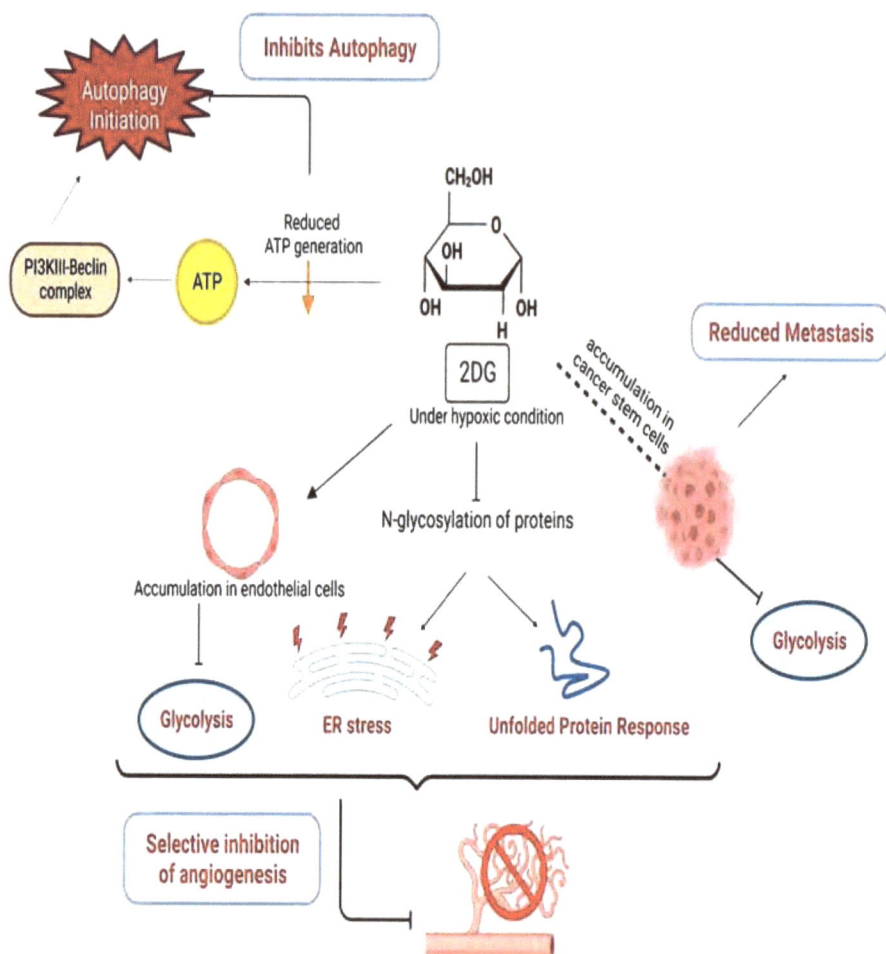

Fig. (5). Effect of 2DG on crucial processes regulating cancer cell proliferation.

Upon treatment with 2DG, it was observed that endothelial cells showed hypersensitivity towards the cytotoxic influence of 2DG, which was much greater as compared to normal or cancerous cells [42]. This angiogenic effect was confirmed through studies in mice models. It only targets actively dividing endothelial cells thereby blocking the formation of new capillaries whereas it does not impose any effect on already established vessels. One of the possible explanations for the hypersensitivity of endothelial cells for 2DG is that it is highly glycolytic, so it accumulates a huge amount of 2DG [32]. It was revealed that 2DG-induced inhibition of N-linked glycosylation caused ER stress and Unfolded Protein Response, ultimately leading to its anti-angiogenic effect. So, it can be used to prevent angiogenesis in tumors.

5.2. Effects on Metastasis

Cancer becomes life-threatening when it becomes metastatic and hence it is considered as a primary cause of death from cancer. *In vitro* study by Sottnik *et al.* [38] reported that 2DG is able to inhibit cancer cell migration and invasion while *in vivo* study of 2DG shows significant delays in tumor metastasis. Although the exact mechanism has not been deciphered, the anti-metastatic effect of 2DG has hypothetically been attributed to its enhanced accumulation in cancer stem cells. Since these cancer stem cells are considered to have the highest metastatic potential (as reported in certain tumors [43, 44], 2DG accumulation in these cells leads to an overall reduction in metastasis of tumors. As 2DG is able to target both primary and metastatic tumors, it can become a valuable drug in cancer.

5.3. Influence of 2DG on Autophagic Cell Death

The term 'autophagy' is derived from the ancient Greek word which means self-devouring. It is a tightly regulated intracellular pathway involved in the degradation and recycling of proteins and cellular organelles [45]. Autophagy in normal cells is involved in maintaining homeostatic function by checking the quality of proteins and organelles and preventing the accumulation of polyubiquitinated and aggregated proteins. Cancer cells suffering from metabolic stress can induce apoptosis but tumor cells with defective apoptotic machinery result in the induction of autophagy and promote their survival [46]. Damaged proteins or organelles are referred to as cargo and their lysis is manifested in specialized cellular structures called autophagosomes. Autophagosomes are double-membrane vesicles that surround the cytoplasmic contents targeted for degradation. Starvation activates autophagy and induces the phagophore formation resulting in the genesis of autophagosomes. Atg proteins are responsible for activating autophagy by inducing the formation of autophagosomes, segregation of intracellular contents, and fusion of autophagosomes to lysosomes finally resulting in degradation and recycling of the content. mTOR regulates autophagy *via* upstream PI3K/AKT pathway [47]. ER stress and glucose starvation act as drivers of autophagy in two ways, first *via* activation of the LKB1-AMPK pathway induced by lowering of ATP level and second, *via* activation of ERK mediated by enhanced ROS levels [48].

Wang *et al.* [49] reported that 2DG causes the activation of AMPK, which results in autophagy in endothelial cells. Further exploration suggests that interference in the glycosylation process by 2DG causes ER stress, which, as a result, induces autophagy. ER is considered the major storage site of intracellular Ca^{+2}. Application of 2DG enhances the ER Ca^{+2} efflux. Thus, the cytoplasmic concentration of Ca^{+2} rises, which, in turn, activates the $Ca^{2+/}$ calmodulin-dependent protein kinase kinase β. As AMPK is its downstream target, its activation induces autophagy. So, based on the above stated facts, it can be said that AMPK, which is known as an energy stress sensor, also acts as a sensor for ER stress [48]. Both glucose starvation and the use of 2DG induce autophagy but with different mechanisms. Cellular ROS gets decreased with the use of 2DG but glucose deprivation increases the ROS and thus activates the autophagy in an extracellular signal-regulated kinase (ERK)-dependent manner.

This entire scenario gets revered in hypoxic conditions as seen in tumor cells growing away from their centre of origin. In hypoxic conditions, treatment of 2DG decreases autophagy activity thereby blocking the pro-survival process in hypoxic tumor cells [48]. 2DG and also glucose starvation are correlated with a tremendous reduction in ATP levels along with the inhibition of several crucial steps of autophagy. Other effects include reduced formation of PI3K III - Beclin1 complex required primarily for the initiation of autophagy, inhibition of ATG12 and ATG5 conjugate formation necessary for autophagosomes to expand together with a constraint opportunity for lysosomal attachment, and autophagic degradation [48].

5.4. Influence of 2DG on Apoptotic Cell Death

Apoptosis is a programmed cell death in which a cell undergoing apoptosis shows a distinct set of morphological changes such as rounding up of cell, shrinkage, chromatin condensation and fragmentation, and blebbing of the plasma membrane [50]. Apoptosis is triggered either by an extracellular receptor-mediated pathway or an intrinsic pathway. In the receptor-mediated pathway, the Fas receptor and tumor necrosis factor receptor on activation recruit caspase-8 and 10 leading to the formation of death-induced signaling complex causing the release of cytochrome C while the intrinsic pathway gets activated by oxidative stress, cytotoxic drugs, or any extra or intracellular stress that causes the release of cytochrome C followed by its binding to the Apoptotic Protease Activating Factor-1 (Apaf-1). It becomes evident that glucose metabolism inhibition promotes apoptosis by activating mitochondrial-dependent and independent pathways [51].

C-myc, a transcription factor with multiple roles, is known for its regulation of cell proliferation, differentiation, and apoptosis and simultaneous inhibition of genes with antiproliferative roles. Lactate dehydrogenase A is upregulated by c-myc and plays an important role in normal anaerobic glycolysis. In non-transformed cells, glucose deprivation causes cell cycle arrest in the Go/G1 phase while c-myc transformed cells show predisposition to cellular proliferation. Upon treatment with 2DG, c-myc-transformed cells underwent extensive apoptosis [52]. 2DG is able to induce apoptosis in Bcl-2/Bcl-X$_L$-deficient neoplasms having high c-Myc or lactate dehydrogenase A expression levels.

Ishino *et al.* [53], reported that 2DG activates ER stress-induced apoptosis in pancreatic cancer cells by interfering in the protein N-glycosylation process through the suppression of glutamine: fructose 6-phosphate aminotransferase 1, an important component of hexosamine biosynthesis pathway involved in glycoprotein maintenance.

TNF-related apoptosis-inducing ligand (TRAIL) selectively induces apoptosis in cancer cells but does not produce any effect on normal cells. Various types of tumors including gastric tumors are resistant to TRAIL-mediated apoptosis. So, it is not majorly used as an anticancer therapy. A study conducted by Xu *et al.* [54] analysed that 2DG enhances the TRAIL sensitivity in various cancers. In response to various stress stimuli, JNK, a stress-activated kinase regulates autophagy in mammalian cells. It is found that 2DG induces apoptosis through TRAIL sensitization by inhibiting the phosphorylation of JNK resulting in recovery from TRAIL resistance. Combining 2DG and TRAIL can be a capable therapeutic target for cancer. 2DG in combination with arsenic trioxide and other anti-tumor agents directs the human myeloid leukemia cell lines toward apoptosis [55]. Cisplatin, a commonly used chemotherapeutic agent when treated on SKOV3 cells in combination with 2DG shows an enhanced antitumor effect due to the induction of ER stress and variation in ATP levels ensuing in the inhibition of cellular proliferation and promotion of apoptosis [56]. The effect of 2DG should be evaluated for its efficacy in combination with several other anti-tumor drugs.

5.5. Effect of 2DG on Virus-Induced Oncogenesis

Kaposi's sarcoma-associated herpesvirus (KSHV), also known as Human herpesvirus 8 is involved in the development of Kaposi sarcoma (KS), endothelial tumor, primary effusion lymphoma, and multicentric Castleman's disease. KS is a common cancer in individuals suffering from HIV/AIDS. KSHV activates the PI3K/Akt/mTOR signaling pathway at different nodes *via* the viral proteins vGPCR, K1, ORF36/vPK, vIL-6, and K15, as well as through virus-mediated upregulation of cellular growth factors, *e.g.*, VEGF and Platelets Derived Growth Factor. KSHV has two distinct phases of the viral life cycle in which the latent or lysogenic phase is characterised by a circular, extra-chromosomal viral genome with no functional infectious viral particles whereas lytic phase of the viral cycle is characterized by viral genome replication and expression of transcripts categorised into immediate-early, early and late transcripts [57]. 2DG inhibits the genome replication of KSHV during the lytic phase of the viral cycle [58]. Along with this, it also decreases the transcriptional expression of virally encoded genes necessary for oncogenesis. N-glycosylation is a protein modification process in which mannose is attached to the nitrogen of an amide group in asparagine. This process occurs early during translation and during its transport to ER trimming and remodeling of oligosaccharide takes place. This process of the host cell is used by viruses to modify the proteins present on their surface, which ultimately helps in providing stability to the viral glycoproteins, antigenicity, and promoting host cell invasion [59]. 2DG is able to inhibit the SARS CoV2 and other coronaviruses by disrupting the glycosylation process of viral proteins [60]. Zika virus for its replication requires concomitant upregulation of glycolysis. The use of 2DG decreased the viral load in HRvEC cells. Thus, 2DG has the potential for effective treatment against Zika virus infection. Large viral surface antigens present in the hepatitis B virus interact with the PKM2, which is actively involved in the regulation of glucose metabolism in hepatocytes thereby increasing glucose utilization and lactate production. Treatment of 2DG inhibits viral replication by suppressing protein synthesis of hepatitis virus [60]. Similarly, 2DG treatment effectively reduced the murine norovirus infection by downregulating the glycolysis [60]. Infection of rhinovirus that causes the common cold and other respiratory tract infections is also reduced by the use of 2DG [60].

CONCLUSION

Glucose is the primary source of energy for all living cells. 2DG as a glucose analog is capable of being taken up by cells but interferes with downstream reactions of glycolysis. The indispensability of cancerous cells for glycolysis as a means of sustenance for proliferating cells and glycolytic inhibition caused by 2DG have together opened a significant therapeutic avenue. 2DG by virtue of its ability to inhibit angiogenesis together with metastatic growth and diversion in mechanisms of cell death happens to curtail cancer cell proliferation. 2DG alone, and in conjunction with other therapeutic agents, needs further testing in order to understand its mechanism of action so as to apply it for widespread use.

ABBREVIATIONS

2DG   2-deoxy-D-glucose

ATP   Adenosine triphosphate

AMPK Adenosine-activated protein kinase

ER   Endoplasmic reticulum

G6P   Glucose 6-phosphate

HK   Hexokinase

HIF-Iα Hypoxia-inducible factor-Iα

KSHV Kaposi's sarcoma-associated herpesvirus

KS	Kaposi sarcoma
PI3K	Phosphoinositide 3-kinase
ROS	Reactive oxygen species
TNF	Tumor necrosis factor
TRAIL	TNF-related apoptosis-inducing ligand
VDAC	Voltage dependent anion channel
VEGF	Vascular endothelial growth factor

ACKNOWLEDGEMENTS

The authors acknowledge the profound support from the Department of Life Science, Central University of South Bihar, for providing the facilities to write and submit this book chapter.

REFERENCES

[1]   Vander Heiden, M.G.; Cantley, L.C.; Thompson, C.B. Understanding the Warburg effect: the metabolic requirements of cell proliferation. *Science,* **2009**, *324*(5930), 1029-1033.
      [http://dx.doi.org/10.1126/science.1160809] [PMID: 19460998]

[2]   Chandel, N.S. Glycolysis. *Cold Spring Harb. Perspect. Biol.,* **2021**, *13*(5), a040535.
      [http://dx.doi.org/10.1101/cshperspect.a040535] [PMID: 33941515]

[3]   Fernie, A.R.; Carrari, F.; Sweetlove, L.J. Respiratory metabolism: glycolysis, the TCA cycle and mitochondrial electron transport. *Curr. Opin. Plant Biol.,* **2004**, *7*(3), 254-261.
      [http://dx.doi.org/10.1016/j.pbi.2004.03.007] [PMID: 15134745]

[4]   Zu, X.L.; Guppy, M. Cancer metabolism: facts, fantasy, and fiction. *Biochem. Biophys. Res. Commun.,* **2004**, *313*(3), 459-465.
      [http://dx.doi.org/10.1016/j.bbrc.2003.11.136] [PMID: 14697210]

[5]   Vazquez, A.; Liu, J.; Zhou, Y.; Oltvai, Z.N. Catabolic efficiency of aerobic glycolysis: The Warburg effect revisited. *BMC Syst. Biol.,* **2010**, *4*(1), 58.
      [http://dx.doi.org/10.1186/1752-0509-4-58] [PMID: 20459610]

[6]   Locasale, J.W.; Cantley, L.C. Altered metabolism in cancer. *BMC Biol.,* **2010**, *8*(1), 88.
      [http://dx.doi.org/10.1186/1741-7007-8-88] [PMID: 20598111]

[7]   Lyons, R.M.; Moses, H.L. Transforming growth factors and the regulation of cell proliferation. *Eur. J. Biochem.,* **1990**, *187*(3), 467-473.
      [http://dx.doi.org/10.1111/j.1432-1033.1990.tb15327.x] [PMID: 2406131]

[8]   Annibaldi, A.; Widmann, C. Glucose metabolism in cancer cells. *Curr. Opin. Clin. Nutr. Metab. Care,* **2010**, *13*(4), 466-470.
      [http://dx.doi.org/10.1097/MCO.0b013e32833a5577] [PMID: 20473153]

[9]   Helmlinger, G.; Yuan, F.; Dellian, M.; Jain, R.K. Interstitial pH and pO2 gradients in solid tumors *in vivo*: High-resolution measurements reveal a lack of correlation. *Nat. Med.,* **1997**, *3*(2), 177-182.
      [http://dx.doi.org/10.1038/nm0297-177] [PMID: 9018236]

[10] Emami Nejad, A.; Najafgholian, S.; Rostami, A.; Sistani, A.; Shojaeifar, S.; Esparvarinha, M.; Nedaeinia, R.; Haghjooy Javanmard, S.; Taherian, M.; Ahmadlou, M.; Salehi, R.; Sadeghi, B.; Manian, M. The role of hypoxia in the tumor microenvironment and development of cancer stem cell: a novel approach to developing treatment. *Cancer Cell Int.,* **2021**, *21*(1), 62.

[http://dx.doi.org/10.1186/s12935-020-01719-5] [PMID: 33472628]

[11]   Pouysségur, J.; Dayan, F.; Mazure, N.M. Hypoxia signalling in cancer and approaches to enforce tumour regression. *Nature,* **2006**, *441*(7092), 437-443.
[http://dx.doi.org/10.1038/nature04871] [PMID: 16724055]

[12]   Rempel, A.; Mathupala, S.P.; Griffin, C.A.; Hawkins, A.L.; Pedersen, P.L. Glucose catabolism in cancer cells: amplification of the gene encoding type II hexokinase. *Cancer Res.,* **1996**, *56*(11), 2468-2471.
[PMID: 8653677]

[13]   Traut, T. *Hexokinase*; Allosteric Regul. Enzymes, **2008**, pp. 179-198.

[14]   Wilson, J.E. Isozymes of mammalian hexokinase: structure, subcellular localization and metabolic function. *J. Exp. Biol.,* **2003**, *206*(12), 2049-2057.
[http://dx.doi.org/10.1242/jeb.00241] [PMID: 12756287]

[15]   Chou, J.Y.; Mansfield, B.C.; Weinstein, D.A. *Renal Disease in Type I Glycogen Storage Disease.* InGenetic Diseases of the Kidney; Academic Press, **2009**, pp. 693-708.

[16]   Nakashima, R.A.; Mangan, P.S.; Colombini, M.; Pedersen, P.L. Hexokinase receptor complex in hepatoma mitochondria: evidence from N,N'-dicyclohexlycarbodiimide-labeling studies for the involvement of the pore-forming protein VDAC. *Biochemistry,* **1986**, *25*(5), 1015-1021.
[http://dx.doi.org/10.1021/bi00353a010] [PMID: 3008816]

[17]   Pedersen, P.L.; Mathupala, S.; Rempel, A.; Geschwind, J.F.; Ko, Y.H. Mitochondrial bound type II hexokinase: a key player in the growth and survival of many cancers and an ideal prospect for therapeutic intervention. *Biochim. Biophys. Acta Bioenerg.,* **2002**, *1555*(1-3), 14-20.
[http://dx.doi.org/10.1016/S0005-2728(02)00248-7] [PMID: 12206885]

[18]   Warburg, O. On the origin of cancer cells. *Science,* **1956**, *123*(3191), 309-314.
[http://dx.doi.org/10.1126/science.123.3191.309] [PMID: 13298683]

[19]   Kim, J.; Tchernyshyov, I.; Semenza, G.L.; Dang, C.V. HIF-1-mediated expression of pyruvate dehydrogenase kinase: A metabolic switch required for cellular adaptation to hypoxia. *Cell Metab.,* **2006**, *3*(3), 177-185.
[http://dx.doi.org/10.1016/j.cmet.2006.02.002] [PMID: 16517405]

[20]   Lunt, S.Y.; Vander Heiden, M.G. Aerobic glycolysis: meeting the metabolic requirements of cell proliferation. *Annu. Rev. Cell Dev. Biol.,* **2011**, *27*(1), 441-464.
[http://dx.doi.org/10.1146/annurev-cellbio-092910-154237] [PMID: 21985671]

[21]   Zois, C.E.; Favaro, E.; Harris, A.L. Glycogen metabolism in cancer. *Biochem. Pharmacol.,* **2014**, *92*(1), 3-11.
[http://dx.doi.org/10.1016/j.bcp.2014.09.001] [PMID: 25219323]

[22]   Richmond, C.S.; Oldenburg, D.; Dancik, G.; Meier, D.R.; Weinhaus, B.; Theodorescu, D.; Guin, S. Glycogen debranching enzyme (AGL) is a novel regulator of non-small cell lung cancer growth. *Oncotarget,* **2018**, *9*(24), 16718-16730.
[http://dx.doi.org/10.18632/oncotarget.24676] [PMID: 29682180]

[23]   Guin, S.; Pollard, C.; Ru, Y.; Ritterson Lew, C.; Duex, J.E.; Dancik, G.; Owens, C.; Spencer, A.; Knight, S.; Holemon, H.; Gupta, S.; Hansel, D.; Hellerstein, M.; Lorkiewicz, P.; Lane, A.N.; Fan, T.W.M.; Theodorescu, D. Role in tumor growth of a glycogen debranching enzyme lost in glycogen storage disease. *J. Natl. Cancer Inst.,* **2014**, *106*(5), dju062.
[http://dx.doi.org/10.1093/jnci/dju062] [PMID: 24700805]

[24]   Favaro, E.; Bensaad, K.; Chong, M.G.; Tennant, D.A.; Ferguson, D.J.P.; Snell, C.; Steers, G.; Turley, H.; Li, J.L.; Günther, U.L.; Buffa, F.M.; McIntyre, A.; Harris, A.L. Glucose utilization *via* glycogen phosphorylase sustains proliferation and prevents premature senescence in cancer cells. *Cell Metab.,* **2012**, *16*(6), 751-764.
[http://dx.doi.org/10.1016/j.cmet.2012.10.017] [PMID: 23177934]

[25]   Chatterjee, A.; Ghosh, R. 2-Deoxy-D-Glucose. *Resonance,* **2022**, *27*(10), 1737-1740.
[http://dx.doi.org/10.1007/s12045-022-1468-1]

[26]   Goel, R. 2-Deoxy-d-glucose: from diagnostics to therapeutics. *Int. J. Basic Clin. Pharmacol.,* **2021**, *10*(6), 732.
[http://dx.doi.org/10.18203/2319-2003.ijbcp20212086]

[27]   Pacák, J.; Cerný, M. History of the first synthesis of 2-deoxy-2-fluoro-D-glucose the unlabeled forerunner of 2-deoxy-2-[18F]fluoro-D-glucose. *Mol. Imaging Biol.,* **2002**, *4*(5), 352-354.
[http://dx.doi.org/10.1016/S1536-1632(02)00083-5] [PMID: 14537109]

[28]   Cramer, F.B.; Woodward, G.E. 2-Desoxy-D-glucose as an antagonist of glucose in yeast fermentation. *J. Franklin Inst.,* **1952**, *253*(4), 354-360.
[http://dx.doi.org/10.1016/0016-0032(52)90852-1]

[29]   Jha, B.; Pohlit, W. Effect of 2-deoxy-D-glucose on DNA double strand break repair, cell survival and energy metabolism in euoxic Ehrlich ascites tumour cells. *Int. J. Radiat. Biol.,* **1992**, *62*(4), 409-415.
[http://dx.doi.org/10.1080/09553009214552291] [PMID: 1357054]

[30]   Bernal, S.D.; Lampidis, T.J.; McIsaac, R.M.; Chen, L.B. Anticarcinoma activity *in vivo* of rhodamine 123, a mitochondrial-specific dye. *Science,* **1983**, *222*(4620), 169-172.
[http://dx.doi.org/10.1126/science.6623064] [PMID: 6623064]

[31]   Jain, V.K.; Kalia, V.K.; Sharma, R.; Maharajan, V.; Menon, M. Effects of 2-deoxy-D-glucose on glycolysis, proliferation kinetics and radiation response of human cancer cells. *Int. J. Radiat. Oncol. Biol. Phys.,* **1985**, *11*(5), 943-950.
[http://dx.doi.org/10.1016/0360-3016(85)90117-8] [PMID: 3988563]

[32]   Xi, H.; Kurtoglu, M.; Lampidis, T.J. The wonders of 2-deoxy- D -glucose. *IUBMB Life,* **2014**, *66*(2), 110-121.
[http://dx.doi.org/10.1002/iub.1251] [PMID: 24578297]

[33]   Cheng, G.; Zielonka, J.; Dranka, B.P.; McAllister, D.; Mackinnon, A.C., Jr; Joseph, J.; Kalyanaraman, B. Mitochondria-targeted drugs synergize with 2-deoxyglucose to trigger breast cancer cell death. *Cancer Res.,* **2012**, *72*(10), 2634-2644.
[http://dx.doi.org/10.1158/0008-5472.CAN-11-3928] [PMID: 22431711]

[34]   Codo, A.C.; Davanzo, G.G.; Monteiro, L.B.; de Souza, G.F.; Muraro, S.P.; Virgilio-da-Silva, J.V.; Prodonoff, J.S.; Carregari, V.C.; de Biagi Junior, C.A.O.; Crunfli, F.; Jimenez Restrepo, J.L.; Vendramini, P.H.; Reis-de-Oliveira, G.; Bispo dos Santos, K.; Toledo-Teixeira, D.A.; Parise, P.L.; Martini, M.C.; Marques, R.E.; Carmo, H.R.; Borin, A.; Coimbra, L.D.; Boldrini, V.O.; Brunetti, N.S.; Vieira, A.S.; Mansour, E.; Ulaf, R.G.; Bernardes, A.F.; Nunes, T.A.; Ribeiro, L.C.; Palma, A.C.; Agrela, M.V.; Moretti, M.L.; Sposito, A.C.; Pereira, F.B.; Velloso, L.A.; Vinolo, M.A.R.; Damasio, A.; Proença-Módena, J.L.; Carvalho, R.F.; Mori, M.A.; Martins-de-Souza, D.; Nakaya, H.I.; Farias, A.S.; Moraes-Vieira, P.M. Elevated Glucose Levels Favor SARS-CoV-2 Infection and Monocyte Response through a HIF-1α/Glycolysis-Dependent Axis. *Cell Metab.,* **2020**, *32*(3), 437-446.e5.
[http://dx.doi.org/10.1016/j.cmet.2020.07.007] [PMID: 32697943]

[35]   Huang, Z.; Chavda, V.P.; Vora, L.K.; Gajjar, N.; Apostolopoulos, V.; Shah, N.; Chen, Z.S. 2-Deoxy-D-Glucose and its Derivatives for the COVID-19 Treatment: An Update. *Front. Pharmacol.,* **2022**, *13*, 899633.
[http://dx.doi.org/10.3389/fphar.2022.899633] [PMID: 35496298]

[36]   Aft, R.L.; Zhang, F.W.; Gius, D. Evaluation of 2-deoxy-D-glucose as a chemotherapeutic agent: mechanism of cell death. *Br. J. Cancer,* **2002**, *87*(7), 805-812.
[http://dx.doi.org/10.1038/sj.bjc.6600547] [PMID: 12232767]

[37]   Kurtoglu, M.; Maher, J.C.; Lampidis, T.J. Differential toxic mechanisms of 2-deoxy-D-glucose *versus* 2-fluorodeoxy-D-glucose in hypoxic and normoxic tumor cells. *Antioxid. Redox Signal.,* **2007**, *9*(9), 1383-1390.
[http://dx.doi.org/10.1089/ars.2007.1714] [PMID: 17627467]

[38]   Sottnik, J.L.; Lori, J.C.; Rose, B.J.; Thamm, D.H. Glycolysis inhibition by 2-deoxy-d-glucose reverts the metastatic phenotype *in vitro* and *in vivo*. *Clin. Exp. Metastasis,* **2011**, *28*(8), 865-875.
[http://dx.doi.org/10.1007/s10585-011-9417-5] [PMID: 21842413]

[39]   Kaplan, O.; Navon, G.; Lyon, R.C.; Faustino, P.J.; Straka, E.J.; Cohen, J.S. Effects of 2-deoxyglucose on drug-sensitive and drug-resistant human breast cancer cells: toxicity and magnetic resonance spectroscopy studies of metabolism. *Cancer Res.,* **1990**, *50*(3), 544-551.
[PMID: 2297696]

[40]   Xie, Y.; Meng, W.Y.; Li, R.Z.; Wang, Y.W.; Qian, X.; Chan, C.; Yu, Z.F.; Fan, X.X.; Pan, H.D.; Xie, C.; Wu, Q.B.; Yan, P.Y.; Liu, L.; Tang, Y.J.; Yao, X.J.; Wang, M.F.; Leung, E.L.H. Early lung cancer diagnostic biomarker discovery by machine learning methods. *Transl. Oncol.,* **2021**, *14*(1), 100907.
[http://dx.doi.org/10.1016/j.tranon.2020.100907] [PMID: 33217646]

[41]   Nishida, N.; Yano, H.; Nishida, T.; Kamura, T.; Kojiro, M. Angiogenesis in cancer. *Vasc. Health Risk Manag.,* **2006**, *2*(3), 213-219.
[http://dx.doi.org/10.2147/vhrm.2006.2.3.213] [PMID: 17326328]

[42]   Merchan, J.R.; Kovács, K.; Railsback, J.W.; Kurtoglu, M.; Jing, Y.; Piña, Y.; Gao, N.; Murray, T.G.; Lehrman, M.A.; Lampidis, T.J. Antiangiogenic activity of 2-deoxy-D-glucose. *PLoS One,* **2010**, *5*(10), e13699.
[http://dx.doi.org/10.1371/journal.pone.0013699] [PMID: 21060881]

[43]   Keith, B.; Simon, M.C. Hypoxia-inducible factors, stem cells, and cancer. *Cell,* **2007**, *129*(3), 465-472.
[http://dx.doi.org/10.1016/j.cell.2007.04.019] [PMID: 17482542]

[44]   Valastyan, S.; Weinberg, R.A. Tumor metastasis: molecular insights and evolving paradigms. *Cell,* **2011**, *147*(2), 275-292.
[http://dx.doi.org/10.1016/j.cell.2011.09.024] [PMID: 22000009]

[45]   Kelekar, A. Autophagy. *Ann. N. Y. Acad. Sci.,* **2006**, *1066*(1), 259-271.
[http://dx.doi.org/10.1196/annals.1363.015] [PMID: 16533930]

[46]   Degenhardt, K.; Mathew, R.; Beaudoin, B.; Bray, K.; Anderson, D.; Chen, G.; Mukherjee, C.; Shi, Y.; Gélinas, C.; Fan, Y.; Nelson, D.A.; Jin, S.; White, E. Autophagy promotes tumor cell survival and restricts necrosis, inflammation, and tumorigenesis. *Cancer Cell,* **2006**, *10*(1), 51-64.
[http://dx.doi.org/10.1016/j.ccr.2006.06.001] [PMID: 16843265]

[47]   Pang, Y.; Lin, W.; Zhan, L.; Zhang, J.; Zhang, S.; Jin, H.; Zhang, H.; Wang, X.; Li, X. Inhibiting Autophagy Pathway of PI3K/AKT/mTOR Promotes Apoptosis in SK-N-SH Cell Model of Alzheimer's Disease. *J. Healthc. Eng.,* **2022**, *2022*, 1-10.
[http://dx.doi.org/10.1155/2022/6069682] [PMID: 35178230]

[48]   Xi, H.; Barredo, J.C.; Merchan, J.R.; Lampidis, T.J. Endoplasmic reticulum stress induced by 2-deoxyglucose but not glucose starvation activates AMPK through CaMKKβ leading to autophagy. *Biochem. Pharmacol.,* **2013**, *85*(10), 1463-1477.
[http://dx.doi.org/10.1016/j.bcp.2013.02.037] [PMID: 23500541]

[49]   Wang, Q.; Liang, B.; Shirwany, N.A.; Zou, M.H. 2-Deoxy-D-glucose treatment of endothelial cells induces autophagy by reactive oxygen species-mediated activation of the AMP-activated protein kinase. *PLoS One,* **2011**, *6*(2), e17234.
[http://dx.doi.org/10.1371/journal.pone.0017234] [PMID: 21386904]

[50]   Lawen, A. Apoptosis—an introduction. *BioEssays,* **2003**, *25*(9), 888-896.
[http://dx.doi.org/10.1002/bies.10329] [PMID: 12938178]

[51]   Muñoz-Pinedo, C.; Ruiz-Ruiz, C.; Ruiz de Almodóvar, C.; Palacios, C.; López-Rivas, A. Inhibition of glucose metabolism sensitizes tumor cells to death receptor-triggered apoptosis through enhancement of death-inducing signaling complex formation and apical procaspase-8 processing. *J. Biol. Chem.,* **2003**, *278*(15), 12759-12768.
[http://dx.doi.org/10.1074/jbc.M212392200] [PMID: 12556444]

[52]   Shim, H.; Chun, Y.S.; Lewis, B.C.; Dang, C.V. A unique glucose-dependent apoptotic pathway induced by c-Myc. *Proc. Natl. Acad. Sci. USA,* **1998**, *95*(4), 1511-1516.
[http://dx.doi.org/10.1073/pnas.95.4.1511] [PMID: 9465046]

[53]   Ishino, K.; Kudo, M.; Peng, W.X.; Kure, S.; Kawahara, K.; Teduka, K.; Kawamoto, Y.; Kitamura, T.; Fujii, T.; Yamamoto, T.; Wada, R.; Naito, Z. 2-Deoxy- d -glucose increases GFAT1 phosphorylation resulting in endoplasmic reticulum-related apoptosis *via* disruption of protein N -glycosylation in pancreatic cancer cells. *Biochem. Biophys. Res. Commun.,* **2018**, *501*(3), 668-673.
[http://dx.doi.org/10.1016/j.bbrc.2018.05.041] [PMID: 29753740]

[54]   Xu, Y.; Wang, Q.; Zhang, L.; Zheng, M. 2-Deoxy-d-glucose enhances TRAIL-induced apoptosis in human gastric cancer cells through downregulating JNK-mediated cytoprotective autophagy. *Cancer Chemother. Pharmacol.,* **2018**, *81*(3), 555-564.
[http://dx.doi.org/10.1007/s00280-018-3526-7] [PMID: 29383484]

[55]   Estañ, M.C.; Calviño, E.; de Blas, E.; Boyano-Adánez, M.C.; Mena, M.L.; Gómez-Gómez, M.; Rial, E.; Aller, P. 2-Deoxy-d-glucose cooperates with arsenic trioxide to induce apoptosis in leukemia cells: Involvement of IGF-1R-regulated Akt/mTOR, MEK/ERK and LKB-1/AMPK signaling pathways. *Biochem. Pharmacol.,* **2012**, *84*(12), 1604-1616.
[http://dx.doi.org/10.1016/j.bcp.2012.09.022] [PMID: 23041229]

[56]   Zhang, L.; Su, J.; Xie, Q.; Zeng, L.; Wang, Y.; Yi, D.; Yu, Y.; Liu, S.; Li, S.; Xu, Y. 2-deoxy- D -glucose sensitizes human ovarian cancer cells to cisplatin by increasing ER stress and decreasing ATP stores in acidic vesicles. *J. Biochem. Mol. Toxicol.,* **2015**, *29*(12), 572-578.
[http://dx.doi.org/10.1002/jbt.21730] [PMID: 26241884]

[57]   Schulz, T.F.; Cesarman, E. Kaposi Sarcoma-associated Herpesvirus: mechanisms of oncogenesis. *Curr. Opin. Virol.,* **2015**, *14*, 116-128.
[http://dx.doi.org/10.1016/j.coviro.2015.08.016] [PMID: 26431609]

[58]   Leung, H.J.; Duran, E.M.; Kurtoglu, M.; Andreansky, S.; Lampidis, T.J.; Mesri, E.A. Activation of the unfolded protein response by 2-deoxy-D-glucose inhibits Kaposi's sarcoma-associated herpesvirus replication and gene expression. *Antimicrob. Agents Chemother.,* **2012**, *56*(11), 5794-5803.
[http://dx.doi.org/10.1128/AAC.01126-12] [PMID: 22926574]

[59]   Vigerust, D.J.; Shepherd, V.L. Virus glycosylation: role in virulence and immune interactions. *Trends Microbiol.,* **2007**, *15*(5), 211-218.
[http://dx.doi.org/10.1016/j.tim.2007.03.003] [PMID: 17398101]

[60]   Pająk, B.; Zieliński, R.; Manning, J.T.; Matejin, S.; Paessler, S.; Fokt, I.; Emmett, M.R.; Priebe, W. The Antiviral Effects of 2-Deoxy-D-glucose (2-DG), a Dual D-Glucose and D-Mannose Mimetic, against SARS-CoV-2 and Other Highly Pathogenic Viruses. *Molecules,* **2022**, *27*(18), 5928.
[http://dx.doi.org/10.3390/molecules27185928] [PMID: 36144664]

CHAPTER 10

2-Deoxy-D-Glucose: A Glycolysis Inhibitor in the Treatment of Cancer

Arunagiri Sivanesan Aruna Poorani[1], Mohamed Ibrahim Mohamed Ismail[1], Pandeeswaran Santhoshkumar[1] and Palaniswamy Suresh[1,*]

[1] *Supramolecular and Catalysis Lab, Department of Natural Products Chemistry, School of Chemistry, Madurai Kamaraj University, Madurai-625021, India*

Abstract: Cancer involves abnormal and rapid cell growth, which requires an increased energy supply for proliferating cells. As the demand for glucose rises in cancer cells, the expression and activity of glucose transporters (GLUTs) also increase to facilitate higher cellular glucose uptake. Cancer cells tend to shift their glucose metabolic pathway from mitochondrial oxidative phosphorylation towards aerobic glycolysis. 2-Deoxy-D-glucose competes with glucose and involves aerobic glycolysis. It leads to the inhibition of HK and PGI, diminishes ATP production, and induces apoptosis. Further, the increase in the AMP/ATP ratio promotes the AMPK signaling, downregulating VEGF, and leading to angiogenesis inhibition and autophagy. As the structural mimic of mannose, 2-DG interferes with the N-linked glycosylation, leading to ER stress, and triggering the mitochondrial apoptotic pathway. 2-DG has been employed as an antiproliferative, antiangiogenic, and antimetastatic drug by being involved in the energy metabolic pathway. Combination therapy shows improved results and reduces chemotherapeutic drug resistance. In this chapter, we will discuss the Warburg effect, the role of 2-DG in the inhibition of aerobic glycolysis, and how 2-DG inhibits the various other cancer hallmarks in energy metabolic pathway. Also, reports on cancer treatment as well as cancer cell-imaging and risks associated with chronic exposure are discussed.

Keywords: Angiogenesis, Autophagy, Apoptosis, Cancer, Glycolysis.

1. INTRODUCTION

Glucose, a monosaccharide sugar molecule, is the primary source of the energy metabolism of living cells. The human body acquires its energy needs *via* food containing carbohydrates, proteins, *etc*. Among these, the carbohydrate is oxidized to ATP (adenosine triphosphate), stored as glycogen, converted into lipids, or utilized to synthesize cellular constituents. There are two processes by

* **Corresponding author Palaniswamy Suresh:** Supramolecular and Catalysis Lab, Dept. of Natural Products Chemistry, School of Chemistry, Madurai Kamaraj University, Madurai-625021, India; Tel: +919790296673; E-mail: suresh.chem@mkuniversity.ac.in

Raman Singh, Antresh Kumar & Kuldeep Singh (Eds.)

which glucose formation occurs. The first is glycogenolysis (glucose formation from glycogen), and the second is gluconeogenesis (formation of glucose from non-carbohydrate sources like lactate, amino acids, and glycerol). The liver is majorly involved in this glucose formation, and the renal cortex of the kidney produces glucose by gluconeogenesis [1]. Glucose is a polar molecule, which means it requires assistance from specialized transporters to cross the lipid bilayer of cell membranes. In the human body, there are fourteen different glucose transporter (GLUT) isoforms. Among these, GLUT1 (present in various tissues including pancreatic beta cells), GLUT2 (found in the intestine, kidney, and liver cells), GLUT3 (expressed in the brain), and GLUT4 (present in the heart, kidney, adipose tissue, and brain) are particularly noteworthy for their roles in glucose uptake and metabolism in different tissues and cell types [2]. After food intake, blood glucose level increases and the GLUTs start their functions. This is how the regular energy metabolism begins [3].

The energy requirement will be higher than expected during malignant tumourigenesis as they have a high proliferation rate. This energy need stimulates more GLUTs to upregulate glucose metabolism [4]. The energy metabolism of cancer cells differs from that of normal cells. It will be discussed in detail in the later part of this chapter under the Warburg Effect. The elevated glucose metabolism in cancer cells can be proven well with the reports of cancer progression under hyperglycemic and hypoglycemic conditions. Cancer patients with chronic hyperglycemia show an elevated level of cell proliferation, angiogenesis, and metastasis than the ones who do not have hyperglycemia [5]. Furthermore, high blood glucose levels can decrease the sensitivity of cancer cells to chemotherapeutic drugs, reducing the drug's effectiveness [6]. In contrast, inducing low blood glucose levels (hypoglycemia) has been shown to inhibit various processes in metastatic breast cancer cells studied in laboratory experiments, including cell differentiation, metastasis, formation of new blood vessels (angiogenesis), and the ability to form colonies [7]. The drug Pioglitazone is used for the treatment of type 2 diabetes and also inhibits breast cancer cell growth [8]. At this point, one can understand the importance of glucose in the survival and progression of cancer cells.

2-DG gets attention in cancer treatment. 2-DG has a vast therapeutic window, and its pharmacokinetics were well studied [9]. Like glucose, 2-DG gets into the cell by GLUTs, crosses the blood-brain barrier, and involves all metabolic pathways [10]. In the succeeding titles, the effect of 2-DG in cancer therapy will be discussed against its natural analogs, glucose, and mannose.

2. WARBURG EFFECT: ENERGY METABOLISM IN CANCER CELLS

The process of glucose metabolism starts in the cytoplasm as soon as GLUTs absorb glucose inside the cell [11]. Glycolysis produces two molecules of pyruvate and two molecules of ATP from one molecule of glucose. When there is enough oxygen present, pyruvate in mitochondria undergoes oxidative phosphorylation, or OXPHOS, which produces thirty molecules of ATP and carbon dioxide. Thirty-two ATP molecules are thus the net energy gained from glycolysis, which is followed by OXPHOS. In case of oxygen scarcity, pyruvate takes the anaerobic glycolysis pathway (lactic acid fermentation pathway). This produces two molecules of ATP and lactate. This is how glucose metabolism happens in normal cells [12].

Otto Heinrich Warburg, a German scientist, discovered that tumor cells affect how glucose is metabolized. Tumor cells are susceptible to hypoxia, which triggers the activation of hypoxia-inducible factor 1-alpha (HIF-1α), which is essential to the energy metabolism of cancer cells [13]. The glucose metabolism shifted from mitochondrial OXPHOS to aerobic glycolysis even when there was adequate oxygen tension. The "Warburg effect" is the name of this mechanism. There is a marked decrease in mitochondrial oxidation, and two molecules of ATP are produced as pyruvate is converted into lactate. Thus, four ATP molecules are the net energy gained during aerobic glycolysis [14]. Warburg effect causes diminished ATP production and the secretion of lactic acid [15]. Fig. (**1**) explains the glucose metabolic pathway of normal and cancer cells.

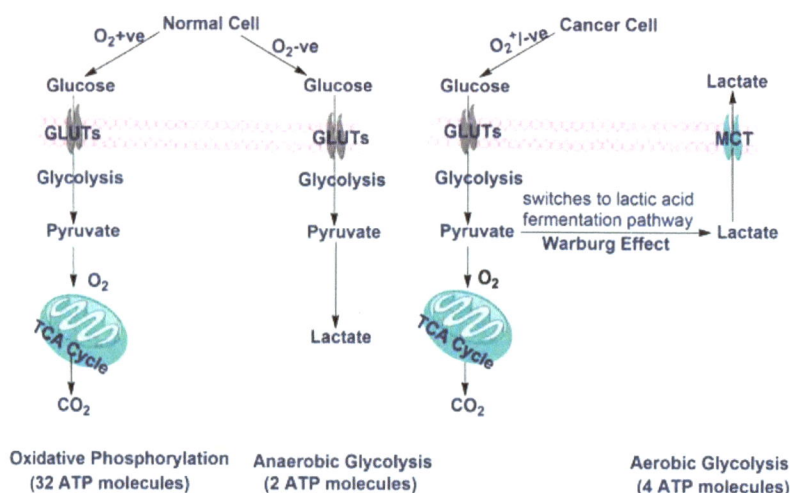

Fig. (1). Glucose Metabolism in Normal Cells *vs* Cancer Cells.

2.1. Causes for the Warburg Effect

Warburg effect is even noticed in early-stage tumors, which do not experience hypoxia [16]. Aside from hypoxia, the majority of tumor cells have mutations in their mitochondrial genomes, which alter the shape and functionality of the mitochondria [17]. However, severe impairment in mitochondria or its irregular function is very rare. Mitochondrial functions throughout this increased aerobic glycolysis and the mechanism of the Warburg effect is still unclear [18]. Although it is uncertain, the four oncogenic factors that are closely related to cancer glycolysis and the Warburg effect will be further discussed.

I. The regulatory gene Myc encodes the transcription factors. It controls apoptosis, cellular transformation, cell cycle progression, glucose metabolism, and cell proliferation [19]. Myc causes the overexpression of Lactate Dehydrogenase A (LDH-A) and other genes related to glucose metabolism and mitochondrial biogenesis in tumors [20].

II. The PI3K/Akt pathway is a signal transduction mechanism that facilitates aerobic glycolysis by blocking β-oxidation, which is the process by which fatty acids convert into acetyl-CoA. As it is a pre-requirement for mitochondrial oxidation (citric acid cycle or TCA Cycle), the energy metabolism through mitochondria gets arrested [21, 22].

III. As a hypoxia sensor, HIF controls the cellular reactions brought on by hypoxia. HIF-1 primarily possesses HIF-1α or HIF-2α, while HIF-1β possesses HIF-1α subunits, both of which are essential for glycolysis. HIF-1α participates in the prolyl hydroxylation process, which is followed by proteasomal breakdown when there is adequate oxygen present. In contrast, proteasomal degradation is inhibited in a hypoxic environment, and HIF-1α binds to hypoxia-responsive elements (HREs) after interacting with HIF-1β. In the end, this directs glycolysis towards the increased synthesis of lactic acid *via* stimulating GLUT1, Hexokinase (HK), Pyruvate kinase M2 (PKM2), LDH-A, Monocarboxylate transporter 4 (MCT4), and Pyruvate dehydrogenase kinase-1 (PDK1) [23, 24].

IV. Tumor suppressor p53, also known as tumor protein p53 or TP53, is activated by a number of events, including telomere erosion, oncogene activation, DNA damage, loss of stromal support, and food and oxygen deprivation. The Warburg effect is intimately linked to p53 inactivation in cancer [25]. The copy of mitochondrial DNA (mtDNA) and mitochondrial bulk are retained by p53. Glycolysis is inhibited and oxidative phosphorylation is maintained by p53 through downregulating GLUTs' expression. Because it inhibits the activity of fructose-2,6-bisphosphate (F-2,6-BP), the p53 transcriptionally activated TIGAR (TP53-induced glycolysis and apoptosis regulator) is essential in reducing the glycolytic rate and increasing the Pentose phosphate pathway (PPP) [26].

Thus, the mutated genes (Myc), deviated regular signaling pathways (PI3K/Akt), modified transcription factors due to the tumor microenvironment (HIF-1α), and inactivation of tumor suppressors (p53) cause the Warburg effect (Fig. **2**).

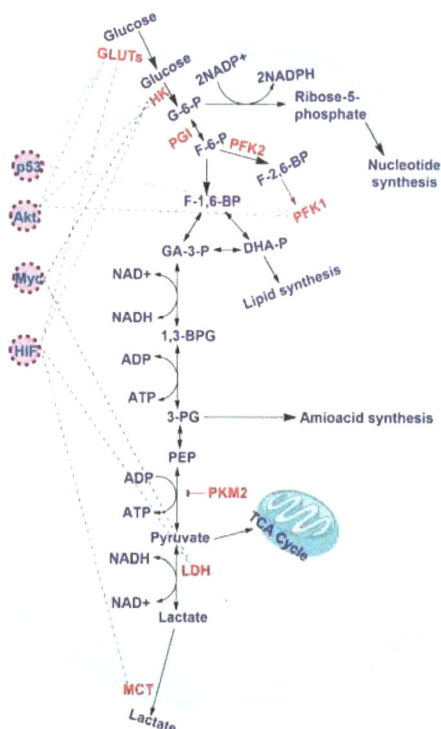

Fig. (2). Glucose Metabolism in Cancer Cells [28].

3. GLUCOSE IN CANCER GLYCOLYSIS

GLUTs transport glucose into the cell cytoplasm, where it is phosphorylated by HK to form glucose-6-phosphate (G-6-P). G-6-phosphate dehydrogenase (G-6-PD) converts G-6-phosphate to ribose-5-phosphate, which is then metabolized further by PPP. Alternatively, phosphoglucose-isomerase (PGI), which is also involved in the glycolysis route, converts G-6-phosphate into fructose-6-phosphate (F-6-P). The phosphorylated glucose gets stranded because cells may need a transport mechanism, and its build-up inhibits HK allosterically. However, the HK attaches itself to the outer membrane of the mitochondria, and a lot of ATP from the mitochondria can quicken the rate-limiting glycolytic phase that the HK catalyzes.

The ATP-dependent phosphorylation of F-6-P is catalyzed by phosphofructokinase (PFK), which is then transformed by PFK-1 to fructose-1, 6-bisphosphate (F-1,6-BP). Furthermore, a high ATP level allosterically inhibits F-1,6-BP. Fructose-2,6-bisphosphate (F-2,6-BP), which is produced by the increased PFK-2, activates PFK-1 and reduces the inhibitory impact of ATP, leading to excessive ATP production.

Dihydroxyacetone phosphate (DHA-P) and glyceraldehyde-3-phosphate (GA-3-P) are the products of the conversion of F-1,6-BP. DHA-P is involved in lipid synthesis and GA-3-P is involved in glycolysis. Pyruvate kinase (PK) catalyzes the conversion of phosphoenol-pyruvate (PEP) to pyruvate in the latter process. PKM2 (isoform of PKM1)-expressed cancer cells show lower affinity for binding PEP. PKM2 disrupts all glycolytic intermediates, causing them to accumulate and starting the synthesis of amino acids, phospholipids, and nucleic acids. Lactate is produced from pyruvate by LDH, whereas NAD^+ is produced concurrently from NADH. High levels of LDH expression maintain high levels of glycolytic flow through NAD^+ regeneration, which is necessary for the conversion of GA-3-P to 1,3-bisphosphoglycerate (1,3-BPG) [27]. Fig. (**2**) illustrates the glucose's aerobic glycolysis route in cancer cells.

Compared to OXPHOS (32 ATP), the net output of this aerobic glycolysis is lower (2 ATP). On the other hand, aerobic glycolysis produces ATP at a rate that is 100 times quicker than OXPHOS [29]. Cancer cells require ten times more glucose than normal and exhibit a thirty-fold increase in the rate of glycolysis to meet the energy requirements for cell development and tumor expansion [30]. MCT elevates lactic acid from the cytoplasm, which causes acidity around the tumor microenvironment as a result of enhanced glycolysis. In contrast to killing cancer cells, this acidic environment encourages angiogenesis, invasion, dissemination, and harm to neighboring cells, including cytotoxic T-cells (immune cells) [31].

4. 2-DG AS A GLUCOSE MIMIC

4.1. 2-DG in Cancer Glycolysis

2-DG shows broad metabolic effects and hinders many biological processes, leading to cellular energy depletion and increasing oxidative stress. PI3K, MAPK, and AMPK signalling pathways are activated and induce autophagy. The results favour 2-DG in anticancer therapy, which combines multiple mechanisms [32, 33].

Similar to glucose, 2-DG is taken in by GLUTs and phosphorylated by HK to form 2-Deoxy-D-glucose-6-phosphate (2-DG-6-P). Moreover, 2-DG-6-P is unable to proceed with the glycolysis pathway; it inhibits PGI competitively and HK non-competitively [34, 35]. As the 2-DG inhibits glucose metabolism in its first step of the glycolysis pathway, it leads to aerobic glycolysis and OXPHOS failure [36]. Reduced ATP synthesis, a disrupted cell cycle, reduced and repressed cell proliferation, and even cell death result from this [37]. The glycolysis inhibition by 2-DG is shown in Fig. (**3**).

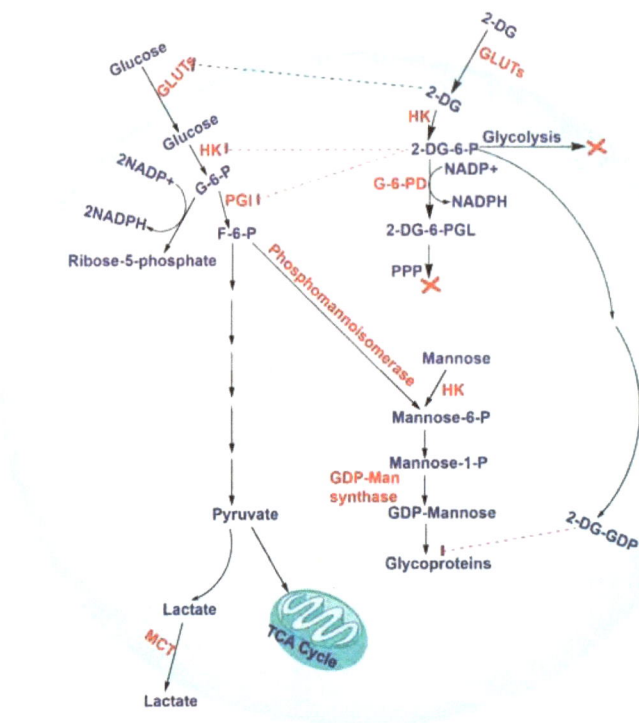

Fig. (3). 2-DG Metabolism in Cancer Cells [28].

4.2. Effect of 2-DG in Cancer Inhibition

4.2.1. Effect of Diminished ATP

Reduced ATP synthesis is the outcome of glycolysis inhibition. Increased AMP/ATP ratios result from ATP depletion, and these ratios encourage the activation of AMP-activated protein kinase (AMPK). It increases the phosphorylation of targets further down the chain, including mTOR (mammalian target of rapamycin) [33]. The decreased ATP induces death receptor-mediated extrinsic apoptosis by binding the tumor necrosis factor (TNF) with their corresponding transmembrane death receptors [36, 38]. The reduced ATP causes defects in p53. As an energy sensor, p53 can repair this energy deprivation by upholding oxidative phosphorylation [26]. Through increasing GLUTs and other glycolytic enzymes, HIF demonstrates resistance to the effects of 2-DG. HIF downregulation is necessary to maintain the 2-DG's impact [34, 39].

4.2.2. Effect of HK Inhibition

HK-1 promotes oncogenic processes beyond its glycolytic function. Specifically, it activates the MAPK/ERK signaling cascade, leading to enhanced cellular proliferation, invasive behavior, and metastatic potential in lung, breast, colorectal, and pancreatic cancers [40]. 2-DG inhibits HK allosterically competitively and leads to diminished lactate and ATP synthesis in glycolysis [41]. Combined treatment with Crizotinib and 2-DG disrupts HK-mediated cancer progression. Specifically, this combination inhibits invasion, colony formation, and proliferation by suppressing the PI3K/Akt/mTOR signaling pathway [42].

4.2.3. Effect of down-regulation of Matrix metalloprotease (MMP)

MMPs are vital in cancer invasion and angiogenesis. MMP-9 and MMP-2 are upregulated in tumor cells and cause invasion [43]. 2-DG exhibits inhibitory effects on the NF-kB signaling pathway, resulting in decreased expression of matrix metalloproteinases MMP-2 and MMP-9. Intriguingly, MMP-9 expression is additionally modulated by the SIRT-1 gene. However, the precise mechanisms by which 2-DG mediates the downregulation of MMP-2 and MMP-9 remain to be fully elucidated [44]. The combined SIRT-1 inhibitor Penfluridol, an antipsychotic drug, and 2-DG therapy for the treatment of lung cancer cells show the blocked mitochondrial ATP production and glycolysis and control cancer progression [45]. VEGF, a pro-angiogenic factor, is an important signaling protein in angiogenesis [46]. The degradation of the basement membrane and other Extracellular matrix (ECM) components is important to release the VEGF from the tumor cells, and MMP does this degradation. So, the downregulation of MMP-9 and MMP-2 by the effect of 2-DG inhibits angiogenesis [44].

4.2.4. Effect of Reactive Oxygen Species (ROS) Upregulation

DCLK-1, a protein kinase family member, exhibits elevated expression in various cancers, including liver, kidney, colon, pancreas, and esophagus. This protein cooperates with the OCT-4 and C-Myc signaling pathways, promoting cancer stem cell (CSC) activity. Furthermore, DCLK-1 is implicated in additional signaling cascades, including Slug, TWIST, NOTCH, NF-κB, and Wnt pathways. Collectively, these interactions contribute to the activation of CSCs and the induction of epithelial-mesenchymal transition (EMT) [47]. 2-DG's ability to increase ROS generation and suppress DCLK-1 activity translates to reduced metastasis, decreased cancer cell survival, and mitigated chemotherapeutic drug resistance [48].

4.2.5. Effect of Inhibition of PPP

The pentose phosphate pathway (PPP) plays a critical role in the synthesis of ribonucleotides. Furthermore, it contributes to cellular antioxidant defense through the production of NADPH, a key scavenger of reactive oxygen species (ROS). 2-DG disrupts the PPP function, consequently leading to elevated ROS formation. This elevation can be attributed to two mechanisms: 1) 2-DG may induce mitochondrial dysfunction, and 2) it can diminish the functional activity of the cellular antioxidant glutathione. The combined effects of increased ROS and compromised antioxidant defenses ultimately culminate in cancer cell death [49].

4.2.6. Effect of Downregulation of FLICE-like Inhibitory Protein (c-FLIP)

The studies found that the receptor-interacting protein (RIP) and the c-FLIP bind with the FADD receptor, inhibit caspase-8 activation, and initiate anti-apoptosis in tumor cells [50]. The 2-DG treatment promotes apoptosis through a dual mechanism: downregulation of anti-apoptotic proteins c-FLIP and RIP, and a reduction in cellular ATP levels. This combined effect sensitizes cells to TRAIL-TNF-mediated cell death pathways [51].

Fig. (**4**) and Table **1** show the overall impact of 2-DG on the metabolism of cancer cells.

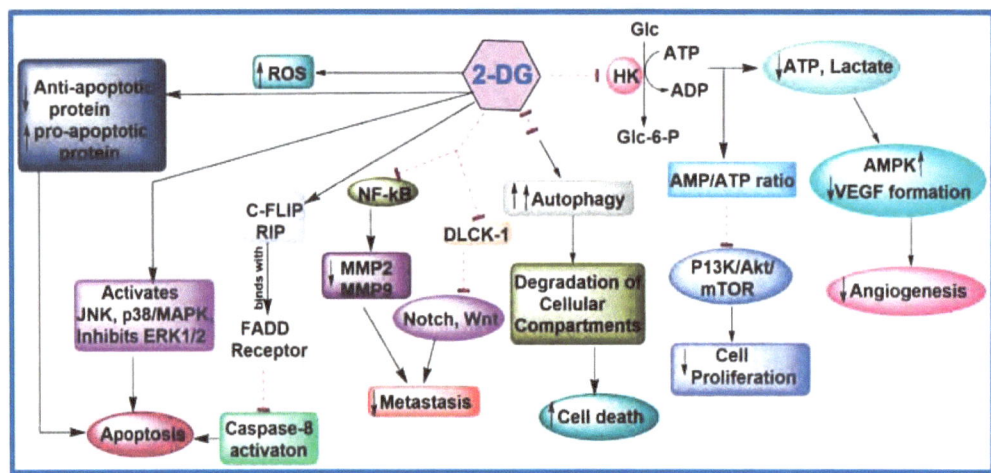

Fig. (4). Effect of 2-DG against the Cancer Cell metabolism [52].

Table 1. Effect of 2-DG on various signalling pathways/molecules involved in cancer cell proliferation [52].

Signaling Pathway / Molecule	Effect of 2DG
PI3K/Akt pathway	- -
EGFR signaling	-
SIRT activation	++
NF-κB	- -
AMPK	++
NOTCH, Wnt pathway	- -
TRAIL/RIP-dependent apoptosis	++
mTOR	- -
MAPK/ p38 Pathway	-
HIF-1 pathway	- -
VEGF level	↓↓
E-cadherin	↑↑
STAT-3 signaling	-
Epithelial mesenchymal transition (EMT)	- -
GLUT1, GLUT3	-
IGF-1, IGFR/ER	-
Ras / Raf/ MAPK pathway	-
ERK Pathway	- -
ULK 1/ 2 pathway	++
Mcl Pathway	-
MMP Expression	- -

* (↑↑)= Upregulation, (↓↓)= Downregulation, (++)= Activation, (- -)= Inhibition

5. 2-DG AS A MANNOSE MIMIC

5.1. N-Linked Glycosylation and 2-DG Participation

An enzymatic process occurs at the lumen of the endoplasmic reticulum (ER), by which glycans (oligosaccharides or carbohydrates) are covalently attached to the hydroxyl (O-linked glycosylation) or N-atom (N-linked glycosylation) of the aminoacid side-chain residues. Glycosylation builds up protein stability, proper folding, and cell adhesion [53, 54]. In the N-linked glycosylation, glycans are attached to the N-atom of the asparagine or arginine side chains of proteins and involve the participation of dolichol phosphate [55]. During the glycosylation, the formation of an oligosaccharide chain is an essential process, where mannose converts into the mannose-GDP by reacting with guanosine diphosphate (GDP) or dolichol phosphate (Dol-P). This mannose-GDP is attached to the N-acetyl-glucosamine residue and GDP-mannosyltransferase and forms an oligosaccharide chain that catalyzes it [56]. In another way, as the epimer of mannose, glucose is also involved in this process. Glucose is converted into glucose-6-phosphate, which can be further converted into mannose-6-phosphate by phosphomannose isomerase (PMI) and then metabolized to mannose-GDP, forming the oligosaccharide chain (Fig. **5**) [57].

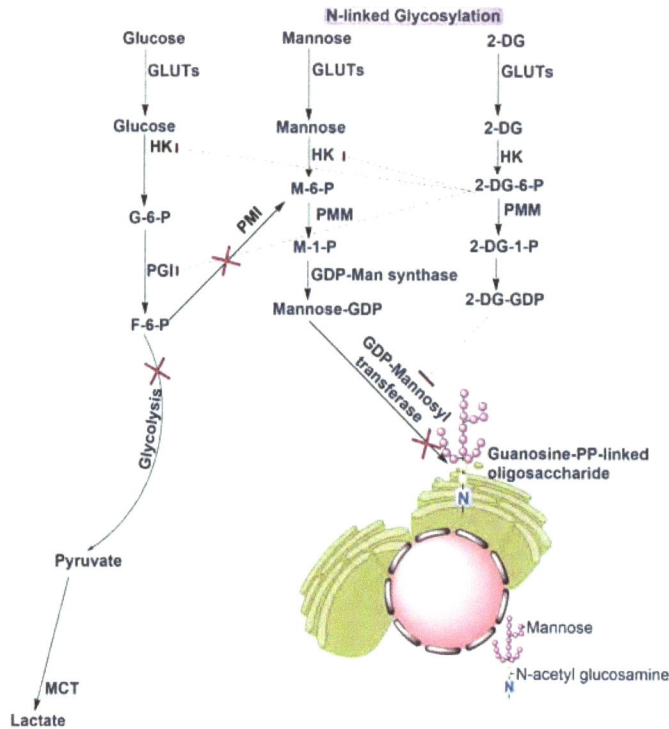

Fig. (5). Effect of 2-DG on N-linked glycosylation.

2-DG mimics mannose forms 2-DG-GDP and further forms a lipid-linked oligosaccharide chain. The formation of 2-DG-GDP leads to the depletion of the chain-forming precursor, and the formation of disrupted oligosaccharides, resulting in the disrupted synthesis of glycoproteins. Despite the fact that glucose is also involved in the N-linked glycosylation through its epimerization to mannose, it does not drive back the toxicity of 2-DG; eventually, 2-DG blocks the conversion from glucose to mannose [58].

5.2. Impact of 2-DG in the N-linked Glycosylation

As 2-DG interferes with N-linked glycosylation, the normal folding of protein gets disrupted and causes the retention of unfolded or misfolded proteins, which results in ER stress. The unfolded proteins activate the unfolded protein response (UPR), which acts as a defensive function to relieve ER stress but is demised [59 - 61]. On the other hand, UPR inhibits protein translation, reduces the amount of proteins entering the ER, and increases the degradation of aberrant proteins [62]. Nevertheless, the prolonged ER stress impairs the organelle. ER stress-specific apoptotic response elements, such as C/EBP homologous protein (CHOP), also known as growth arrest, DNA damage-inducible gene 153 (GADD153), glucose-regulated protein of 78 kDa, and glucose-regulated protein of 94 kDa are activated [63]. Cells with poorer CHOP are unaffected by the ER stress, which shows that CHOP is a hallmark of ER stress-induced cell death [64 - 66].

In the N-linked glycosylation, 2-DG causes ER stress, which actuates the mitochondrial apoptotic pathway by activating the proapoptotic Bcl-2 proteins such as Bax and Bak [67 - 69]. Many research supports that 2-DG-induced cell death under aerobic conditions is mainly caused by the inhibition of glycosylation rather than glycolysis [69, 70].

5.3. ER Stress-Induced Autophagy (self-eating)

Whenever the cell or tissue experiences starvation, hypoxia, hyperthermia, radiotherapy, hormone or growth factor deprivation, and cytotoxic agents, the cellular response triggers autophagy. During autophagy, the cellular organelles and bulk cytoplasm are encompassed in the autophagosome. Then, it gets fused to the lysosome to form the autophagolysosome, where its contents are degraded and provide an alternate energy source for cells [71 - 74]. Autophagy is involved in the degradation of defective proteins and organelles. 2-DG in N-linked glycosylation generates UPR, which causes ER stress. This leads to autophagic engulfment, hence preserving the ER [75 - 77]. Regardless of this self-preservation by autophagy, the prolonged ER stress causes depletion in the tumorigenesis [78]. The transformation of microtubule-associated protein 1A/1B-light chain 3 (LC3), a soluble protein, is a hallmark of autophagy. Whenever autophagy is actuated, the cytoplasmic form of LC3 (LC3-I) is converted into the autophagosome, and instantly, it conjugated to phosphatidylethanolamine to produce LC3-phosphatidylethanolamine conjugate (LC3-II), LC3-II aligned to the autophagosomal membrane and further proceeds autophagy. The exposure to 2-DG shows the significant positivity of LC3-II, which is evident in autophagy [79]. The 2-DG intake induces autophagy by N-linked glycosylation (ER stress) and its mimicking in glycolysis causes ATP depletion [80, 81].

6. 2-DG: IS IT A POTENT ANTICANCER DRUG?

The increased glycolysis results in the acidification of tumour microenvironment due to lactate production. The inhibition of lactate production by 2-DG reduces the drug resistance of other anticancer agents [82]. The 2-DG causes ATP depletion, and ATP-dependent efflux pumps get interrupted, which would remove the cytotoxic agents. This leads to intracellular drug accumulation and cell death [83]. As expected, the high glucose-consuming cancer cells facilitate their death by accumulating 2-DG. As it reduces drug resistance, 2-DG opens the window for combination therapy. The simultaneous inhibition of glycolysis with 2-DG and oxidative phosphorylation with either chemical (mitochondrial inhibitors), mitochondrial electron transport chain blockers, genetic, or environmental (hypoxia) methods show the inhibition of cellular energy generation and causes cell death [84, 85]. These examples demonstrate the promising scope of combination therapy.

6.1. Associated Risk, Dose-Response Study and Combination Therapy

The 2-DG follows the same metabolic pathway as glucose, as discussed above. Like cancer cells, tissues with high metabolic or growth factors like heart, brain, kidney and hair follicles also have an upregulated glucose metabolism [86]. So, the toxicity associated with 2-DG must be a concern. *In vivo* studies on rats revealed that the chronic administration of 2-DG (200mg/kg) caused reduced food intake, toxicity, and increased mortality [87].

2-DG has been practiced in the treatment of diseases like COVID-19, psychiatric disorders, prostate cancer, and glioma [88 - 90]. Side effects such as fatigue, dizziness, restlessness, and asymptomatic continuation of QTc (irregular heart rhythm - ECG) were common [91].

Preclinical and clinical studies indicate that 2-DG administration, both as monotherapy and in combination with chemotherapy or radiotherapy, yields favorable therapeutic responses and demonstrates acceptable tolerability in patients. The preclinical and clinical studies of 2-DG in cancer therapy are listed in Table **2** [92], and a few examples were discussed in detail.

Table 2. Preclinical and clinical studies of combined therapy with 2-DG [92].

Combined Therapy with 2DG	Cancer Type
Preclinical Studies	
Cisplatin	Head and Neck carcinoma, Glioblastoma multiforme (GBM), Bladder cancer

(Table 2) cont.....

Combined Therapy with 2DG	Cancer Type
Metformin	Breast cancer, B cell lymphoma cells, Ovarian cancer, GBM
NCL-240	Melanoma, Small lung carcinomas, Ovarian cancer, Breast cancer
Doxorubicin	Papillary thyroid carcinoma, Breast cancer, Bladder cancer
Daunorubicin	Colon cancer, Breast cancer
Gemcitabine	Bladder cancer
Sorafenib	Papillary thyroid carcinoma, Hepatocellular carcinoma
Adriamycin	Osteosarcoma, Non-small cell lung cancer
Barasertib and Everolimus	Leukemia
Salirasib	Pancreatic cancer
Paclitaxel	Osteosarcoma, Non-small cell lung cancer
Berberine	Lung cancer
Fenofibrate (FF)	Breast cancer, Melanoma, Osteosarcoma
Resveratrol	Neuroblastoma
Mito-Q, Mito-CP, Dec-TPP+	Breast cancer
Methylprednisolone	Non-Hodgkin lymphoma
Alpha-tocopheryl succinate	Colon adenocarcinoma, Cervical carcinoma, Lung adenocarcinoma
Afatinib	Non-small cell lung cancer
Etoposide	Ehrlich ascites tumor bearing mice
Oligomycin	Small cell lung cancer, GBM
Bevacizumab	GBM
5'-Fluorouracil	Pancreatic cancer
Trastuzumab	Breast cancer
Ferulic acid with irradiation	Non-small cell lung carcinoma
Radiotherapy	Breast cancer, Prostate cancer, Cervical cancer
Virotherapy (avian Newcastle disease virus (NDV))	Breast cancer
Clinical Studies	
-	Prostate cancer (Phase – II, terminated)
Docetaxel	Breast cancer, Lung cancer, Head and Neck cancers (Phase – I, completed)
Dehydroepiandrosterone (DHEA)	Breast cancer, Prostate cancer (Phase – I)

(Table 2) cont.....

Combined Therapy with 2DG	Cancer Type
Radiotherapy	Glioblastoma multiforme (Phase – I), Cerebral gliomas (Phase – II)

6.1.1. 2-DG in Combination with Adezmapimod (SB203580)

Adezmapimod (Fig. **6**) is a selective and ATP-competitive p38 MAPK inhibitor. In the treatment of lymphoma, Adezmapimod along with 2-DG exhibited the additive anti-proliferative effect [93].

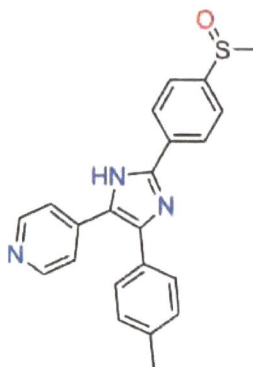

Fig. (6). Structure of Adezmapimod (SB203580).

6.1.2. 2-DG in Combination with PD98059

PD98059 (Fig. **7**) is a specific ERK1/2 signalling inhibitor. Like Adezmapimod, PD98059 with 2-DG showed an additive antiproliferative effect in Lymphoma [93].

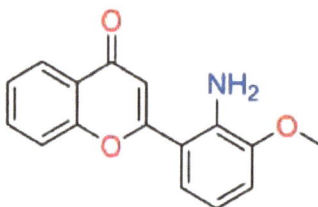

Fig. (7). Structure of PD98059.

6.1.3. 2-DG in Combination with LY294002 and 10058-F4

LY294002 (Fig. **8A**) is an Akt inhibitor, and 10058-F4 (Fig. **8B**) is a c-Myc inhibitor. 2-DG, a glycolysis inhibitor in combination with Akt and c-Myc inhibitors, exposed the additive anti-proliferative effect in Lymphoma [93].

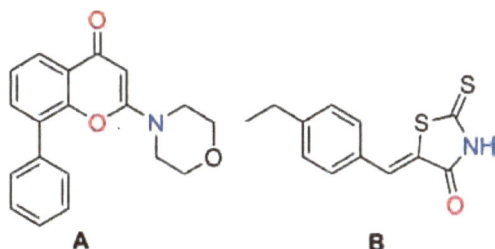

Fig. (8). Structure of (**A**) LY294002 and (**B**) 10058-F4.

6.1.4. 2-DG in Combination with Erlotinib

Erlotinib (Fig. **9**) is an EGFR tyrosine kinase inhibitor. Its oral administration with 2-DG showed synergistic effects by downregulating GLUT1, EGFR, and LDH-A [94].

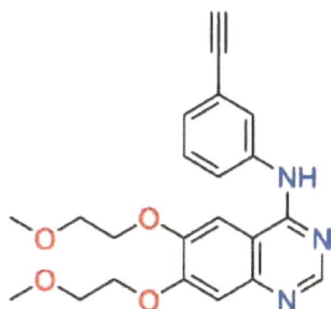

Fig. (9). Structure of Erlotinib.

6.1.5. 2-DG in Combination with Mibefradil

Mibefradil (Posicor) (Fig. **10**) is a tetralol calcium channel-blocking agent used to treat hypertension. In the treatment of breast cancer, 2-DG and Mibefradil together cause cell cycle synchronization, synergistic antiproliferative effects, and cell cycle arrest [95].

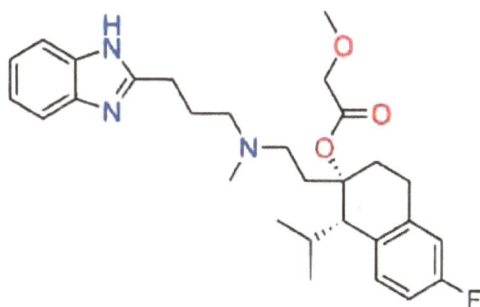

Fig. (10). Structure of Mibefradil.

7. 2-DG IN CANCER CELL IMAGING

7.1. NIR Optical Imaging Probe

Joy L. Kovar *et al.* reported the NIR (Near-infrared) optical imaging probe for detecting cancer in mouse models. As discussed earlier, cancer cells exhibit upregulated glycolysis and also the GLUTs. This was exploited for the optical imaging of tumors in mice. An NIR fluorophore, IRDye 800CW (emission max - 794 nm), was conjugated to 2-deoxyglucose (2-DG) (Fig. **11**). Epithelial and prostate carcinomas were clearly imaged with good signal-to-noise characteristics, which indicates that IRDye 800CW 2-DG is a broadly applicable optical imaging agent. Highly sensitive NIR fluorescent glucose analogue implicates the GLUT1 in the mechanism of enhanced detection *in vitro* and *in vivo*, which overcomes cell penetration issues [96].

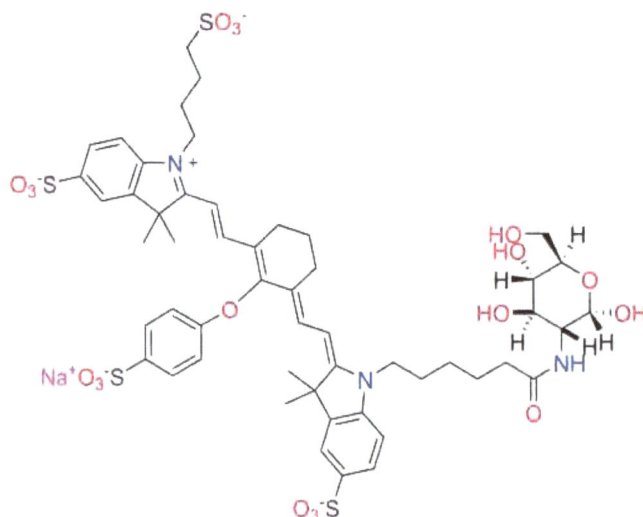

Fig. (11). Structure of the NIR optical imaging probe.

7.2. Radioactive Diagnostic Agent in PET

In Positron Emission Tomography (PET) and Computed Tomography (CT), the application of the fluorinated derivative of 2-DG, ^{18}F-Fluro-2-deoxy-D-glucose (FDG) (Fig. **12**), has shown tremendous results, particularly in the field of oncology. In PET, FDG is used as a radioactive tracer to localize the tissues with altered glucose metabolism, and it does not have any therapeutic application. Aberrations in glucose metabolism are increasingly recognized as hallmarks of various pathologies, including malignancies, epilepsy, and myocardial ischemia. This phenomenon extends to inflammatory conditions and neurodegenerative diseases like Alzheimer's, highlighting the broad utility of FDG-PET in their exploration. Within oncology, FDG stands as a cornerstone diagnostic tool. Approved by the FDA, it serves a multifaceted role in cancer management. FDG-PET is employed for the detection, staging, and monitoring of treatment response across a wide range of cancers, including non-small cell lung cancer, lymphomas, colorectal carcinomas, malignant melanomas, esophageal carcinomas, head and neck cancers, thyroid carcinomas, and breast cancers [97]. Along with PET, CT also delivers a distinct indication in the staging and therapy monitoring of various malignancies [98].

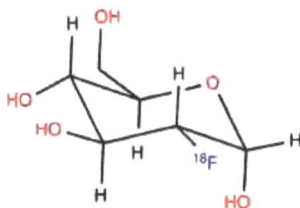

Fig. (12).   Structure of the ^{18}F-Fluro-2-deoxy-D-glucose.

8. 2-DG RESISTANCE

A seminal 1962 study demonstrated the potential to induce 2-DG resistance in Hela cell lines. Researchers observed adaptation in Hela cells by gradually escalating 2-DG concentrations within the culture medium over 2-3 weeks. While exhibiting diminished growth rates (approximately half that of the 2-DG-sensitive control), the resistant cells demonstrated tolerance to the compound [99]. Similar 2-DG resistance has been documented in pig kidney cell lines. Intriguingly, these resistant cells display an enhanced growth capacity compared to their sensitive counterparts when maintained in environments with limited glucose availability. This finding implies the presence of metabolic reprogramming within resistant cells [100]. The process by which mammalian cells potentially detoxify 2-DG remains unclear. This suggests the potential for diverse resistance mechanisms, which require further investigation, as existing theories lack strong supporting evidence. Further research is needed to elucidate 2-DG detoxification mechanisms and potential resistance pathways.

CONCLUSION

2-deoxy-D-glucose (2-DG), a glucose-mimicking drug, is a potential weapon against cancer. Energy metabolism of cancer cells, reasons for its altered metabolism, and 2-DG in cancer energy metabolic pathway were delivered in detail. Glycolysis inhibition, ATP depletion, PPP inhibition, and interference in the N-linked glycosylation were well pictured. Its concordant effect on the various signaling pathways such as AMPK, PI3K/Akt/mTOR, signaling or sensing proteins HIF-1α, and genes such as p53 were discussed. Further, this chapter deals with the risk associated with its therapeutic application and the promising results of the combination therapy. Other than the therapeutic use, it also has applications in bioimaging. The 2-DG conjugated NIR probe and ^{18}F-2-DG in the PET/CT imaging techniques were discussed. Though the 2-DG detoxification has less evidence, it was noted in concern with its future need. The effect of 2-DG is too multifaceted, and its implications on various cancer hallmarks were jumbled. Although it is unbiased, its anti-proliferative effect was noticeably proven; hence, the combination therapy would provide the support for successful treatment.

LIST OF ABBREVIATIONS

1,3-BPG	1,3-Bisphosphoglycerate
2-DG	2-deoxy-D-Glucose
2-DG-6-P	2-deoxy-D-Glucose-6-Phosphate
2-DG-6-PGL	2-deoxy-D-Glucose-6-phosphogluconolactone
2-DG-GDP	2-deoxy-D-Glucose-Guanosine diphosphate
3-PG	3-Phosphoglycerate
AMP	Adenosine monophosphate
AMPK	Adenosine monophosphate (AMP)-activated protein kinase
ATP	Adenosine triphosphate
Bcl-2	B-cell lymphoma 2
c-FLIP	FLICE -like inhibitory protein
CHOP	C/EBP homologous protein
C-Myc	Cellular Myc
CSC	Cancer Stem Cells
CT	Computed Tomography
DCLK-1	Doublecortin-like kinase 1
DHA-P	Dihydroxyacetone Phosphate
Dol-P	Dolicholphosphate
ECM	Extracellular Matrix
EGFR	Epidermal Growth Factor Receptor
EMT	Epithelial-mesenchymal transition
ER	Endoplasmic Reticulum
F-1,6-BP	Fructose-1,6-Bisphosphate
F-2,6-BP	Fructose-2,6-Bisphosphate
F-6-P	Fructose-6-Phosphate
FADD	Fas-associated death domain
FDG	^{18}F-Fluro-2-deoxy-D-glucose

G-6-P	Glucose-6-Phosphate
G-6-PD	Glucose-6-Phosphate dehydrogenase
GA-3-P	Glyceraldehyde-3-Phosphate
GADD153	DNA damage-inducible gene 153
GDP	Guanosine diphosphate
GDP-Man synthase	Guanosine diphosphate mannose synthase
GLUT	Glucose Transporters
HIF-1α	Hypoxia-inducible factor 1-alpha
HK	Hexokinase
HREs	Hypoxia-responsive elements
LC3	Microtubule-associated Protein 1A/1B Light Chain 3 or MAP1LC3
LDH-A	Lactate dehydrogenase A
Mannose-GDP	Mannose Guanosine diphosphate
MAPK	Mitogen-activated protein kinase
MAPK/ERK1/2	Mitogen activated protein kinase/ Extracellular
Mcl	Myeloid Cell Leukemia - 1
MCT	Monocarboxylate Transporter
MCT4	Monocarboxylate Transporter-4
MMP	Matrix Mettalloprotease
mtDNA	Mitochondrial DNA
mTOR	Mammalin Target of Rapamycin
NAD	Nicotinamide Adenine Dinucleotide
NADPH	Nicotinamide Adenine Dinucleotide Phosphate
NF-KB	Nuclear factor kappa-light-chain-enchancer of activated B cell
NIR	Near Infra Red
NOTCH	Neurogenic locus notch homolog protein
OCT-4	Octamer Transcription Factor - 4
OXPHOS	Oxidative Phosphorylation
p53	Tumor protein p53
PEP	Phosphoenol pyruvate
PET	Positron Emission Tomography
PFK	Phosphofructokinase
PGI	Phosphoglucoisomerase
PI3K/Akt	Phosphoinositide-3-kinase
PK	Pyruvate Kinase

PKM2	Pyruvate Kinase M2
PMI	Phosphomannoseisomerase
PMM	Phosphomannomutase
PPP	Pentose Phosphate Pathway
QTc	Irregular Heart Rhythm (in ECG)
RIP	Receptor Interacting Protein
ROS	Reactive Oxygen Species
SIRT-1	Silent mating type information-2-homologue 1
Slung	a Zinc finger transcription factor
STAT-3	Signal transducer and Activator of transcription 3
TCA Cycle	Tricarboxylicacid Cycle/ Citricacid Cycle
TNF	Tumor Necrosis Factor
TRAIL	Tumor Necrosis Factor (TNF) related apoptosis-inducing ligand
TWIST	Basic helix-loop-helix transcription factor
ULK 1/2	Unc-51-like autophagy-activating kinase 1 and 2
UPR	Unfolded Protein Response
VEGF	Vascular Endothelial Growth Factor
Wnt	Wingless-related Integration Site

ACKNOWLEDGEMENTS

We gratefully acknowledge the financial support from MKU-RUSA 2.0, India and TANSCHE & TNSCST, Tamil Nadu. Also, we thank DST-FIST-II, New Delhi.

FUNDING INFORMATION

This work was funded by Madurai Kamaraj University- Rashtriya Uchchatar Shiksha Abhiyan (MKU-RUSA) Ref No. 007-R2/MKU/SOC/2020-2021, Tamil Nadu State Council for Higher Education (TANCSHE) Ref No. 131/2019A dated 23-06-22, Tamil Nadu State Council for Science and Technology Ref No. TNSCST/STP/Covid-19/2020-21-3682 and Department of Science and Technology Ref No. SR/FST/CS-II/2017/35(C).

REFERENCES

[1]   Mitrakou, A. Kidney: Its impact on glucose homeostasis and hormonal regulation. *Diabetes Res. Clin. Pract.,* **2011**, *93* Suppl. 1, S66-S72.
[http://dx.doi.org/10.1016/S0168-8227(11)70016-X] [PMID: 21864754]

[2]   Mueckler, M.; Thorens, B. The SLC2 (GLUT) family of membrane transporters. *Mol. Aspects Med.,* **2013**, *34*(2-3), 121-138.
[http://dx.doi.org/10.1016/j.mam.2012.07.001] [PMID: 23506862]

[3] Giri, B.; Dey, S.; Das, T.; Sarkar, M.; Banerjee, J.; Dash, S.K. Chronic hyperglycemia mediated physiological alteration and metabolic distortion leads to organ dysfunction, infection, cancer progression and other pathophysiological consequences: An update on glucose toxicity. *Biomed. Pharmacother.*, **2018**, *107*, 306-328.
[http://dx.doi.org/10.1016/j.biopha.2018.07.157] [PMID: 30098549]

[4] Liu, Y.; Zhang, W.; Cao, Y.; Liu, Y.; Bergmeier, S.; Chen, X. Small compound inhibitors of basal glucose transport inhibit cell proliferation and induce apoptosis in cancer cells *via* glucose-deprivatio--like mechanisms. *Cancer Lett.*, **2010**, *298*(2), 176-185.
[http://dx.doi.org/10.1016/j.canlet.2010.07.002] [PMID: 20678861]

[5] Ryu, T.Y.; Park, J.; Scherer, P.E. Hyperglycemia as a risk factor for cancer progression. *Diabetes Metab. J.*, **2014**, *38*(5), 330-336.
[http://dx.doi.org/10.4093/dmj.2014.38.5.330] [PMID: 25349819]

[6] Ma, Y.S.; Yang, I.P.; Tsai, H.L.; Huang, C.W.; Juo, S.H.H.; Wang, J.Y. High glucose modulates antiproliferative effect and cytotoxicity of 5-fluorouracil in human colon cancer cells. *DNA Cell Biol.*, **2014**, *33*(2), 64-72.
[http://dx.doi.org/10.1089/dna.2013.2161] [PMID: 24283362]

[7] Adham, S.A.I.; Al Rawahi, H.; Habib, S.; Al Moundhri, M.S.; Viloria-Petit, A.; Coomber, B.L. Modeling of hypo/hyperglycemia and their impact on breast cancer progression related molecules. *PLoS One*, **2014**, *9*(11), e113103.
[http://dx.doi.org/10.1371/journal.pone.0113103] [PMID: 25401697]

[8] Kole, L.; Sarkar, M.; Deb, A.; Giri, B. Pioglitazone, an anti-diabetic drug requires sustained MAPK activation for its anti-tumor activity in MCF7 breast cancer cells, independent of PPAR-γ pathway. *Pharmacol. Rep.*, **2016**, *68*(1), 144-154.
[http://dx.doi.org/10.1016/j.pharep.2015.08.001] [PMID: 26721366]

[9] Aghaee, F.; Pirayesh Islamian, J.; Baradaran, B. Enhanced radiosensitivity and chemosensitivity of breast cancer cells by 2-deoxy-d-glucose in combination therapy. *J. Breast Cancer*, **2012**, *15*(2), 141-147.
[http://dx.doi.org/10.4048/jbc.2012.15.2.141] [PMID: 22807930]

[10] Aft, R.L.; Zhang, F.W.; Gius, D. Evaluation of 2-deoxy-D-glucose as a chemotherapeutic agent: mechanism of cell death. *Br. J. Cancer*, **2002**, *87*(7), 805-812.
[http://dx.doi.org/10.1038/sj.bjc.6600547] [PMID: 12232767]

[11] Wilson, D.F. Oxidative phosphorylation: regulation and role in cellular and tissue metabolism. *J. Physiol.*, **2017**, *595*(23), 7023-7038.
[http://dx.doi.org/10.1113/JP273839] [PMID: 29023737]

[12] Vander Heiden, M.G.; Cantley, L.C.; Thompson, C.B. Understanding the Warburg effect: the metabolic requirements of cell proliferation. *Science*, **2009**, *324*(5930), 1029-1033.
[http://dx.doi.org/10.1126/science.1160809] [PMID: 19460998]

[13] Mole, D.R.; Blancher, C.; Copley, R.R.; Pollard, P.J.; Gleadle, J.M.; Ragoussis, J.; Ratcliffe, P.J. Genome-wide association of hypoxia-inducible factor (HIF)-1α and HIF-2α DNA binding with expression profiling of hypoxia-inducible transcripts. *J. Biol. Chem.*, **2009**, *284*(25), 16767-16775.
[http://dx.doi.org/10.1074/jbc.M901790200] [PMID: 19386601]

[14] Fukuda, R.; Zhang, H.; Kim, J.; Shimoda, L.; Dang, C.V.; Semenza, G.L. HIF-1 regulates cytochrome oxidase subunits to optimize efficiency of respiration in hypoxic cells. *Cell*, **2007**, *129*(1), 111-122.
[http://dx.doi.org/10.1016/j.cell.2007.01.047] [PMID: 17418790]

[15] Semenza, G.L. HIF-1: upstream and downstream of cancer metabolism. *Curr. Opin. Genet. Dev.*, **2010**, *20*(1), 51-56.
[http://dx.doi.org/10.1016/j.gde.2009.10.009] [PMID: 19942427]

[16] Moreno-Sánchez, R.; Rodríguez-Enríquez, S.; Marín-Hernández, A.; Saavedra, E. Energy metabolism

in tumor cells. *FEBS J.,* **2007**, *274*(6), 1393-1418.
[http://dx.doi.org/10.1111/j.1742-4658.2007.05686.x] [PMID: 17302740]

[17]   Mizutani, S.; Miyato, Y.; Shidara, Y.; Asoh, S.; Tokunaga, A.; Tajiri, T.; Ohta, S. Mutations in the mitochondrial genome confer resistance of cancer cells to anticancer drugs. *Cancer Sci.,* **2009**, *100*(9), 1680-1687.
[http://dx.doi.org/10.1111/j.1349-7006.2009.01238.x] [PMID: 19555391]

[18]   Hamanaka, R.B.; Chandel, N.S. Targeting glucose metabolism for cancer therapy. *J. Exp. Med.,* **2012**, *209*(2), 211-215.
[http://dx.doi.org/10.1084/jem.20120162] [PMID: 22330683]

[19]   Dang, C.V. MYC, metabolism, cell growth, and tumorigenesis. *Cold Spring Harb. Perspect. Med.,* **2013**, *3*(8), a014217-a014217.
[http://dx.doi.org/10.1101/cshperspect.a014217] [PMID: 23906881]

[20]   Dang, C.V.; Le, A.; Gao, P. MYC-induced cancer cell energy metabolism and therapeutic opportunities. *Clin. Cancer Res.,* **2009**, *15*(21), 6479-6483.
[http://dx.doi.org/10.1158/1078-0432.CCR-09-0889] [PMID: 19861459]

[21]   Icard, P.; Lincet, H. A global view of the biochemical pathways involved in the regulation of the metabolism of cancer cells. *Biochim. Biophys. Acta Rev. Cancer,* **2012**, *1826*(2), 423-433.
[http://dx.doi.org/10.1016/j.bbcan.2012.07.001] [PMID: 22841746]

[22]   Kroemer, G.; Pouyssegur, J. Tumor cell metabolism: cancer's Achilles' heel. *Cancer Cell,* **2008**, *13*(6), 472-482.
[http://dx.doi.org/10.1016/j.ccr.2008.05.005] [PMID: 18538731]

[23]   Semenza, G.L. HIF-1 mediates metabolic responses to intratumoral hypoxia and oncogenic mutations. *J. Clin. Invest.,* **2013**, *123*(9), 3664-3671.
[http://dx.doi.org/10.1172/JCI67230] [PMID: 23999440]

[24]   Maher, J.C.; Savaraj, N.; Priebe, W.; Liu, H.; Lampidis, T.J. Differential sensitivity to 2-deoxy-D-glucose between two pancreatic cell lines correlates with GLUT-1 expression. *Pancreas,* **2005**, *30*(2), e34-e39.
[http://dx.doi.org/10.1097/01.mpa.0000153327.46945.26] [PMID: 15714127]

[25]   Gottlieb, E.; Vousden, K.H. p53 regulation of metabolic pathways. *Cold Spring Harb. Perspect. Biol.,* **2010**, *2*(4), a001040-a001040.
[http://dx.doi.org/10.1101/cshperspect.a001040] [PMID: 20452943]

[26]   Sinthupibulyakit, C.; Ittarat, W.; St Clair, W.H.; St Clair, D.K. p53 Protects lung cancer cells against metabolic stress. *Int. J. Oncol.,* **2010**, *37*(6), 1575-1581.
[http://dx.doi.org/10.3892/ijo_00000811] [PMID: 21042727]

[27]   Christofk, H.R.; Vander Heiden, M.G.; Harris, M.H.; Ramanathan, A.; Gerszten, R.E.; Wei, R.; Fleming, M.D.; Schreiber, S.L.; Cantley, L.C. The M2 splice isoform of pyruvate kinase is important for cancer metabolism and tumour growth. *Nature,* **2008**, *452*(7184), 230-233.
[http://dx.doi.org/10.1038/nature06734] [PMID: 18337823]

[28]   Zhang, D.; Li, J.; Wang, F.; Hu, J.; Wang, S.; Sun, Y. 2-Deoxy-D-glucose targeting of glucose metabolism in cancer cells as a potential therapy. *Cancer Lett.,* **2014**, *355*(2), 176-183.
[http://dx.doi.org/10.1016/j.canlet.2014.09.003] [PMID: 25218591]

[29]   Koppenol, W.H.; Bounds, P.L.; Dang, C.V. Otto Warburg's contributions to current concepts of cancer metabolism. *Nat. Rev. Cancer,* **2011**, *11*(5), 325-337.
[http://dx.doi.org/10.1038/nrc3038] [PMID: 21508971]

[30]   Priebe, A.; Tan, L.; Wahl, H.; Kueck, A.; He, G.; Kwok, R.; Opipari, A.; Liu, J.R. Glucose deprivation activates AMPK and induces cell death through modulation of Akt in ovarian cancer cells. *Gynecol. Oncol.,* **2011**, *122*(2), 389-395.
[http://dx.doi.org/10.1016/j.ygyno.2011.04.024] [PMID: 21570709]

[31]   Swietach, P.; Vaughan-Jones, R.D.; Harris, A.L. Regulation of tumor pH and the role of carbonic anhydrase 9. *Cancer Metastasis Rev.,* **2007**, *26*(2), 299-310.
[http://dx.doi.org/10.1007/s10555-007-9064-0] [PMID: 17415526]

[32]   Yamaguchi, R.; Janssen, E.; Perkins, G.; Ellisman, M.; Kitada, S.; Reed, J.C. Efficient elimination of cancer cells by deoxyglucose-ABT-263/737 combination therapy. *PLoS One,* **2011**, *6*(9), e24102.
[http://dx.doi.org/10.1371/journal.pone.0024102] [PMID: 21949692]

[33]   Kim, S.M.; Yun, M.R.; Hong, Y.K.; Solca, F.; Kim, J.H.; Kim, H.J.; Cho, B.C. Glycolysis inhibition sensitizes non-small cell lung cancer with T790M mutation to irreversible EGFR inhibitors *via* translational suppression of Mcl-1 by AMPK activation. *Mol. Cancer Ther.,* **2013**, *12*(10), 2145-2156.
[http://dx.doi.org/10.1158/1535-7163.MCT-12-1188] [PMID: 23883584]

[34]   Kurtoglu, M.; Maher, J.C.; Lampidis, T.J. Differential toxic mechanisms of 2-deoxy-D-glucose *versus* 2-fluorodeoxy-D-glucose in hypoxic and normoxic tumor cells. *Antioxid. Redox Signal.,* **2007**, *9*(9), 1383-1390.
[http://dx.doi.org/10.1089/ars.2007.1714] [PMID: 17627467]

[35]   Urakami, K.; Zangiacomi, V.; Yamaguchi, K.; Kusuhara, M. Impact of 2-deoxy-D-glucose on the target metabolome profile of a human endometrial cancer cell line. *Biomed. Res.,* **2013**, *34*(5), 221-229.
[http://dx.doi.org/10.2220/biomedres.34.221] [PMID: 24190234]

[36]   Robinson, G.L.; Dinsdale, D.; MacFarlane, M.; Cain, K. Switching from aerobic glycolysis to oxidative phosphorylation modulates the sensitivity of mantle cell lymphoma cells to TRAIL. *Oncogene,* **2012**, *31*(48), 4996-5006.
[http://dx.doi.org/10.1038/onc.2012.13] [PMID: 22310286]

[37]   Golding, J.P.; Wardhaugh, T.; Patrick, L.; Turner, M.; Phillips, J.B.; Bruce, J.I.; Kimani, S.G. Targeting tumour energy metabolism potentiates the cytotoxicity of 5-aminolevulinic acid photodynamic therapy. *Br. J. Cancer,* **2013**, *109*(4), 976-982.
[http://dx.doi.org/10.1038/bjc.2013.391] [PMID: 23860536]

[38]   Wood, T.E.; Dalili, S.; Simpson, C.D.; Hurren, R.; Mao, X.; Saiz, F.S.; Gronda, M.; Eberhard, Y.; Minden, M.D.; Bilan, P.J.; Klip, A.; Batey, R.A.; Schimmer, A.D. A novel inhibitor of glucose uptake sensitizes cells to FAS-induced cell death. *Mol. Cancer Ther.,* **2008**, *7*(11), 3546-3555.
[http://dx.doi.org/10.1158/1535-7163.MCT-08-0569] [PMID: 19001437]

[39]   Maher, J.C.; Wangpaichitr, M.; Savaraj, N.; Kurtoglu, M.; Lampidis, T.J. Hypoxia-inducible factor-1 confers resistance to the glycolytic inhibitor 2-deoxy- D -glucose. *Mol. Cancer Ther.,* **2007**, *6*(2), 732-741.
[http://dx.doi.org/10.1158/1535-7163.MCT-06-0407] [PMID: 17308069]

[40]   Amendola, C.R.; Mahaffey, J.P.; Parker, S.J.; Ahearn, I.M.; Chen, W.C.; Zhou, M.; Court, H.; Shi, J.; Mendoza, S.L.; Morten, M.J.; Rothenberg, E.; Gottlieb, E.; Wadghiri, Y.Z.; Possemato, R.; Hubbard, S.R.; Balmain, A.; Kimmelman, A.C.; Philips, M.R. KRAS4A directly regulates hexokinase 1. *Nature,* **2019**, *576*(7787), 482-486.
[http://dx.doi.org/10.1038/s41586-019-1832-9] [PMID: 31827279]

[41]   Li, Y.; Tian, H.; Luo, H.; Fu, J.; Jiao, Y.; Li, Y. Prognostic significance and related mechanisms of nexokinase 1 in ovarian cancer. *OncoTargets Ther.,* **2020**, *13*, 11583-11594.
[http://dx.doi.org/10.2147/OTT.S270688] [PMID: 33204111]

[42]   Lin, C.; Chen, H.; Han, R.; Li, L.; Lu, C.; Hao, S.; Wang, Y.; He, Y. Hexokinases II -mediated glycolysis governs susceptibility to crizotinib in ALK -positive non-small cell lung cancer. *Thorac. Cancer,* **2021**, *12*(23), 3184-3193.
[http://dx.doi.org/10.1111/1759-7714.14184] [PMID: 34729938]

[43]   Kessenbrock, K.; Plaks, V.; Werb, Z. Matrix metalloproteinases: regulators of the tumor microenvironment. *Cell,* **2010**, *141*(1), 52-67.
[http://dx.doi.org/10.1016/j.cell.2010.03.015] [PMID: 20371345]

[44] Zhao, E.; Hou, J.; Ke, X.; Abbas, M.N.; Kausar, S.; Zhang, L.; Cui, H. The roles of sirtuin family proteins in cancer progression. *Cancers (Basel)*, **2019**, *11*(12), 1949.
[http://dx.doi.org/10.3390/cancers11121949] [PMID: 31817470]

[45] Lai, T.C.; Lee, Y.L.; Lee, W.J.; Hung, W.Y.; Cheng, G.Z.; Chen, J.Q.; Hsiao, M.; Chien, M.H.; Chang, J.H. Synergistic tumor inhibition *via* energy elimination by repurposing penfluridol and 2-deoxy-D-glucose in lung cancer. *Cancers (Basel)*, **2022**, *14*(11), 2750.
[http://dx.doi.org/10.3390/cancers14112750] [PMID: 35681729]

[46] Chuang, I.C.; Yang, C.M.; Song, T.Y.; Yang, N.C.; Hu, M.L. The anti-angiogenic action of 2-deoxyglucose involves attenuation of VEGFR2 signaling and MMP-2 expression in HUVECs. *Life Sci.*, **2015**, *139*, 52-61.
[http://dx.doi.org/10.1016/j.lfs.2015.08.002] [PMID: 26285173]

[47] P, C.; J, P. Regulatory roles of dclk1 in epithelial mesenchymal transition and cancer stem cells. *J. Carcinog. Mutagen.*, **2016**, *7*(2)
[http://dx.doi.org/10.4172/2157-2518.1000257]

[48] Zhao, H.; Duan, Q.; Zhang, Z.; Li, H.; Wu, H.; Shen, Q.; Wang, C.; Yin, T. Up-regulation of glycolysis promotes the stemness and EMT phenotypes in gemcitabine-resistant pancreatic cancer cells. *J. Cell. Mol. Med.*, **2017**, *21*(9), 2055-2067.
[http://dx.doi.org/10.1111/jcmm.13126] [PMID: 28244691]

[49] Qiao, L.; Shao, X.; Gao, S.; Ming, Z.; Fu, X.; Wei, Q. Research on endoplasmic reticulum–targeting fluorescent probes and endoplasmic reticulum stress–mediated nanoanticancer strategies: A review. *Colloids Surf. B Biointerfaces*, **2021**, *208*(112046), 112046.
[http://dx.doi.org/10.1016/j.colsurfb.2021.112046] [PMID: 34419809]

[50] Ivanisenko, N.V.; Seyrek, K.; Hillert-Richter, L.K.; König, C.; Espe, J.; Bose, K.; Lavrik, I.N. Regulation of extrinsic apoptotic signaling by c-FLIP: towards targeting cancer networks. *Trends Cancer*, **2022**, *8*(3), 190-209.
[http://dx.doi.org/10.1016/j.trecan.2021.12.002] [PMID: 34973957]

[51] Xu, R.; Pelicano, H.; Zhou, Y.; Carew, J.S.; Feng, L.; Bhalla, K.N.; Keating, M.J.; Huang, P. Inhibition of glycolysis in cancer cells: a novel strategy to overcome drug resistance associated with mitochondrial respiratory defect and hypoxia. *Cancer Res.*, **2005**, *65*(2), 613-621.
[http://dx.doi.org/10.1158/0008-5472.613.65.2] [PMID: 15695406]

[52] Dey, S.; Murmu, N.; Mondal, T.; Saha, I.; Chatterjee, S.; Manna, R.; Haldar, S.; Dash, S.K.; Sarkar, T.R.; Giri, B. Multifaceted entrancing role of glucose and its analogue, 2-deoxy-D-glucose in cancer cell proliferation, inflammation, and virus infection. *Biomed. Pharmacother.*, **2022**, *156*(113801), 113801.
[http://dx.doi.org/10.1016/j.biopha.2022.113801] [PMID: 36228369]

[53] Csala, M.; Kereszturi, É.; Mandl, J.; Bánhegyi, G. The endoplasmic reticulum as the extracellular space inside the cell: role in protein folding and glycosylation. *Antioxid. Redox Signal.*, **2012**, *16*(10), 1100-1108.
[http://dx.doi.org/10.1089/ars.2011.4227] [PMID: 22149109]

[54] Schedin-Weiss, S.; Winblad, B.; Tjernberg, L.O. The role of protein glycosylation in Alzheimer disease. *FEBS J.*, **2014**, *281*(1), 46-62.
[http://dx.doi.org/10.1111/febs.12590] [PMID: 24279329]

[55] Breitling, J.; Aebi, M. N-linked protein glycosylation in the endoplasmic reticulum. *Cold Spring Harb. Perspect. Biol.*, **2013**, *5*(8), a013359-a013359.
[http://dx.doi.org/10.1101/cshperspect.a013359] [PMID: 23751184]

[56] Qin, J.Z.; Xin, H.; Nickoloff, B.J. 2-Deoxyglucose sensitizes melanoma cells to TRAIL-induced apoptosis which is reduced by mannose. *Biochem. Biophys. Res. Commun.*, **2010**, *401*(2), 293-299.
[http://dx.doi.org/10.1016/j.bbrc.2010.09.054] [PMID: 20851102]

[57]   Varki, A. *Essentials of Glycobiology*; Cold Spring Harbor Laboratory Press: New York, NY, **2009**.

[58]   Yoshida, H. ER stress and diseases. *FEBS J.,* **2007**, *274*(3), 630-658.
         [http://dx.doi.org/10.1111/j.1742-4658.2007.05639.x] [PMID: 17288551]

[59]   Oyadomari, S.; Mori, M. Roles of CHOP/GADD153 in endoplasmic reticulum stress. *Cell Death Differ.,* **2004**, *11*(4), 381-389.
         [http://dx.doi.org/10.1038/sj.cdd.4401373] [PMID: 14685163]

[60]   Cheng, Y.; Diao, D.; Zhang, H.; Song, Y.C.; Dang, C.X. Proliferation enhanced by NGF-NTRK1 signaling makes pancreatic cancer cells more sensitive to 2DG-induced apoptosis. *Int. J. Med. Sci.,* **2013**, *10*(5), 634-640.
         [http://dx.doi.org/10.7150/ijms.5547] [PMID: 23569426]

[61]   Schröder, M.; Kaufman, R.J. ER stress and the unfolded protein response. *Mutat. Res.,* **2005**, *569*(1-2), 29-63.
         [http://dx.doi.org/10.1016/j.mrfmmm.2004.06.056] [PMID: 15603751]

[62]   Tajiri, S.; Yano, S.; Morioka, M.; Kuratsu, J.; Mori, M.; Gotoh, T. CHOP is involved in neuronal apoptosis induced by neurotrophic factor deprivation. *FEBS Lett.,* **2006**, *580*(14), 3462-3468.
         [http://dx.doi.org/10.1016/j.febslet.2006.05.021] [PMID: 16716308]

[63]   Andresen, L.; Skovbakke, S.L.; Persson, G.; Hagemann-Jensen, M.; Hansen, K.A.; Jensen, H.; Skov, S. 2-deoxy D-glucose prevents cell surface expression of NKG2D ligands through inhibition of *N*-linked glycosylation. *J. Immunol.,* **2012**, *188*(4), 1847-1855.
         [http://dx.doi.org/10.4049/jimmunol.1004085] [PMID: 22227571]

[64]   Liu, L.; Chowdhury, S.; Fang, X.; Liu, J.L.; Srikant, C.B. Attenuation of unfolded protein response and apoptosis by mReg2 induced GRP78 in mouse insulinoma cells. *FEBS Lett.,* **2014**, *588*(11), 2016-2024.
         [http://dx.doi.org/10.1016/j.febslet.2014.04.030] [PMID: 24801175]

[65]   Yu, S.M.; Kim, S.J. Endoplasmic reticulum stress (ER-stress) by 2-deoxy-D-glucose (2DG) reduces cyclooxygenase-2 (COX-2) expression and N-glycosylation and induces a loss of COX-2 activity *via* a Src kinase-dependent pathway in rabbit articular chondrocytes. *Exp. Mol. Med.,* **2010**, *42*(11), 777-786.
         [http://dx.doi.org/10.3858/emm.2010.42.11.079] [PMID: 20926918]

[66]   Bandugula, V.R.; N, R.P. 2-Deoxy-d-glucose and ferulic acid modulates radiation response signaling in non-small cell lung cancer cells. *Tumour Biol.,* **2013**, *34*(1), 251-259.
         [http://dx.doi.org/10.1007/s13277-012-0545-6] [PMID: 23065571]

[67]   Giammarioli, A.M.; Gambardella, L.; Barbati, C.; Pietraforte, D.; Tinari, A.; Alberton, M.; Gnessi, L.; Griffin, R.J.; Minetti, M.; Malorni, W. Differential effects of the glycolysis inhibitor 2-deoxy- D -glucose on the activity of pro-apoptotic agents in metastatic melanoma cells, and induction of a cytoprotective autophagic response. *Int. J. Cancer,* **2012**, *131*(4), E337-E347.
         [http://dx.doi.org/10.1002/ijc.26420] [PMID: 21913183]

[68]   Ramírez-Peinado, S.; Alcázar-Limones, F.; Lagares-Tena, L.; El Mjiyad, N.; Caro-Maldonado, A.; Tirado, O.M.; Muñoz-Pinedo, C. 2-deoxyglucose induces Noxa-dependent apoptosis in alveolar rhabdomyosarcoma. *Cancer Res.,* **2011**, *71*(21), 6796-6806.
         [http://dx.doi.org/10.1158/0008-5472.CAN-11-0759] [PMID: 21911456]

[69]   Xi, H.; Kurtoglu, M.; Liu, H.; Wangpaichitr, M.; You, M.; Liu, X.; Savaraj, N.; Lampidis, T.J. 2-Deoxy-d-glucose activates autophagy *via* endoplasmic reticulum stress rather than ATP depletion. *Cancer Chemother. Pharmacol.,* **2011**, *67*(4), 899-910.
         [http://dx.doi.org/10.1007/s00280-010-1391-0] [PMID: 20593179]

[70]   Zagorodna, O.; Martin, S.M.; Rutkowski, D.T.; Kuwana, T.; Spitz, D.R.; Knudson, C.M. 2-Deoxyglucose-induced toxicity is regulated by Bcl-2 family members and is enhanced by antagonizing Bcl-2 in lymphoma cell lines. *Oncogene,* **2012**, *31*(22), 2738-2749.

[http://dx.doi.org/10.1038/onc.2011.454] [PMID: 21986940]

[71]   Hamasaki, M.; Yoshimori, T. Where do they come from? Insights into autophagosome formation. *FEBS Lett.,* **2010**, *584*(7), 1296-1301.
[http://dx.doi.org/10.1016/j.febslet.2010.02.061] [PMID: 20188731]

[72]   Klionsky, D.J.; Abeliovich, H.; Agostinis, P.; Agrawal, D.K.; Aliev, G.; Askew, D.S.; Baba, M.; Baehrecke, E.H.; Bahr, B.A.; Ballabio, A.; Bamber, B.A.; Bassham, D.C.; Bergamini, E.; Bi, X.; Biard-Piechaczyk, M.; Blum, J.S.; Bredesen, D.E.; Brodsky, J.L.; Brumell, J.H.; Brunk, U.T.; Bursch, W.; Camougrand, N.; Cebollero, E.; Cecconi, F.; Chen, Y.; Chin, L.S.; Choi, A.; Chu, C.T.; Chung, J.; Clark, R.S.B.; Clarke, P.G.H.; Clarke, S.G.; Clavé, C.; Cleveland, J.L.; Codogno, P.; Colombo, M.I.; Coto-Montes, A.; Cregg, J.M.; Cuervo, A.M.; Debnath, J.; Dennis, P.B.; Dennis, P.A.; Demarchi, F.; Deretic, V.; Devenish, R.J.; Di Sano, F.; Dice, J.F.; Distelhorst, C.W.; Dinesh-Kumar, S.P.; Eissa, N.T.; DiFiglia, M.; Djavaheri-Mergny, M.; Dorsey, F.C.; Dröge, W.; Dron, M.; Dunn, W.A., Jr; Duszenko, M.; Elazar, Z.; Esclatine, A.; Eskelinen, E.L.; Fésüs, L.; Finley, K.D.; Fuentes, J.M.; Fueyo-Margareto, J.; Fujisaki, K.; Galliot, B.; Gao, F.B.; Gewirtz, D.A.; Gibson, S.B.; Gohla, A.; Goldberg, A.L.; Gonzalez, R.; González-Estévez, C.; Gorski, S.M.; Gottlieb, R.A.; Häussinger, D.; He, Y.W.; Heidenreich, K.; Hill, J.A.; Høyer-Hansen, M.; Hu, X.; Huang, W.P.; Iwasaki, A.; Jäättelä, M.; Jackson, W.T.; Jiang, X.; Jin, S.V.; Johansen, T.; Jung, J.U.; Kadowaki, M.; Kang, C.; Kelekar, A.; Kessel, D.H.; Kiel, J.A.K.W.; Kim, H.P.; Kimchi, A.; Kinsella, T.J.; Kiselyov, K.; Kitamoto, K.; Knecht, E.; Komatsu, M.; Kominami, E.; Kondo, S.; Kovács, A.L.; Kroemer, G.; Kuan, C.Y.; Kumar, R.; Kundu, M.; Landry, J.; Laporte, M.; Le, W.; Lei, H.Y.; Levine, B.; Lieberman, A.P.; Lim, K-L.; Lin, F-C.; Liou, W.; Liu, L.F.; Lopez-Berestein, G.; López-Otín, C.; Lu, B.; Macleod, K.F.; Malorni, W.; Martinet, W.; Matsuoka, K.; Mautner, J.; Meijer, A.J.; Meléndez, A.; Michels, P.; Miotto, G.; Mistiaen, W.P.; Mizushima, N.; Mograbi, B.; Moore, M.N.; Moreira, P.I.; Moriyasu, Y.; Motyl, T.; Münz, C.; Murphy, L.O.; Naqvi, N.I.; Neufeld, T.P.; Nishino, I.; Nixon, R.A.; Noda, T.; Nürnberg, B.; Ogawa, M.; Oleinick, N.L.; Olsen, L.J.; Ozpolat, B.; Paglin, S.; Palmer, G.E.; Papassideri, I.S.; Parkes, M.; Perlmutter, D.H.; Perry, G.; Piacentini, M.; Pinkas-Kramarski, R.; Prescott, M.; Proikas-Cezanne, T.; Raben, N.; Rami, A.; Reggiori, F.; Rohrer, B.; Rubinsztein, D.C.; Ryan, K.M.; Sadoshima, J.; Sakagami, H.; Sakai, Y.; Sandri, M.; Sasakawa, C.; Sass, M.; Schneider, C.; Seglen, P.O.; Seleverstov, O.; Settleman, J.; Shacka, J.J.; Shapiro, I.M.; Sibirny, A.A.; Silva-Zacarin, E.C.M.; Simon, H-U.; Simone, C.; Simonsen, A.; Smith, M.A.; Spanel-Borowski, K.; Srinivas, V.; Steeves, M.; Stenmark, H.; Stromhaug, P.E.; Subauste, C.S.; Sugimoto, S.; Sulzer, D.; Suzuki, T.; Swanson, M.S.; Tabas, I.; Takeshita, F.; Talbot, N.J.; Tallóczy, Z.; Tanaka, K.; Tanaka, K.; Tanida, I.; Taylor, G.S.; Taylor, J.P.; Terman, A.; Tettamanti, G.; Thompson, C.B.; Thumm, M.; Tolkovsky, A.M.; Tooze, S.A.; Truant, R.; Tumanovska, L.V.; Uchiyama, Y.; Ueno, T.; Uzcátegui, N.L.; van der Klei, I.J.; Vaquero, E.C.; Vellai, T.; Vogel, M.W.; Wang, H-G.; Webster, P.; Xi, Z.; Xiao, G.; Yahalom, J.; Yang, J-M.; Yap, G.S.; Yin, X-M.; Yoshimori, T.; Yue, Z.; Yuzaki, M.; Zabirnyk, O.; Zheng, X.; Zhu, X.; Deter, R.L.; Zabirnyk, O.; Zheng, X.; Zhu, X.; Deter, R.L. Guidelines for the use and interpretation of assays for monitoring autophagy in higher eukaryotes. *Autophagy,* **2008**, *4*(2), 151-175.
[http://dx.doi.org/10.4161/auto.5338] [PMID: 18188003]

[73]   Shi, Z.; Li, C.; Zhao, S.; Yu, Y.; An, N.; Liu, Y.; Wu, C.; Yue, B.; Bao, J. A systems biology analysis of autophagy in cancer therapy. *Cancer Lett.,* **2013**, *337*(2), 149-160.
[http://dx.doi.org/10.1016/j.canlet.2013.06.004] [PMID: 23791881]

[74]   Zhou, S.; Zhao, L.; Kuang, M.; Zhang, B.; Liang, Z.; Yi, T.; Wei, Y.; Zhao, X. Autophagy in tumorigenesis and cancer therapy: Dr. Jekyll or Mr. Hyde? *Cancer Lett.,* **2012**, *323*(2), 115-127.
[http://dx.doi.org/10.1016/j.canlet.2012.02.017] [PMID: 22542808]

[75]   Mei, Y.; Thompson, M.D.; Cohen, R.A.; Tong, X. Autophagy and oxidative stress in cardiovascular diseases. *Biochim. Biophys. Acta Mol. Basis Dis.,* **2015**, *1852*(2), 243-251.
[http://dx.doi.org/10.1016/j.bbadis.2014.05.005] [PMID: 24834848]

[76]   Yorimitsu, T.; Nair, U.; Yang, Z.; Klionsky, D.J. Endoplasmic reticulum stress triggers autophagy. *J. Biol. Chem.,* **2006**, *281*(40), 30299-30304.
[http://dx.doi.org/10.1074/jbc.M607007200] [PMID: 16901900]

[77]   Ciechomska, I.A.; Gabrusiewicz, K.; Szczepankiewicz, A.A.; Kaminska, B. Endoplasmic reticulum

stress triggers autophagy in malignant glioma cells undergoing cyclosporine A-induced cell death. *Oncogene*, **2013**, *32*(12), 1518-1529.
[http://dx.doi.org/10.1038/onc.2012.174] [PMID: 22580614]

[78]   Liu, L.L.; Long, Z.J.; Wang, L.X.; Zheng, F.M.; Fang, Z.G.; Yan, M.; Xu, D.F.; Chen, J.J.; Wang, S.W.; Lin, D.J.; Liu, Q. Inhibition of mTOR pathway sensitizes acute myeloid leukemia cells to aurora inhibitors by suppression of glycolytic metabolism. *Mol. Cancer Res.*, **2013**, *11*(11), 1326-1336.
[http://dx.doi.org/10.1158/1541-7786.MCR-13-0172] [PMID: 24008673]

[79]   Tanida, I.; Ueno, T.; Kominami, E. LC3 and Autophagy. In: *Autophagosome and Phagosome*; Humana Press: Totowa, NJ, **2008**; pp. 77-88.
[http://dx.doi.org/10.1007/978-1-59745-157-4_4]

[80]   Kurtoglu, M.; Gao, N.; Shang, J.; Maher, J.C.; Lehrman, M.A.; Wangpaichitr, M.; Savaraj, N.; Lane, A.N.; Lampidis, T.J. Under normoxia, 2-deoxy- D -glucose elicits cell death in select tumor types not by inhibition of glycolysis but by interfering with N-linked glycosylation. *Mol. Cancer Ther.*, **2007**, *6*(11), 3049-3058.
[http://dx.doi.org/10.1158/1535-7163.MCT-07-0310] [PMID: 18025288]

[81]   Ben Sahra, I.; Laurent, K.; Giuliano, S.; Larbret, F.; Ponzio, G.; Gounon, P.; Le Marchand-Brustel, Y.; Giorgetti-Peraldi, S.; Cormont, M.; Bertolotto, C.; Deckert, M.; Auberger, P.; Tanti, J.F.; Bost, F. Targeting cancer cell metabolism: the combination of metformin and 2-deoxyglucose induces p53-dependent apoptosis in prostate cancer cells. *Cancer Res.*, **2010**, *70*(6), 2465-2475.
[http://dx.doi.org/10.1158/0008-5472.CAN-09-2782] [PMID: 20215500]

[82]   Sottnik, J.L.; Lori, J.C.; Rose, B.J.; Thamm, D.H. Glycolysis inhibition by 2-deoxy-d-glucose reverts the metastatic phenotype *in vitro* and *in vivo*. *Clin. Exp. Metastasis*, **2011**, *28*(8), 865-875.
[http://dx.doi.org/10.1007/s10585-011-9417-5] [PMID: 21842413]

[83]   Maschek, G.; Savaraj, N.; Priebe, W.; Braunschweiger, P.; Hamilton, K.; Tidmarsh, G.F.; De Young, L.R.; Lampidis, T.J. 2-deoxy-D-glucose increases the efficacy of adriamycin and paclitaxel in human osteosarcoma and non-small cell lung cancers *in vivo*. *Cancer Res.*, **2004**, *64*(1), 31-34.
[http://dx.doi.org/10.1158/0008-5472.CAN-03-3294] [PMID: 14729604]

[84]   Kennedy, C.R.; Tilkens, S.B.; Guan, H.; Garner, J.A.; Or, P.M.Y.; Chan, A.M. Differential sensitivities of glioblastoma cell lines towards metabolic and signaling pathway inhibitions. *Cancer Lett.*, **2013**, *336*(2), 299-306.
[http://dx.doi.org/10.1016/j.canlet.2013.03.020] [PMID: 23523615]

[85]   Liu, H.; Hu, Y.P.; Savaraj, N.; Priebe, W.; Lampidis, T.J. Hypersensitization of tumor cells to glycolytic inhibitors. *Biochemistry*, **2001**, *40*(18), 5542-5547.
[http://dx.doi.org/10.1021/bi002426w] [PMID: 11331019]

[86]   Minor, R.K.; Smith, D.L., Jr; Sossong, A.M.; Kaushik, S.; Poosala, S.; Spangler, E.L.; Roth, G.S.; Lane, M.; Allison, D.B.; de Cabo, R.; Ingram, D.K.; Mattison, J.A. Chronic ingestion of 2-deoxy-d-glucose induces cardiac vacuolization and increases mortality in rats. *Toxicol. Appl. Pharmacol.*, **2010**, *243*(3), 332-339.
[http://dx.doi.org/10.1016/j.taap.2009.11.025] [PMID: 20026095]

[87]   Sandoval, D.A.; Ryan, K.K.; de Kloet, A.D.; Woods, S.C.; Seeley, R.J. Female rats are relatively more sensitive to reduced lipid *versus* reduced carbohydrate availability. *Nutr. Diabetes*, **2012**, *2*(2), e27-e27.
[http://dx.doi.org/10.1038/nutd.2011.23] [PMID: 23169552]

[88]   Kalyanaraman, B. Reactive oxygen species, proinflammatory and immunosuppressive mediators induced in COVID-19: overlapping biology with cancer. *RSC Chemical Biology*, **2021**, *2*(5), 1402-1414.
[http://dx.doi.org/10.1039/D1CB00042J] [PMID: 34704045]

[89]   Raez, L.E.; Papadopoulos, K.; Ricart, A.D.; Chiorean, E.G.; DiPaola, R.S.; Stein, M.N.; Rocha Lima, C.M.; Schlesselman, J.J.; Tolba, K.; Langmuir, V.K.; Kroll, S.; Jung, D.T.; Kurtoglu, M.; Rosenblatt,

J.; Lampidis, T.J. A phase I dose-escalation trial of 2-deoxy-d-glucose alone or combined with docetaxel in patients with advanced solid tumors. *Cancer Chemother. Pharmacol.,* **2013**, *71*(2), 523-530.
[http://dx.doi.org/10.1007/s00280-012-2045-1] [PMID: 23228990]

[90]   Yamaguchi, R.; Perkins, G. Finding a Panacea among combination cancer therapies. *Cancer Res.,* **2012**, *72*(1), 18-23.
[http://dx.doi.org/10.1158/0008-5472.CAN-11-3091] [PMID: 22052464]

[91]   Dwarakanath, B.S.; Singh, D.; Banerji, A.; Sarin, R.; Venkataramana, N.K.; Jalali, R.; Vishwanath, P.N.; Mohanti, B.K.; Tripathi, R.P.; Kalia, V.K.; Jain, V. Clinical studies for improving radiotherapy with 2-deoxy-D-glucose: Present status and future prospects. *J. Cancer Res. Ther.,* **2009**, *5*(9) Suppl. 1, 21.
[http://dx.doi.org/10.4103/0973-1482.55136] [PMID: 20009289]

[92]   Pajak, B.; Siwiak, E.; Sołtyka, M.; Priebe, A.; Zieliński, R.; Fokt, I.; Ziemniak, M.; Jaśkiewicz, A.; Borowski, R.; Domoradzki, T.; Priebe, W. 2-deoxy-d-glucose and its analogs: From diagnostic to therapeutic agents. *Int. J. Mol. Sci.,* **2019**, *21*(1), 234.
[http://dx.doi.org/10.3390/ijms21010234] [PMID: 31905745]

[93]   Broecker-Preuss, M.; Becher-Boveleth, N.; Bockisch, A.; Dührsen, U.; Müller, S. Regulation of glucose uptake in lymphoma cell lines by c-MYC- and PI3K-dependent signaling pathways and impact of glycolytic pathways on cell viability. *J. Transl. Med.,* **2017**, *15*(1), 158.
[http://dx.doi.org/10.1186/s12967-017-1258-9] [PMID: 28724379]

[94]   Liang, L-M.; Feng, L.; Zhang, Z-G.; Wei, B. https://e-century.us/files/ijcem/10/2/ijcem0036766.pdf

[95]   Lee, S.J.; Park, B.N.; Roh, J.H.; an, Y.S.; Hur, H.; Yoon, J.K. Enhancing the therapeutic efficacy of 2-deoxyglucose in breast cancer cells using cell-cycle synchronization. *Anticancer Res.,* **2016**, *36*(11), 5975-5980.
[http://dx.doi.org/10.21873/anticanres.11185] [PMID: 27793923]

[96]   Kovar, J.L.; Volcheck, W.; Sevick-Muraca, E.; Simpson, M.A.; Olive, D.M. Characterization and performance of a near-infrared 2-deoxyglucose optical imaging agent for mouse cancer models. *Anal. Biochem.,* **2009**, *384*(2), 254-262.
[http://dx.doi.org/10.1016/j.ab.2008.09.050] [PMID: 18938129]

[97]   Ashraf, M.A.; Goyal, A. *Fludeoxyglucose (18F)*; StatPearls Publishing, **2023**.

[98]   Mittal, B.R.; Manohar, K.; Bhattacharya, A.; Malhotra, P.; Varma, S. Fluoro-deoxy-glucose positron emission tomography/computed tomography in lymphoma: A pictorial essay. *Indian J. Nucl. Med.,* **2013**, *28*(2), 85-92.
[http://dx.doi.org/10.4103/0972-3919.118256] [PMID: 24163512]

[99]   Barban, S. Mechanism of resistance to 2-deoxy-d-glucose in HeLa cells. *Biochim. Biophys. Acta,* **1961**, *47*(3), 604-605.
[http://dx.doi.org/10.1016/0006-3002(61)90561-3] [PMID: 13686732]

[100]   Bailey, P.J.; Harris, M. Patterns of resistance to 2-deoxy-D-glucose in pig kidney cells. *J. Cell. Physiol.,* **1968**, *71*(1), 23-32.
[http://dx.doi.org/10.1002/jcp.1040710105] [PMID: 5663112]

CHAPTER 11

Dual Role of 2-Deoxy-D-Glucose in Seizure Modulation

Shaurya Prakash[1], Kuldeep Singh[2] and **Antresh Kumar[1,*]**

[1] *Department of Biochemistry, Central University of Haryana, Mahendergarh-123031, India*

[2] *Department of Applied Chemistry, Amity University Madhya Pradesh, Gwalior-474005, India*

Abstract: 2-Deoxy-D-glucose (2-DG) is a glucose analog that inhibits glycolysis. Conflicting evidence exists regarding the effects of 2-DG on seizure activity. The effects of 2-deoxy-D-glucose (2-DG) on seizures and epileptogenesis have been a subject of interest in the field of neuroscience and epilepsy research. In the 6-Hz seizure threshold test, 2-DG significantly increased the seizure threshold, indicating anticonvulsant properties. However, in other models, such as the mouse electroshock seizure threshold test, intravenous pentylenetetrazol test, and intravenous kainic acid test, 2-DG decreased the seizure threshold and exhibited proconvulsant effects. Similarly, the related compound 3-methylglucose reduced seizure threshold when administered intravenously with pentylenetetrazol. In contrast, 2-DG administered chronically retarded the progression of kindled seizures in rats, suggesting antiepileptic effects. The anticonvulsant actions of 2-DG may be mediated through the inhibition of glycolysis and diversion of glucose metabolism towards the pentose phosphate pathway. Meanwhile, its acute proconvulsant effects are likely due to reduced glucose uptake. In summary, 2-DG displays both anticonvulsant and proconvulsant actions on seizures, which depend on the model system and mechanisms involved, including glycolytic inhibition and decreased glucose uptake. Further study is needed to fully elucidate the contradictory effects of 2-DG on seizure activity in different experimental models.

Keywords: Anticonvulsant, Epilepsy, Proconvulsant, Seizure, Synaptic excitation, Seizure threshold, 2-Deoxy-D-glucose.

1. INTRODUCTION

Epilepsy is a chronic non-communicable neurological disorder of the brain that affects over 50 million people worldwide. The defining features of epilepsy include a brief period of uncontrollable movement of a part of or the whole body. Such sudden abnormal behavior of the patients is termed a seizure. The recurrent

---

* **Corresponding author Antresh Kumar:** Department of Biochemistry, Central University of Haryana, Mahendergarh-123031, India; E-mail: antreshkumar@cuh.ac.in

Raman Singh, Antresh Kumar & Kuldeep Singh (Eds.)
All rights reserved-© 2024 Bentham Science Publishers

epileptic seizure is due to impulsive neuronal excitability at the synapse, resulting in the loss of consciousness and control over bladder or bowel movements. Various structures and processes related to neurons, ion channels, receptors, glia, and inhibitory and excitatory synapses are associated with the development of a seizure. Antiseizure drugs are used to regulate neural excitability for the treatment of epilepsy. Different groups of studies have revealed that various metabolic factors also affect neural excitability, which gained more attention for targeting a promising source for the prevention of epileptic episodes. The clinical observations suggest that ketogenic diets containing high fat, low-carbohydrate, and rich proteins are proven to control seizures and prevent epilepsy. However, the underlying mechanism of the ketogenic diet's role in controlling seizures is still not well-defined. The clinical studies noted that a low carbohydrate diet remarkably controls seizures which led to the hypothesis that restriction in the glycolysis and carbohydrate metabolism might have an anticonvulsant activity. The purpose of this chapter is to review the evidence on 2-DG to explore the action mechanism and its therapeutic activity both anticonvulsant and pro-convulsant agents.

2. ROLE OF 2-DG IN EPILEPSY

2-deoxy-D-glucose (2-DG) is a glucose analog that inhibits glycolysis which has been extensively studied for its potential as a chemotherapeutic agent against different health disorders. The detailed mechanism of 2-DG in glycolysis inhibition has been discussed earlier in this book. Interestingly, 2-DG has also demonstrated conflicting effects on seizures in different experimental models. The effects of 2-deoxy-D-glucose (2-DG) on seizures and epileptogenesis have been the subject of intense interest in the field of neuroscience and epilepsy research. The effects of 2-DG involved different mechanisms, such as the inhibition of glycolysis *versus* reduced glucose uptake. The anticonvulsant and proconvulsant actions of 2-deoxy-D-glucose (2-DG) have been extensively studied in various experimental models. These findings highlight the need for further investigation to elucidate the precise mechanisms underlying its actions and to explore its therapeutic potential in various neurological and oncological conditions. Elucidating the contradictory impacts of 2-DG on seizures in different models may provide insights into glucose metabolism in epilepsy and alternative glycolytic inhibitors for treatment. In the 6-Hz seizure threshold test, 2-DG elevates the seizure threshold and displays anticonvulsant properties. However, in other models like the mouse electroshock seizure threshold test and pentylenetetrazol or kainic acid models, 2-DG reduces the seizure threshold and acts as a proconvulsant. Clinical studies on kindling models also suggest that 2-DG can retard the progression of kindled seizures and have antiepileptic effects. The research on 2-DG's anticonvulsant and proconvulsant actions, its potential as a chemotherapeutic agent, and its applications in neuroimaging collectively demonstrate the diverse effects of this glycolytic inhibitor. The anti and pro-convulsant properties of 2-DG are determined by its effects on glucose metabolism and its subsequent impact on seizure susceptibility. The metabolic changes due to this antimetabolite lead to both anticonvulsant and proconvulsant effects, depending on specific seizure models. In some tests, 2-DG has been shown to elevate the seizure threshold indicating its anticonvulsant activity. However, in other seizure models, it has been found to reduce the seizure threshold, demonstrating the proconvulsant properties [1].

3. ANTICONVULSANT EFFECTS

2-DG, a glycolytic inhibitor, has shown promising anticonvulsant effects in the rat kindling model of temporal lobe epilepsy [2]. It effectively suppresses spontaneous neuronal firing and epileptiform bursts in hippocampal slices, indicating its potential as an anticonvulsant agent [3]. Additionally, acute anticonvulsant actions of 2-DG were observed in experimental models of seizures and epilepsy, suggesting its potential therapeutic use in these conditions [2]. 2-Deoxy-d-glucose (2-DG) is being developed as a potential anticonvulsant and disease-modifying agent for patients with epilepsy. The anticonvulsant role of 2-DG is based on its ability to interfere with glucose metabolism by inhibiting the glycolytic enzymes. This interference leads to anticonvulsant actions. 2-DG is avidly taken up into the cells by GLUT transporters and is phosphorylated by hexokinase to form 2-DG-6-phosphate. This compound competitively inhibits the downstream process in glycolysis, preventing the progression of glycolytic pathway, since 2-DG-6-P cannot undergo the downstream steps of the pathway. Consequently, 2-DG shunts glucose metabolism into the pentose phosphate pathway (PPP), limiting glycolysis and increasing the glucose flux through the PPP. This metabolic alteration is believed to contribute to the anticonvulsant activity of 2-DG. 2-DG has shown suppressive effects on interictal-like epileptiform discharge (IED) but at the same time, promotes the induction of seizure-like epileptiform discharge (SLE). It has been shown that acute exposure to 2-DG or severe hypoglycemia decreases spontaneous IED induced by certain conditions, while also inducing seizure-like discharge. Findings suggest that the inhibitory effect of 2-DG on IED is linked to the impairment of glycolysis, while the proconvulsant effects are caused by an excitatory mechanism that depends on the impairment of mitochondrial oxidative phosphorylation [4]. The dual nature of 2-DG on seizure susceptibility suggests a complex interplay between its metabolic actions and the specific mechanisms underlying different seizure models. Additionally, 2-DG has been found to elevate the seizure threshold in the 6-Hz seizure test, indicating its anticonvulsant action. Among various studies, 2-DG has demonstrated acute anticonvulsive and chronic antiepileptic properties, both *in vitro* and *in vivo*. It has shown its potential in the reduction of the frequency of interictal epileptiform bursts and ictal electrographic seizures in hippocampal slices and chronic antiepileptic action against kindling progression [1 - 7]. However, during preclinical development, cardiac toxicity has been encountered in rats [8].

3.1. Evidence from 6-Hz Seizure Threshold Test

The anticonvulsant effect of 2-DG can be evaluated by the 6-Hz model, implied to evaluate the potential of anticonvulsant agents in seizure induction. 6-Hz test in mice performed by Gasior *et al.* demonstrated that acute treatment with 2-DG significantly elevated the seizure threshold, indicating the anticonvulsant action [1]. Another similar study performed by Xiao *et al.* found that pre-treatment of the subjects with 2-DG was effective in reducing the seizure activity and decreased seizure severity. The findings of both the above-stated studies collectively suggest that 2-DG has a potential anticonvulsant effect by reducing the seizure severity in the 6-Hz model [9]. Using the 6-Hz model, another study provides substantial evidence for the anticonvulsive effect of 2-DG. In the study, it was observed that 2-DG demonstrated acute anticonvulsant properties against minimal clonic seizures evoked by 6-Hz stimulation in mice. Protection against 6-Hz evoked seizures was observed 15 minutes after the administration of 2-DG at various doses, with a calculated dose that resulted in protection for 50% of rats (ED50) being 79.7mg/kg. The time to peak action of 2-DG was 15 minutes at a dose of 75mg/kg i.p. and 1 hour at a dose of 100mg/kg i.p. Collectively, these findings suggest that 2-DG has an anticonvulsive effect in the 6-Hz model, suggesting its potential as a therapy for epilepsy [2]. Although 2-DG protects against seizures in the 6-Hz seizure test, it promotes seizures in some other models. The proconvulsant action may relate to reduced glucose uptake, whereas the anticonvulsant action may require inhibition of glycolysis and shunting of glucose metabolism through the pentose phosphate pathway (PPP).

3.2. Evidence from Kindling Models

In the study performed by Xiao *et al.*, it was observed that 2-DG was unable to affect the simulation threshold to induce the electrographic seizures or the expression of either electrographic or behavioural seizures in fully amygdala kindled rats. This suggests that 2-DG did not confer seizure protection in fully kindled animals [9]. Though limited, but the study provides some evidence about the anticonvulsant activity of 2-DG in kindling model. Another study by Stafstrom *et al.* provides conclusive evidence about the anticonvulsive effect of 2-DG in kindling model. The study demonstrated that 2-DG exerted chronic antiepileptic action by increasing the after discharge threshold (AFT) in the performant path kindling that resulted in a 2-fold slowing of the kindled seizure progression. This effect was uniform in both the performant path and olfactory bulb stimulation. Additionally, they showed that 2-DG has anticonvulsive effects against seizures evoked by 6-Hz stimulation in mice and audiogenic stimulation in Fring's mice [2]. These findings indicate that 2-DG has a novel pattern of effectiveness in preclinical screening models, suggesting its potential as a therapy for epilepsy with distinctive mechanisms of action compared to currently available anticonvulsants.

4. PROCONVULSANT EFFECTS

The proconvulsant role of 2-DG is related to its ability to reduce glucose uptake and inhibit glycolysis, leading to increase seizures susceptibility in certain seizure models. When 2-DG is taken up into the cells, it is phosphorylated to form 2-DG-6-phosphate (2-DG-6-P), which competitively inhibits the downstream cascade in the glycolysis pathway. This inhibition prevents the entry of glucose in the glycolysis pathway and shunts it for metabolism through the PPP. This shift in glucose metabolism is thought to contribute to the proconvulsant role of 2-DG. Additionally, 2-DG has been found to reduce the seizure threshold in various seizure tests such as the mouse electroshock seizure threshold (MEST) test and intravenous pentylenetetrazol (PTZ) and kainic acid (KA) seizure threshold tests, indicating its procovulsant action. Similar documentations have been done over time that argue about the proconvulsive properties of 2-DG [10]. Gąsior *et al.*, reported that 2-DG, as a glucose analog, accumulates in cells and interferes with carbohydrate metabolism, leading to proconvulsant actions [1]. Furthermore, Shao & Stafstrom investigated the effects of glycolytic inhibition with 2-DG on basal membrane properties, spontaneous neuronal firing, and epileptiform network bursts in hippocampal slices, providing insights into the mechanisms underlying the proconvulsant effects of 2-DG [3]. Moreover, Samokhina *et al.* highlighted that chronic inhibition of brain glycolysis by 2-DG initiates epileptogenesis, indicating a potential role of long-term glycolytic inhibition in the development of seizures [11]. Additionally, Nedergaard and Andreasen discussed the opposing effects of 2-DG on interictal- and ictal-like activity when K^+ currents and GABAA receptors are blocked in the rat hippocampus, shedding light on the complex interplay between glycolytic inhibition and seizure activity [4].

4.1. Evidence from MEST, PTZ, and KA Models

The evidence for the proconvulsive effect of 2-DG could be validated by the findings obtained by MEST, PTZ and kainic acid models. In a series of experiments, i.v. the administration of PTZ and KA was done and corneal simulation at 60Hz for 0.2s for MEST was performed. Thirty minutes prior to the seizure tests, the models were treated with variable doses of 2-DG (250 or 500 mg/kg), intra peritoneal. The measurement of the seizure threshold revealed reduced threshold which indicated a proconvulsant effect [1].

4.2. Related Evidence from 3-methylglucose

Similar to 2-DG, 3-MG also has been found to have a proconvulsant role in different seizure models. The convulsive effect of 3-MG on the mice model was assessed by the 6-Hz test and i.v. PTZ test. Pre-treatment of the subjects was performed at 250 and 500mg/kg doses of 3-MG. In the 6-Hz test, there was no effect on the seizure threshold at any tested concentration. However, in the i.v. PTZ test, the same doses significantly decreased the seizure threshold for the induction of tail twitch and clonic seizures. These findings indicate that 3-MG also exhibits a proconvulant role in specific seizure models in the i.v. PTZ test [1].

5. 2-DG MECHANISMS INVOLVED IN THE EPILEPSY TREATMENT

5.1. Inhibition of Glycolysis

As previously discussed, glucose-deficient diet (ketogenic diet, atkins diet, *etc.*) has been widely employed for control of seizures and epilepsy, it becomes evident that employing a glucose deficient condition could be a promising approach. Administration of 2-DG effectively inhibits the glycolytic pathway, which suppresses the downstream pathways. The limitation of glucose metabolism, restricts the amount of ATP present in the neuronal region and thus restricts the neuronal excitation which is responsible for seizures. In humans, PET imaging has revealed very significant contribution of glycolysis in the dynamic metabolic shifts observed in the epileptic brain [12]. In the normal scenario of seizure, increase in the extracellular potassium in the hippocampal CA3 neurons leads to the establishment of epileptiform (high-frequency interictal bursting). The administration of 2-DG in the epileptic mice model reduced the burst frequency to about half [2]. The glycolytic inhibition by 2-DG was shown to play a crucial role in the inhibition of neuronal firing as it was reduced by 67% in the CA3 neurons. By intracellular administration of 2-DG, it was found that glycolytic inhibition of individual neurons was not sufficient for the inhibition of neuronal firing [13]. As per the studies to validate the role of glycolysis inhibition in the control of seizure events, the treatment of lactate to the 2-DG treated models, completely reversed its anticonvulsant role, which suggested that 2-DG mediated glycolysis inhibition was involved in its role as an anticonvulsant. Lactate supplementation was done to provide the substrate beyond the point of glycolytic inhibition by 2-DG *i.e.* inhibition of hexokinase activity [9].

The mechanisms associated with the anticonvulsant role of 2-DG *via* glycolytic inhibition is variable. Primarily, 2-DG administration leads to the activation of K_{ATP} channel [14], a potassium gradient channel that is sensitive to and regulated by intracellular ATP concentration. The high or low ATP concentration due to the interference of 2-DG in the glucose metabolism leads to regulation of these channels resulting in hyperpolarization of the neuronal cell membrane by the outflow of potassium ions and reducing the neuronal excitation [14, 15]. Secondly, 2-DG reduces the seizure progression by the downregulation of brain-derived neurotrophic factor (BDNF) and its receptor TrkB. This reduced expression is facilitated by the decrease in transcription factor NRSF catalyzed by the 2-DG administration [16]. Apart from these, it is speculated that the energy-deprived state in the neurons lowers the energy availability which results in lower synaptic excitation and thus, less frequent events of epileptic attacks.

5.2. Shunting of Glucose Metabolism Through Pentose Phosphate Pathway

Apart from the inhibition of glycolysis, pentose phosphate pathway (PPP) is another glucose metabolism pathway that has been speculated to exhibit anticonvulsant role. The shunting of glucose-6-phosphate (G6P) from glycolysis to PPP triggers the synthesis of ribose-5-phosphate, GSH and NADP, all of which in a way or other, contribute to the anticonvulsant activity. Interactions between 2-DG and the Pentose Phosphate Pathway play a crucial role in its anticonvulsant properties. The Pentose Phosphate Pathway is a metabolic pathway that operates parallel to glycolysis and is involved in the production of NADPH and ribose-5-phosphate, both of which have significant implications in neuronal health and function. This pathway is associated with the production of reduced glutathione (GSH), an important free radical scavenger in the nervous system and an endogenous anticonvulsant [17 - 19]. The shift of glucose metabolism from glycolysis to the PPP, leads to increased GSH levels and this increase facilitated by PPP is believed to contribute to the anticonvulsant efficacy. The diversion of glucose metabolism to the PPP not only increases the GSH levels, but also maintains the energy source for the brain by the production of NADPH, thereby providing significant anticonvulsant efficacy [9]. NADPH is a key molecule in various biochemical processes, including the regulation of oxidative stress, detoxification reactions, and the maintenance of cellular redox balance. Moreover, NADPH is a critical cofactor in the defense against oxidative stress in neurons, which can contribute to epileptic seizures. Increased NADPH concentration also potentiates the biosynthesis of neurosteroids *via* enhancing the activity of 5α-reductase, which is a crucial enzyme that catalyses steroid precursors into neurosteroids and results in the potentiation of GABAergic tonic inhibition [14, 20]. In addition, the pentose phosphate pathway generates ribose-5-phosphate, a precursor for nucleotide synthesis, which plays a crucial role in maintaining neuronal integrity and function. By promoting nucleotide synthesis, 2-DG can help replenish the cellular pool of nucleotides that may be depleted during seizures, thereby supporting the recovery and repair of damaged neurons.

CONCLUSION

In conclusion, this chapter has delved into the intricate exploration of 2-DG's impact on proconvulsant and anticonvulsant activities across various test models such as MEST, PTZ, KA, and 6-Hz. The comprehensive analysis of these models has shed light on the diverse mechanisms through which 2-DG interacts with the epileptic processes. Through a meticulous literature review, we have compiled its proconvulsant effects under specific conditions, as well as its potential as an anticonvulsant agent in other scenarios. The findings, presented here underscore the complexity of 2-DG's actions, emphasizing the need for a detailed understanding of its role in different epileptic contexts. The insights gained from the chapter contribute not only to the expanding body of knowledge regarding 2-DG but also hold potential implications for the development of targeted therapeutic interventions in epilepsy. As we navigate the intricate landscape of proconvulsant and anticonvulsant properties, further research is required to elucidate the underlying mechanisms and to explore the translational potential of 2-DG in clinical settings. This chapter serves as a stepping stone, laying the groundwork for future investigations that may ultimately contribute to the advancement of epilepsy treatment strategies. Continuous exploration and understanding of 2-DG's role in seizure modulation can help pave the way for innovative approaches in the management of epileptic disorders.

LIST OF ABBREVIATIONS

2-DG	2-deoxy-D-glucose
3-MG	3- methyl glucose
AFT	Aftercharge Threshold
ATP	Adenosine Triphosphate
AP-1	Activator protein-1
G6P	Glucose-6-Phosphate
GLUT	Glucose Transporter
KA	Kainic Acid
i.v.	intra venous
i.p.	intraperitoneal
MEST	Mouse Electroshock Seizure Threshold
NADPH	Nictotinamide Adenosine Diphosphate

PPP   Pentose Phosphate Pathway

PTZ   Pentylenetetrazol

REFERENCES

[1]   Shao, L.R.; Stafstrom, C.E. Glycolytic inhibition by 2-deoxy- D -glucose abolishes both neuronal and network bursts vitro seizure model. J.
[http://dx.doi.org/10.1152/jn.00100.2017] [PMID: 28404824]

[2]   Nedergaard, S.; Andreasen, M. Opposing effects of 2-deoxy- D -glucose on interictal- and ictal-like activity when K $^+$ currents and GABA $_A$ receptors are blocked in rat hippocampus *in vitro*. *J. Neurophysiol.,* **2018**, *119*(5), 1912-1923.
[http://dx.doi.org/10.1152/jn.00732.2017] [PMID: 29412775]

[3]   Aft, R.L.; Zhang, F.W.; Gius, D. Evaluation of 2-deoxy-D-glucose as a chemotherapeutic agent: mechanism of cell death. *Br. J. Cancer,* **2002**, *87*(7), 805-812.
[http://dx.doi.org/10.1038/sj.bjc.6600547] [PMID: 12232767]

[4]   Pan, Y.Z.; Sutula, T.P.; Rutecki, P.A. 2-Deoxy- D -glucose reduces epileptiform activity by presynaptic mechanisms. *J. Neurophysiol.,* **2019**, *121*(4), 1092-1101.
[http://dx.doi.org/10.1152/jn.00723.2018] [PMID: 30673364]

[5]   Benedek, K.; Juhász, C.; Muzik, O.; Chugani, D.C.; Chugani, H.T. Metabolic changes of subcortical structures in intractable focal epilepsy. *Epilepsia,* **2004**, *45*(9), 1100-1105.
[http://dx.doi.org/10.1111/j.0013-9580.2004.43303.x] [PMID: 15329075]

[6]   Gasior, M.; Yankura, J.; Hartman, A.L.; French, A.; Rogawski, M.A. Anticonvulsant and proconvulsant actions of 2-deoxy- D -glucose. *Epilepsia,* **2010**, *51*(8), 1385-1394.
[http://dx.doi.org/10.1111/j.1528-1167.2010.02593.x] [PMID: 20491877]

[7]   Stafstrom, C.E.; Ockuly, J.C.; Murphree, L.; Valley, M.T.; Roopra, A.; Sutula, T.P. Anticonvulsant and antiepileptic actions of 2-deoxy-D-glucose in epilepsy models. *Ann. Neurol.,* **2009**, *65*(4), 435-447.
[http://dx.doi.org/10.1002/ana.21603] [PMID: 19399874]

[8]   Terse, P.S.; Joshi, P.S.; Bordelon, N.R.; Brys, A.M.; Patton, K.M.; Arndt, T.P.; Sutula, T.P. 2-deox--d-glucose (2-DG)-induced cardiac toxicity in rat: NT-proBNP and BNP as potential early cardiac safety biomarkers. *Int. J. Toxicol.,* **2016**, *35*(3), 284-293.
[http://dx.doi.org/10.1177/1091581815624397] [PMID: 26838190]

[9]   Lian, X.Y.; Khan, F.A.; Stringer, J.L. Fructose-1,6-bisphosphate has anticonvulsant activity in models of acute seizures in adult rats. *J. Neurosci.,* **2007**, *27*(44), 12007-12011.
[http://dx.doi.org/10.1523/JNEUROSCI.3163-07.2007] [PMID: 17978042]

[10]   Forte, N.; Medrihan, L.; Cappetti, B.; Baldelli, P.; Benfenati, F. 2-Deoxy- D -glucose enhances tonic inhibition through the neurosteroid-mediated activation of extrasynaptic GABA$_A$ receptors. *Epilepsia,* **2016**, *57*(12), 1987-2000.
[http://dx.doi.org/10.1111/epi.13578] [PMID: 27735054]

[11]   Nichols, C.G. KATP channels as molecular sensors of cellular metabolism. *Nature,* **2006**, *440*(7083), 470-476.
[http://dx.doi.org/10.1038/nature04711] [PMID: 16554807]

[12]   Garriga-Canut, M.; Schoenike, B.; Qazi, R.; Bergendahl, K.; Daley, T.J.; Pfender, R.M.; Morrison, J.F.; Ockuly, J.; Stafstrom, C.; Sutula, T.; Roopra, A. 2-Deoxy-D-glucose reduces epilepsy progression by NRSF-CtBP–dependent metabolic regulation of chromatin structure. *Nat. Neurosci.,* **2006**, *9*(11), 1382-1387.
[http://dx.doi.org/10.1038/nn1791] [PMID: 17041593]

[13]   Vexler, Z.S.; Wong, A.; Francisco, C.; Manabat, C.; Christen, S.; Täuber, M.; Ferriero, D.M.;

Gregory, G. Fructose-1,6-bisphosphate preserves intracellular glutathione and protects cortical neurons against oxidative stress. *Brain Res.,* **2003**, *960*(1-2), 90-98.
[http://dx.doi.org/10.1016/S0006-8993(02)03777-0] [PMID: 12505661]

[14]   Albright, J.C.; Henke, M.T.; Soukup, A.A.; McClure, R.A.; Thomson, R.J.; Keller, N.P.; Kelleher, N.L. Large-scale metabolomics reveals a complex response of Aspergillus nidulans to epigenetic perturbation. *ACS Chem. Biol.,* **2015**, *10*(6), 1535-1541.
[http://dx.doi.org/10.1021/acschembio.5b00025] [PMID: 25815712]

[15]   Ponomareva, D.; Ivanov, A.; Bregestovski, P. *Analysis of Pentose Phosphate Pathway Inhibition on Generation of Reactive Oxygen Species and Epileptiform Activity in Hippocampal Slices.,* **2023**.
[http://dx.doi.org/10.20944/preprints202312.1373.v1]

[16]   Reddy, D.S. Role of hormones and neurosteroids in epileptogenesis. *Front. Cell. Neurosci.,* **2013**, *7*, 115.
[http://dx.doi.org/10.3389/fncel.2013.00115] [PMID: 23914154]

[17]   Yao, X.; Ye, F.; Zhang, M.; Cui, C.; Huang, B.; Niu, P.; Liu, X.; Zhao, L.; Dong, E.; Song, C.; Zhan, S.; Lu, R.; Li, H.; Tan, W.; Liu, D. *In vitro* antiviral activity and projection of optimized dosing design of hydroxychloroquine for the treatment of severe acute respiratory syndrome coronavirus 2 (SARS-CoV-2). *Clin. Infect. Dis.,* **2020**, *71*(15), 732-739.
[http://dx.doi.org/10.1093/cid/ciaa237] [PMID: 32150618]

[18]   Samokhina, E.; Popova, I.; Malkov, A.; Ivanov, A.I.; Papadia, D.; Osypov, A.; Molchanov, M.; Paskevich, S.; Fisahn, A.; Zilberter, M.; Zilberter, Y. Chronic inhibition of brain glycolysis initiates epileptogenesis. *J. Neurosci. Res.,* **2017**, *95*(11), 2195-2206.
[http://dx.doi.org/10.1002/jnr.24019] [PMID: 28150440]

[19]   Cendes, F.; Theodore, W.H.; Brinkmann, B.H.; Sulc, V.; Cascino, G.D. Neuroimaging of epilepsy. *Handb. Clin. Neurol.,* **2016**, *136*, 985-1014.
[http://dx.doi.org/10.1016/B978-0-444-53486-6.00051-X] [PMID: 27430454]

[20]   Shao, L.R.; Rho, J.M.; Stafstrom, C.E. Glycolytic inhibition: A novel approach toward controlling neuronal excitability and seizures. Epilepsia Open, **2018**, 3(S2) Suppl. 2, 191-197.
[http://dx.doi.org/10.1002/epi4.12251] [PMID: 30564778]

ANNEXURE

Lipinski's Rule of Five

Raman Singh[1] and **Kuldeep Singh**[1,*]

[1] Department of Applied Chemistry, Amity University Madhya Pradesh, Gwalior-474005, India

Abstract: Christopher A. Lipinski formulated a rule based on his observation that most drugs administered orally are relatively small and moderately lipophilic molecules. This rule serves as a guideline to determine whether a molecule with specific pharmacological or biological activity possesses properties that would make it a viable orally active drug in humans. Lipinski's Rule of Five functions as a powerful screening tool in the initial phases of drug discovery, enabling researchers to pick molecules with ideal attributes for subsequent development and testing.

Keywords: Absorption, Acceptors, Biological activity, Donors, Exceptions drugability, Lipinski's rule of five.

1. INTRODUCTION

Lipinski's Rule of Five, also known as the Rule of Five (RO5), is an approach utilized in drug discovery that aids in assessing the drug-likeness of chemical compounds. In 1997, Christopher A. Lipinski, a scientist at Pfizer, formulated this rule based on his observation that most drugs administered orally are relatively small and moderately lipophilic molecules [1].

Lipinski and his coworkers at Pfizer analyzed a database of compounds that successfully passed Phase I clinical trials and entered into Phase II studies. They correlated the computed physicochemical properties of these molecules to their observed aqueous solubility, permeability, and oral bioavailability using graphing software JMP [2].

Lipinski used JMP to generate plots of Pfizer compounds that successfully cleared the clinical trial hurdle between Phase I and Phase II. Through this analysis, he noted some common trends in the physicochemical properties of these successful

*[*] **Corresponding author Kuldeep Singh:** Department of Applied Chemistry, Amity University Madhya Pradesh, Gwalior-474005, India; E-mail: singh@orgsyn.in

Raman Singh, Antresh Kumar & Kuldeep Singh (Eds.)

drug candidates [2]. This led him to propose the Rule of Five as a guideline to determine whether a molecule with specific pharmacological or biological activity possesses properties that would make it a viable orally active drug in humans [3].

2. LIPINSKI'S RULE OF FIVE

The name "rule of five" comes from the fact that all the conditions have multiples of five as the determinant conditions. According to Lipinski's rule, an orally active drug should have no more than one violation of these four conditions [4, 5].

The Rule of Five states that, for a compound to have a reasonable probability of being membrane permeable and easily absorbed, it should meet the following criteria [4, 6]:

1. Molecular Weight < 500 Da
2. logP < 5
3. Hydrogen Bond Donors < 5
4. Hydrogen Bond Acceptors < 10

Poor absorption or permeation is more likely when a compound violates two or more of the following:

1. Molecular weight > 500 Da
2. Calculated logP > 5
3. More than 5 hydrogen bond donors
4. More than 10 hydrogen bond acceptors

This set of criteria helps filter out compounds with poor oral absorption and low permeation, ensuring potential drug candidates have favorable physicochemical properties for effective delivery and action within the body. The Rule of Five is a valuable tool in drug discovery for assessing chemical libraries and prioritizing promising drug candidates [7].

3. ROLE OF LIPINSKI'S RULE OF FIVE IN DETERMINATION OF DRUG-LIKENESS

Lipinski's Rule of Five has been instrumental in the design and evaluation of various classes of compounds, ranging from antimicrobial agents to anticancer drugs [8]. The rule provides a straightforward framework for determining the drug-likeness of molecules, enabling researchers to prioritize compounds with higher probabilities of success in terms of absorption, distribution, metabolism, and excretion (ADME) properties [9]. By considering parameters such as molecular weight, hydrogen bond donors, hydrogen bond acceptors, and lipophilicity, Lipinski's Rule of Five aids in the rational selection of compounds with favourable pharmacokinetic profiles [10].

The most critical aspect in drug development is to verify that potential drug candidates exhibit the requisite physicochemical qualities for effective therapeutic action. The majority of drug candidates fail while moving clinical trial phase 1 to phase 2. When there are multiple violations of Lipinski's Rule of Five, it might result in issues with the bioavailability of a substance. This demonstrates the significance of these parameters in determining the suitability of a chemical compounds for oral delivery. Therefore, RO5 functions as a powerful screening tool in the initial phases of drug discovery, enabling researchers to pick molecules with ideal attributes for subsequent development and testing [11].

4. EXCEPTIONS OF THE RULE OF FIVE

The RO5 is derived from a distribution of estimated qualities among thousands of medications. Consequently, certain medications will inherently fall outside of the rule's parameter cutoffs. Most USAN (United States Adopted Name) medications with characteristics not covered by the Lipinski criterion can be grouped into a relatively small number of therapeutic groups. These oral active medicinal classes include cardiac glycosides, vitamins, antifungals, and antibiotics.

Because of the molecular characteristics of these molecules, the medications can function as substrates for naturally occurring transporters. There won't be many instances of chemicals that break the RO5 if these classes are removed from the USAN library [4, 6]. Drugs or clinical candidates having good bioavailability may be termed as Beyond Rule-of-5 (bRo5) compounds [12]. RO5 should not be hard and fast. It is important to note that to break a rule it is necessary to understood why there is a rule [2].

CONCLUSION

Lipinski's rule of five plays a pivotal role in drug discovery by providing a set of criteria to assess the drug-likeness of chemical compounds. By considering parameters such as molecular weight, lipophilicity, and hydrogen-bond donors and acceptors, this rule aids researchers in identifying potential drug candidates with favorable pharmacokinetic properties. Adherence to Lipinski's rule of five helps select compounds that are more likely to exhibit optimal oral absorption and bioavailability, thereby enhancing the efficiency of the drug development process. Although there are many exceptions, this rule helps to flag compounds.

LIST OF ABBREVIATIONS

bRo5 Beyond Rule-of-5

Da Dalton

HBA Hydrogen Bond Acceptors

HBD Hydrogen Bond donors

PSA Polar Surface Area

RO5 Rule of Five

RotB Rotatable Bond

USAN United States Adopted Name

ACKNOWLEDGEMENT

The authors extend their heartfelt gratitude to the management of Amity University Madhya Pradesh, Gwalior, Madhya Pradesh, India, for providing the facilities that enabled the writing and submission of the book chapter for publication.

REFERENCES

[1] Georgieva, M.; Mitkov, J.; Zlatkov, A. Synthesis and druglikeness estimation of amide derivatives of 1-benzyltheobromine- 8-thioglycolic acid. *Scripta Scientifica Pharmaceutica,* **2014**, *1*(1), 28.
[http://dx.doi.org/10.14748/ssp.v1i1.602]

[2] Bethany Halford, Wrestling with the rule of 5. *C&EN Global Enterprise,* **2023**, *101*(8), 16-19.
[http://dx.doi.org/10.1021/cen-10108-feature1]

[3] Sampat, G.; Suryawanshi, S.S.; Palled, M.S.; Patil, A.S.; Khanal, P.; Salokhe, A.S. Drug likeness screening and evaluation of physicochemical properties of selected medicinal agents by computer aided drug design tools. *Advances in Pharmacology and Pharmacy,* **2022**, *10*(4), 234-246.
[http://dx.doi.org/10.13189/app.2022.100402]

[4] Lipinski, C.A.; Lombardo, F.; Dominy, B.W.; Feeney, P.J. Experimental and computational approaches to estimate solubility and permeability in drug discovery and development settings 1PII of original article: S0169-409X(96)00423-1. The article was originally published in Advanced Drug Delivery Reviews 23 (1997) 3–25. 1. *Adv. Drug Deliv. Rev.,* **2001**, *46*(1-3), 3-26.
[http://dx.doi.org/10.1016/S0169-409X(00)00129-0] [PMID: 11259830]

[5] Benet, L.Z.; Hosey, C.M.; Ursu, O.; Oprea, T.I. BDDCS, the Rule of 5 and drugability. *Adv. Drug Deliv. Rev.,* **2016**, *101*, 89-98.
[http://dx.doi.org/10.1016/j.addr.2016.05.007] [PMID: 27182629]

[6] Lipinski, C.A. Lead- and drug-like compounds: the rule-of-five revolution. *Drug Discov. Today. Technol.,* **2004**, *1*(4), 337-341.
[http://dx.doi.org/10.1016/j.ddtec.2004.11.007] [PMID: 24981612]

[7] Nguyen, V.B.; Wang, S.L.; Phan, T.Q.; Pham, T.H.T.; Huang, H.T.; Liaw, C.C.; Nguyen, A.D. Screening and elucidation of chemical structures of novel mammalian α-glucosidase inhibitors targeting anti-diabetes drug from herbals used by E de ethnic tribe in Vietnam. *Pharmaceuticals (Basel),* **2023**, *16*(5), 756.
[http://dx.doi.org/10.3390/ph16050756] [PMID: 37242539]

[8] Prijadi, S.M.; Aulia, S.; Afinasari, A.; Aristawidya, L.; Syahrul Hikam, M.D.; Muchtaridi, M. *In silico*

study of sesquiterpene and monoterpene compounds from valerian roots (valerian officinalis) as acetylcholinesterase inhibitor. *Indonesian Journal of Computational Biology (IJCB),* **2022**, *1*(1), 1. [http://dx.doi.org/10.24198/ijcb.v1i1.35898]

[9]   Jha, S.K.; Kumar, P. Molecular Docking Study of Neuroprotectiveplant-Derived Biomolecules in Parkinson'S Disease. *Int. J. Pharm. Pharm. Sci.,* **2017**, *9*(9), 149. [http://dx.doi.org/10.22159/ijpps.2017v9i9.20445]

[10] Sakkiah, S.; Meganathan, C.; Sohn, Y.S.; Namadevan, S.; Lee, K.W. Identification of important chemical features of 11β-hydroxysteroid dehydrogenase type1 inhibitors: application of ligand based virtual screening and density functional theory. *Int. J. Mol. Sci.,* **2012**, *13*(4), 5138-5162. [http://dx.doi.org/10.3390/ijms13045138] [PMID: 22606035]

[11] Kang, H.; Tang, K.; Liu, Q.; Sun, Y.; Huang, Q.; Zhu, R.; Gao, J.; Zhang, D.; Huang, C.; Cao, Z. HIM-herbal ingredients *in-vivo* metabolism database. *J. Cheminform.,* **2013**, *5*(1), 28. [http://dx.doi.org/10.1186/1758-2946-5-28] [PMID: 23721660]

[12] Egbert, M.; Whitty, A.; Keserű, G.M.; Vajda, S. Why some targets benefit from beyond rule of five drugs. *J. Med. Chem.,* **2019**, *62*(22), 10005-10025. [http://dx.doi.org/10.1021/acs.jmedchem.8b01732] [PMID: 31188592]

SUBJECT INDEX

A

Abnormal glycolytic flux in cancer cells 186
Abrogated viral effects 75
Acid(s) 13, 33, 58, 62, 71, 77, 86, 89, 94, 111, 112, 205, 206, 216, 232, 233, 236, 239
  acetic 13
  aminobutyric 111
  ascorbic 94
  degradation 33
  ferulic 216
  hydrobromic 77
  hydrochloric 62
  hydrolysis 62
  kainic (KA) 111, 112, 232, 233, 236, 239
  lactic 205, 206
  -mediated invasion hypothesis 89
  tricarboxylic 71, 86
Acidosis 89
Action, anti-inflammatory 107
Activation 95, 100, 108, 111, 131, 167, 187, 188, 191, 192, 194, 195, 205, 206, 209, 210, 212
  immune 167
  macrophage 108
  mediated protein kinase 192
  neuronal 111
  oncogene 206
  -related neuronal loss 131
  transcriptional 191
Activity 73, 88, 90, 91, 92, 94, 95, 96, 98, 99, 100, 110, 111, 186, 206, 233, 236, 238
  abnormal high-voltage 110
  anabolic 88
  oncogenic 186
  therapeutic 233
  tumor cell 94
Acute 99, 103
  myeloid leukemia (AML) 99
  respiratory distress syndrome (ARDS) 103
Adaptations 86, 94
  metabolic 86, 94

Adeno-associated virus 132
Adenosine 130, 148, 184, 192, 203
  monophosphate 192
  triphosphate 130, 148, 184, 203
Aerobic glycolysis 86, 87, 88, 89, 90, 162, 183, 184, 185, 187, 203, 205, 206, 208, 209
Aliphatic diastereotopic protons 38
Alkaline phosphatase (AP) 25
Alzheimer's disease 131, 158, 159
Amidotransferase 100
Amino acid synthesis 93
AMPK 7, 76, 96, 102, 106, 108, 138, 188, 194, 195, 208, 209, 212, 220
  downregulation 138
  pathway 106, 108
  phosphorylation 76
  signalling pathways 208
Analogs, radioisotope 192
Angiogenesis 102, 185, 192, 193, 197, 203, 204, 208, 210
Angiography 160
Anti-apoptosis 211
Anti-COVID-19 agent 73
Anti-epileptic agent 104
Anti-inflammatory 106, 107
  cytokine 106
  effect 107
Anti-proliferative effect 221
Anti-viral agent 73
Antibody-mediated neutralization 73
Anticancer 25, 130, 131, 183, 190, 215
  agents 190, 215
  effects 25
Anticonvulsant 232, 233, 234, 235, 237, 238, 239
  actions 232, 234, 235
  effect 234, 235
  properties 233, 238, 239
Antigen-presenting cells (APCs) 105
Antiseizure drugs 233
Antitumor agent 183

www.ingramcontent.com/pod-product-compliance
Lightning Source LLC
Chambersburg PA
CBHW050821220326
41598CB00006B/276